ECOTOXICOLOGY

Perspectives on Key Issues

ECOTOXICOLOGY
Perspectives on Key Issues

Editors

Rachel Ann Hauser-Davis

Centro de Estudos da Saúde do Trabalhador e Ecologia Humana (CESTEH)
Escola Nacional de Saúde Pública Sérgio Arouca (ENSP)
Fundação Oswaldo Cruz – FIOCRUZ
Rio de Janeiro, RJ
Brazil

Thiago Estevam Parente

Instituto Oswaldo Cruz (IOC)
Fundação Oswaldo Cruz – FIOCRUZ
Rio de Janeiro, RJ
Brazil

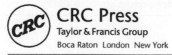

CRC Press
Taylor & Francis Group
Boca Raton London New York

CRC Press is an imprint of the
Taylor & Francis Group, an **informa** business

A SCIENCE PUBLISHERS BOOK

Cover credit:
Adult *Daphnia magna*: Right hand side photograph (Figure 3) from Chapter 8. Reproduced with kind courtesy of the authors of the chapter.

CRC Press
Taylor & Francis Group
6000 Broken Sound Parkway NW, Suite 300
Boca Raton, FL 33487-2742

First issued in paperback 2021

© 2018 by Taylor & Francis Group, LLC
CRC Press is an imprint of Taylor & Francis Group, an Informa business

No claim to original U.S. Government works

Version Date: 20180221

ISBN-13: 978-0-367-78124-8 (pbk)
ISBN-13: 978-1-138-19682-7 (hbk)

Library of Congress Cataloging-in-Publication Data

Names: Hauser-Davis, Rachel Ann, editor. | Parente, Thiago Estevam, editor.
Title: Ecotoxicology : perspectives on key issues / editors Rachel Ann
 Hauser-Davis, Centro de Estudos da Saúde do Trabalhador e Ecologia Humana
 (CESTEH), Escola Nacional de Saúde Pública Sérgio Arouca (ENSP),
 Fundação Oswaldo Cruz, Fiocruz Rio de Janeiro, RJ, Brazil, Thiago
 Estevam Parente, Instituto Oswaldo Cruz, Fiocruz, Rio de Janeiro, Brazil.
Description: Boca Raton, FL : Taylor & Francis Group, [2018] | Includes
 bibliographical references and index.
Identifiers: LCCN 2018006391 | ISBN 9781138196827 (hardback)
Subjects: LCSH: Environmental toxicology.
Classification: LCC RA1226 .E258 2018 | DDC 615.9/02--dc23
LC record available at https://lccn.loc.gov/2018006391

Visit the Taylor & Francis Web site at
http://www.taylorandfrancis.com

and the CRC Press Web site at
http://www.crcpress.com

Preface

Ecotoxicology is a vast and fast evolving transdisciplinary area of research, with multiple intersections with the productive and governmental sectors. Although several published books provide an in-depth coverage of Ecotoxicology, none of these books cover the topic exhaustively due to its amplitude. Nonetheless, most of these books are capable to transmit to an interested reader the "*essence of Ecotoxicology*". Likewise, this book does not attempt to provide an in-depth coverage of each of the Ecotoxicology facets, of which there are many. Instead, we opted to provide readers with a diverse array of practical questions faced and addressed on a daily basis by ecotoxicologists from different parts of the world. In doing so, we hope to transmit the same essence and to provide fresh perspectives on key issues of Ecotoxicology. Our goal would not be fulfilled if we had not provided the authors of each chapter, to whom we are deeply grateful, the freedom to express their personal points of view. Finally, we strongly encourage each of you to read the seminal paper from René Truhaut entitled "Ecotoxicology: Objectives, Principles and Perspectives" (Ecotoxicol. Environ. Saf. 1977, 1: 151–173), which marks the formal establishment of Ecotoxicology as an independent area of investigation.

Rachel Ann Hauser-Davis
Thiago Estevam Parente

Contents

1

What Can Proteomics and Metalloproteomics Add to Aquatic Toxicology and Public Health?

Rachel Ann Hauser-Davis

Introduction

Anthropogenic activities are increasingly causing significant impacts on the aquatic environment, leading to several changes in their ecological processes. The relationship between the health of these environments, anthropogenic activities and public health is already a consensus; however, the mechanisms involved are not yet fully known due to their complexity (Andersen 1997, Fleming and Laws 2006, Moura et al. 2011, NRC 1999).

Among the many important aspects concerning human health, aquatic environment represents a significant source of water, biomass and oxygen production and biological diversity, and the quality of these ecosystems is indispensable for the maintenance of the planet and public health (Moura et al. 2011, NRC 1999, Sandifer et al. 2004). Unfortunately, anthropogenic activities have led to several negative impacts on these ecosystems, such as habitat destruction and the consequent extinction of several species, changes in sedimentation rates, mobilization of different contaminants (Andersen 1997), diseases in the human population due to chemical pollutants (Bassil et al. 2007, Dhillon et al. 2008) and infectious agents present in marine hosts, including bacterial, viral and protozoan agents (Santos et al. 2017), with repercussions on socioeconomic and cultural activities and, finally, on public health (Fleming and Laws 2006, PNUMA 2004).

Centro de Estudos da Saúde do Trabalhador e Ecologia Humana (CESTEH), Escola Nacional de Saúde Pública Sérgio Arouca (ENSP), Fundação Oswaldo Cruz, Av. Leopoldo Bulhões, 1480, Manguinhos, CEP: 21041210, Rio de Janeiro, RJ, Brazil.
E-mail: rachel.hauser.davis@gmail.com

Approximately 65% of the world's human population lives close to coastal regions, at distances of up to 159 km from the coastline, and it is estimated that this figure will increase to 75% by 2025 (Cohen 1995). This demonstrates the growing importance of the relationship between public health and the health of aquatic environments, owing to the increasing number of human population living in these areas, especially in tropical and subtropical regions (Moura et al. 2011). In these regions, water bodies are important sources of protein, recreation and economic activities (Dewailly and Knap 2006). This leads to extreme socio-environmental vulnerability of the local human inhabitants since possible harmful effects arising from the relationship between aquatic environments and human health have a direct impact on these populations.

In addition, an increasing trend to include economic values over natural resources is observed, where ecosystem conservation is seen as more economically profitable than the economic value derived from the acquisition and use of its resources which, most of the time, results in severe environmental impacts (Moura et al. 2011). In this context, it is important to note that although coastal regions account for only 8% of the world's continental surface, services and benefits from these areas account for approximately 43% of the estimated total value of global ecosystem services, valued at 12.6 trillion dollars (Costanza et al. 1997).

One of the major damaging effects that occur in aquatic environments due to anthropogenic activities is contamination by chemical pollutants. Approximately 80% of aquatic contamination comes from continents, and this problem is aggravated by the fact that most human activities are concentrated in coastal regions (Cohen 1995). These contaminants continuously enter the aquatic environment from both anthropogenic activities and inadequate waste disposal, and many of them are not completely removed by sewage treatment plants. They are also introduced by the untreated sewage discharges and dumped into water bodies due to the absence of adequate collection and treatment networks. Among the several environmental contaminants present in these ecosystems, those of greatest concern are the pollutants that show environmental persistence, bioavailability, a tendency to bioaccumulate in the food chain which may cause toxic effects, such as persistent organic pollutants (POPs) (Jones and de Voogt 1999), polycyclic aromatic hydrocarbons (PAHS) (Abdel-Shafy and Mansour 2016), metals (Singh et al. 2011) and, more recently, emerging contaminants originating from substances used daily by the human population, such as pharmaceutical formulations and personal care products, most of which have the potential to cause toxic effects and/or interfere with the normal functioning of the human and animal endocrine system (Burkhardt-Holm 2010).

However, despite the increasing pollution of aquatic environments, the biochemistry of the intoxication of organisms living in these ecosystems still suffers from gaps in basic knowledge. Such information, if available, would serve to anticipate the impact of environmental contamination on the local fauna, since biochemical alterations precede pathological damages, as well as allow for decision-making processes aiming at the mitigation of harmful effects on both biota and human health, which are directly linked to public health.

Assessment of Toxic Effects of Environmental Pollutants on Aquatic Organisms

Aquatic organisms are recognized bioindicators of environmental contamination, and their behavioral, physiological and biochemical responses are of great relevance in this regard. In addition, they are particularly useful for the evaluation of xenobiotics in water and sediments, providing early warnings about the potential danger of new chemical compounds and the possibility of environmental contamination. Finally, they also play an extremely important ecological role in the trophic webs as energy carriers to higher trophic levels, and are also important links between the environment, contaminants and human population, through aquaculture activities and their consumption by both other organisms and humans (Espino 2000, Powers 1989). In this context, it is important to mention that certain organisms, such as marine mammals, have been increasingly recognized as important aquatic ecosystem health sentinels, and may indicate toxic pollutant effects directly related to human health since they are mammals and top-chain predators (Gulland and Hall 2007, Moura et al. 2011).

Often, the classification of a chemical pollutant as harmful or not applies the criterion of organism death. However, this is a very extreme criterion where it is not possible to take preventive actions to avoid exposure. Therefore, from an ecological and human health risk perspective, it is more interesting to measure sublethal effects of pollutants, which arise before the organism dies. This ensures not only the protection of wild species, in a biodiversity conservation scope, but also the health of human populations that depend on species consumed and used in economic activities. This is performed through the use of biomarkers, defined as measurements of biochemical changes in cells or tissues as a response to exposure to contaminants (Parente and Hauser-Davis 2013). Investigations regarding these responses have been increasingly used in the study and identification of deleterious effects on aquatic biota and provide information that serves to anticipate the impact of pollutants on aquatic fauna. Biomarkers of response, in this regard, are more adequate for the evaluation of deleterious effects at the molecular level than only the detection of xenobiotics in tissues and fluids since many contaminants can be quickly metabolized and eliminated, resulting in low residual tissue concentrations (Galgani et al. 1992), thus limiting the usefulness of these organisms as bioindicators or sentinel species.

This makes it possible, in the long run, to perform environmental management decisions that may also be anticipated in order to avoid harmful effects on biota before the cellular and molecular biochemical changes that precede the pathological damage of xenobiotics to organs, which may subsequently lead to effects on populations and, later, communities, in a direct mitigation of both biota and human risks and of importance in a public health context.

The investigation of biomarkers of exposure to environmental contaminants in aquatic organisms is varied and includes biotransformation enzymes, oxidative stress endpoints and linked metabolism proteins, haematological, immunological, endocrine, reproductive, physiological, morphological and histological parameters, among others (Bunton and Frazier 1994, Dijkstra et al. 1996, Snape et al. 2004). However, the advent of more advanced technologies has allowed the investigation of biomarkers that are, increasingly, being considered more appropriate in the evaluation of toxic effects of environmental pollutants, namely proteomic and metalloproteomic biomarkers (Hauser-Davis et al. 2017).

Application of "Omics" Techniques in the Identification of Toxic Effects of Environmental Pollutants

The large amount of information on the molecular level obtained from "omics" technologies, mainly in the genomic, proteomic and metalloproteomic fields, presents great potential in addressing the toxic effects of environmental pollutants in more detail, discovering underlying mechanisms of action and identifying new biomarkers of exposure and effect (Dowling and Sheehan 2006, López-Barea and Gómez-Ariza 2006, Quackenbush 2001). For example, biomarkers may comprise an integrated set of genes or proteins expressed simultaneously, and alterations in their expression may provide important information regarding the characterization of related functions of genes and gene products with profiles of similar activity or common mechanisms of regulation (Snape et al. 2004), the classification of compounds with similar modes of action when observing their toxicological effects (Miracle and Ankley 2005, Oberemm et al. 2005) and indications of different levels of stress, integrating general and highly specific markers in one assay.

Proteomic techniques in the identification of toxic effects of environmental pollutants

Proteomic techniques have, mainly, benefited research on well-characterized species, such as certain fish species used as model organisms, rats, humans and yeasts, and few proteomic studies are available in relation to organisms present in natural ecosystems (Karim et al. 2011). Unfortunately, however, well-characterized species may be environmentally and ecotoxicologically inadequate since they may not be useful as sentinel species concerning environmental contamination (Hogstrand et al. 2002), demonstrating the importance of further studies.

The most promising path used in this area of research to find relevant biomarkers in environmental contamination is the investigation of changes in the expression of proteins in complex field situations. In this context, the comparison between the proteomes of organisms in different situations is very attractive, since alterations in the proteomic expression in complex field situations may be able to point out which gene products, metabolites or proteins merit further and more in-depth investigations (Albertsson et al. 2007). For example, studies have investigated differences in protein expression in fish caught in unpolluted and polluted sites, and metabolic and proteomic differences in the liver of wild fish with and without tumors (Stentiford et al. 2005, Williams et al. 2003). These types of studies provide a link between traditional studies of a single biological marker gene and those regarding environmental contamination, and demonstrate the application of proteomic analyses in relation to the actual environment, and not model organisms, with a completely sequenced genome, exposed to environmental contaminants in the laboratory.

In this regard, proteomic studies have been increasingly performed to investigate metal effects on aquatic organisms since, among environmental pollutants, metals are of particular concern because, besides causing potential toxic effects, they also display the ability to bioaccumulate in the aquatic trophic web (Censi et al. 2006, MacFarlane and Burchett 2000, Miller et al. 2002). For example, in one study, the economically relevant *Mytilus galloprovincialis* mussels were exposed to copper and copper nanoparticles, both environmentally important pollutants, and significant changes in the proteomic expressions of several tissues were observed (Gomes et al. 2014). Copper nanoparticles showed a trend of up-regulation proteins in gills and down-regulation in the digestive gland, while the opposite was observed for copper alone. Different toxicity mechanisms were postulated for copper alone and bound to nanoparticles, since distinctive sets of differentially expressed proteins were found for each contaminant. However, common response mechanisms (cytoskeleton and cell structure, stress response, transcription regulation and energy metabolism) were also observed that, after confirmation and validation, could be used as putative new biomarkers. The authors, however, indicate that the absence of the mussel genome prevented the identification of other proteins relevant to clarify the effects of both contaminants. As cited previously, this is one of the drawbacks of evaluating non-model organisms, although this practice is more environmentally realistic.

In another study, short-term cadmium toxicity was evaluated in the European bullhead *Cottus gobio*, a candidate sentinel species. After analysis by the 2D-DIGE technique, several differentially expressed hepatic and gill proteins were identified, categorized into different functional classes, related to metabolic process, general stress response, protein fate, and cell structure, providing new insights into the biochemical and molecular events in cadmium induced toxicity in fish (Dorts et al. 2011). Thus, proteomics also shows potential in identifying novel sentinel species that may have been previously overlooked by classical toxicological studies.

Another study with the extremely relevant environmental contaminant Hg observed that quantitative analyses of the hepatic proteome of methylmercury-exposed Atlantic cod (*Gadus morhua*) suggest oxidative stress-mediated effects on cellular energy metabolism (Yadetie et al. 2016). Specifically, a more pronounced effect of methylmercury on amino acid, glucose and fatty acid metabolic pathways was observed, which the authors postulate as suggesting possible interactions of the cellular energy metabolism and antioxidant defense pathways. Again, this demonstrates that proteomics is a valuable tool in the in-depth elucidation of metabolism pathways and contaminant modes of action, previously not possible by other techniques.

Differential proteomic analyses can also be applied to investigate the effects of biological, and not chemical, contamination such as viruses and bacteria that can be found in the aquatic environment. In this context, an interesting study evaluated the effects of a marine bacterium, *Vibrio harveyi*, in shrimp, through proteomic techniques

(Somboonwiwat et al. 2010). Several hemocyte proteins were up-regulated upon *V. harveyi* infection, such as hemocyanin, arginine kinase, as well as down-regulated, including alpha-2-macroglobulin, calmodulin and 14-3-3 protein epsilon. The authors concluded that this proteomic approach was useful for understanding the immune system of shrimp against pathogenic bacteria. In a similar study conducted on the commercially important crab *Scylla paramamosain*, the effects of a *Vibrio alginolyticus* infection were evaluated by proteomic techniques (Sun et al. 2017). A total of 43 proteins were differentially expressed during *V. alginolyticus* infection, 121 up-regulated and 122 down-regulated after infection. As in the previous study, many proteins linked to crab immune system were identified, which the authors indicated will contribute to the understanding of the molecular mechanisms of crab immune response to *V. alginolyticus* infection. These types of study are interesting because they display direct applicability in aquaculture activities and regarding public health, since these organisms are highly consumed by both other animals and by humans.

Another biological contaminant of interest is bacteria that excrete toxic substances known to cause deleterious effects on aquatic organisms. For example, microcystins have been shown to significantly alter the proteome expression of several aquatic organisms. In one study, adult medaka fish fed mycrocistins displayed significant alterations in the liver proteome after only 2 hours (Mezhoud et al. 2008), with the identified proteins involved in cell structure, signal transduction, enzyme regulation and oxidative stress. In this context, proteomics have also been applied to the investigation of the cyanotoxins themselves, since little is known about microcystin synthesis by cyanobacteria, and the elucidation of this metabolism would aid in decision-making processes regarding environmental contamination by these toxins in several countries. In one study, two *M. aeruginosa* strains were compared by proteomic tools (Tonietto et al. 2012), leading to the discovery of 11 protein spots unique to the toxin producing strain and eight in the non-toxin producing strain. Approximately 57% of the identified proteins in that study were related to energy metabolism, and 14 proteins up-regulated in the toxin producing strain. The authors concluded that these results indicated the presence of higher amounts of metabolic enzymes related to microcystin metabolism in the toxic strain, and that the production of microcystin could also be related to other proteins than those directly involved in its production, such as the enzymes involved in the energy metabolism.

In another study, proteome differences of six toxic and nontoxic *M. aeruginosa* strains were compared (Alexova et al. 2011). Several significant differences were observed, with many strain-specific proteins identified. No proteins were produced only by toxic or nontoxic strains, and nine proteins were differentially expressed, linked to the carbon-nitrogen metabolism and redox balance maintenance. The involvement of the global nitrogen regulator NtcA in toxicity and the switching of a previously inactive toxin-producing strain for microcystin synthesis were also reported, allowing for novel mechanism of action knowledge in cytotoxin production in this species.

The effects of organic contamination have also been investigated by proteomic techniques. For example, the authors of a recent study exposed the decapod crustacean *Macrobrachium rosenbergii* to chlordecone, an organochlorine insecticide at environmentally relevant concentrations, for the first time (Lafontaine et al. 2017). Many significantly up- or down-regulated proteins were observed in the hepatopancreas compared to non-exposed controls, involved in several important physiological processes such as ion transport, defense mechanisms and immune system, cytoskeleton dynamics, or protein synthesis and degradation. Interestingly, 6% of the down-regulated proteins are involved in the endocrine system and in the hormonal control of reproduction or development processes, indicating that chlordecone is a potential endocrine disruptor for decapods, as has been observed in vertebrates. The authors, thus, suggest that these protein modifications could lead to the disruption of *M. rosenbergii* growth and reproduction and, consequently, to modification in population fitness. This, in turn, may significantly impact aquaculture activities, leading to economic losses, since this is a commercially important species. In addition to these conclusions, public health issues may also be cited since the same endocrine disruptor effects may also occur in other crustaceans after chlordecone exposure. As many crustaceans are consumed by other animals and also by humans, the possible endocrine effects of this insecticide could reach higher hierarchical levels, thus further demonstrating proteomic applicability in the public health context regarding anticipating the impact of environmental contamination in the biota and allowing for decision-making processes for remediation projects.

Other organic contaminants also show importance in the aquatic environment, such as polycyclic aromatic hydrocarbons (PAH), and proteomic studies evaluating the effects of these compounds have increased in the last years. For example, the plasma proteome of Atlantic cod (*Gadus morhua*) was evaluated in a recent study after exposure to single PAHs (naphthalene or chrysene) and their corresponding metabolites (dihydrodiols) (Enerstvedt et al. 2017). A total of 12 differentially expressed proteins were found significantly altered in PAH exposed fish and were proposed as new biomarker candidates. Interestingly, the authors suggest that the uniformity of the identified up-regulated proteins indicates a triggered immune response in the exposed fish, furthering the understanding of the mechanisms of action of these environmental contaminants. In another study, the peroxisomal proteomes (purified subcellular fractions containing only peroxisomes) of blue mussels (*Mytilus edulis*) exposed to two different crude oil mixtures were evaluated by two-dimensional fluorescence difference electrophoresis and mass spectrometry (Mi et al. 2007). Results indicated 22 differentially exposed peroxisomal proteins, and the authors suggest that due to the consistency, comparing the protein patterns of that study to those obtained in previous field experiments, specific peroxisomal proteomics could be used to assess oil exposure in marine pollution assessments. This leads the way to the study of specific subcellular fractions (microsomal, peroxisomal, thermostable, and soluble, among others) in the search for biomarkers of environmental exposure, thus broadening proteomic applications in this regard.

Some aquatic organisms also display interesting differences in temporal protein expression profiles which may be important in ecological field studies, since organism proteomes at different time-points may show different effects concerning environmental pollutants, and differential sensitive developmental stages to contaminants (Sveinsdottir et al. 2008, Tay et al. 2006). These differences may also be useful for analyzing the expression of altered proteins during organism development in order to understand the molecular mechanisms underlying normal and abnormal development after contaminant exposure (Kanaya et al. 2000, Kultz and Somero 1996).

In a broader view, man-made alterations to the environment, such as climate change, have also been increasingly studied *via* proteomic techniques. For example, increased levels of atmospheric CO_2 leads to ocean acidification and warming to which marine organisms are exposed simultaneously (de Souza et al. 2014). However, although the effects of temperature on fish have been investigated thoroughly over the last century, the long-term effects of moderate CO_2 exposure and the combination of both stressors on these organisms are almost entirely unknown (de Souza et al. 2014).

In the study conducted by de Souza et al. (2014), a proteomics approach was applied to assess physiological and biochemical changes after exposure to these environmental stressors in the gills and blood plasma of Atlantic halibut (*Hippoglossus hippoglossus*) exposed to the control temperatures of 12°C and 18°C (impaired growth) in combination with control or high-CO_2 water for 14 weeks. The results of that study demonstrated that high-CO_2 treatment induced the up-regulation of immune system-related proteins, in both temperatures, while changes in gill proteome in the high-CO_2 (18°C) group were mostly related to increased energy metabolism proteins, which the authors postulate may be due to a higher energy demand. Gills from fish exposed to high-CO_2 at both temperature treatments, on the other hand, showed changes in proteins associated with increased cellular turnover and apoptosis signaling. The authors, thus, concluded that moderate CO_2-driven significant acidification, alone and combined with high temperature, can elicit biochemical changes that may affect fish health.

In another study in the same context, the global protein expression pattern of oyster larvae four days post-fertilization exposed to ambient and to high-CO_2 was evaluated (Dineshram et al. 2012) by bioanalytical proteomic techniques. A significant reduction of global protein expression was observed, with the expression of 71 out of 379 proteins either decreased or completely lost or expressed below the detection limit of the applied method.

In another study, the molecular responses of the fish brain to increased CO_2 and the expression of parental tolerance to high CO_2 levels in the offspring molecular phenotype of juvenile spiny damselfish, *Acanthochromis polyacanthus*, were evaluated by proteomic techniques (Schunter et al. 2016). Differential regulation of 109 and 68 proteins in the tolerant and sensitive groups were observed, with the most differences found between offspring of tolerant and sensitive parents occurring in high CO_2 conditions. The authors concluded that the transgenerational molecular signature observed in their study suggests that individual variation in CO_2 sensitivity could facilitate adaptation of fish populations to ocean acidification.

It is, thus, quite clear that comparative proteomic approaches allow discrimination between differential environmental situations, ultimately providing a molecular understanding of the effects of environmental contaminants or variables on organism health and leading to the identification of biomarkers of exposure.

Metalloproteomics in the identification of toxic effects of environmental pollutants

Within proteomics, the very recently developed field of metalloproteomics considers that biomolecules that bind metals and metalloids constitute a substantial part of molecules involved in cell metabolism and behavior, and that identifying a metal cofactor in a protein may aid in the functional assignment and positioning in the context of known cellular pathways (Haraguchi 2004a).

This is a field being developed in conjunction with genomics and proteomics, as well as structural biology (Fig. 1), as the molecular basis of many of the metal-dependent biochemical processes are not yet known, and the mechanisms by which metals are perceived, stored or incorporated as co-factors in cells are also often unknown (Haraguchi 2004b, Williams et al. 2003). First, however, it is necessary to locate, identify and quantify metal-binding molecules to subsequently analyze their role in the organism (Gao et al. 2007, Szokefalvi-Nagy et al. 1999).

Metalloproteins are defined as proteins whose functions are conferred by their binding to metals, such as catalytic activity, implication in electron transfer reactions or stabilization of the tertiary or quaternary structure of proteins (Garcia et al. 2006, Mounicou et al. 2009). They have been identified as one of the most important groups of biomarkers present in physiological differentiations or alterations in cells or biological tissues, involving metal or semi-metallic ions bound to proteins (Mounicou et al. 2009). A significant number of proteins and enzymes (approximately 30%) contain metal or metalloid species in their structures (Banci 2003, Gao et al. 2007).

These metal-bound proteins, or metalloproteins, are increasingly being used as biomarkers of environmental exposure (López-Barea and Gómez-Ariza 2006),

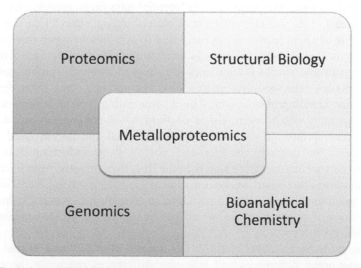

Fig. 1. Interrelationships between metalloproteomics and diverse fields of knowledge.

although the number of discoveries and studies in the metalloproteomic area is still much lower than in the proteomic area, due to the unique issues that must be considered when dealing with metalloproteins. These include, mainly, the difficulty in preserving the native states of metalloproteins during the analysis (Lothian et al. 2013), the low concentration of trace elements present in biological tissues and the complexity of the matrices (Gomez-Ariza et al. 2004). In addition, traditional proteomic approaches may also be incompatible in investigating metal-protein interactions, since denaturing conditions and enzymatic digestion are the norm for these types of applications, leading to the disruption of the weak ionic interactions present in most metalloprotein bonds (Hauser-Davis et al. 2017). Thus, the analysis of metal-bound biomolecules has traditionally been considered difficult and challenging. However, the continuous development of atomic spectroscopy combining biochemical or proteomic techniques, such as gel electrophoresis, capillary chromatography or multidimensional nanoflow, and the development of strategies for the complementary application of specific elements and molecule detection techniques, such as mass spectrometry coupled to inductively coupled plasma (ICP-MS) and electrospray (ESI-MS) have led to new possibilities in this field of research (Prange and Profrock 2005). Using these techniques, extremely large amounts of data can be collected with potential for the identification of adverse effects in organisms exposed to environmental contaminants (Kling et al. 2008).

Several environmental studies linking metalloproteomics and public health have been recently published. One such study characterized the metalloprotein fraction of fish and mussels of differentially-exposed organisms in the environment (Hauser-Davis et al. 2014, Lavradas et al. 2016), through screening by different bioanalytical techniques, such as size exclusion high performance chromatography coupled with inductively coupled plasma mass spectrometry (SEC-HPLC-ICP-MS). These studies highlight the presence of differential intra-organ expression of several metalloproteins. This includes differential metal-binding behavior in the case of liver and bile of *Oreochromis nilotics* exposed to sub-lethal copper concentrations (Hauser-Davis et al. 2014). This study is interesting in this regard since differences between organs are usually present only with regard to quantification, not metal-binding behavior (Hauser-Davis et al. 2014). In addition, data from that study indicated that metalloproteomics may be an interesting tool to provide adequate choices regarding which organ, tissue or fluid to investigate, since differences between metalloproteomic profiles groups of exposed and non-exposed animals were present, for example, in bile and not in liver, indicating that certain metalloproteins accumulate more slowly in the liver than excreted from liver to bile. This demonstrates that biliary analysis may be more adequate than liver with regard to recent environmental exposure to pollutants, as organism responses in this regard are more quickly observed in bile, which has been increasingly investigated in an environmental context.

In the study by Lavradas et al. (2016) conducted in different mussel tissues, several inter-organ differences and inter-site differences regarding thermostable protein content were verified, indicating metal accumulation and disruption of homeostasis of essential elements, toxic-metal detoxification attempts by metal-bound proteins, and proving that a historically uncontaminated site is now contaminated by toxic metals, again proving the value of metalloproteomics in both biomonitoring and public health contexts, since these organisms are highly consumed by humans.

It is important to note that thermostable fractions have also been recently reported as containing several potential biomarker metalloproteins (Hauser-Davis et al. 2012, Lavradas et al. 2016), although studies in this context are still incipient. This is also interesting since, as discussed previously, the study of specific subcellular fractions has been increasingly noted as rich sources of potential biomarkers for environmental contamination, displaying several advantages, such as a "cleaner" matrix with lower amounts of proteins to be analyzed, making them somewhat easier to investigate.

Ecotoxicological inferences can also be made from these types of studies. For example, one study observed a possible protective effect of selenium (Se) against mercury (Hg) and arsenic (As) toxicity in bighead carp liver from a polluted area in China by identifying metal after separation by thin layer isoelectric focusing by synchrotron radiation x-ray fluorescence (Li et al. 2008). This was postulated due to the presence of Se in As- and Hg-containing protein bands. In addition, the authors state that the fact that Hg and As were found in the same protein bands suggest that both elements may be involved in the same metabolic processes, furthering knowledge regarding molecular effects of these environmentally relevant contaminants.

Low molecular weight mercury-binding proteins were also identified in the marine mussel *Mytilus edulis* environmentally exposed to mercury (Roesijadi 1986). The mercury-binding proteins were isolated from gills and were shown to occur as two molecular weight variants when separated by Sephadex G-75 chromatography. Further purification of these proteins by DEAE-cellulose ion-exchange chromatography resulted in the resolution of three major mercury-binding protein peaks with similar amino acid compositions. Further chromatographic separation by anion-exchange high-performance liquid chromatography resulted in the resolution of six peaks, indicating a more complex situation than evident from DEAE-cellulose separations. This type of study indicates the complexity of metal-binding proteins and how much is still unknown in this regard.

In another study, endogenous levels of metal binding proteins (MBP) were determined in three species of Chesapeake Bay fish. All species exhibited measurable but varied levels of endogenous MBPs in the molecular weight range of 5 to 20 kdalton. Two species showed increased total MBP content upon induction with cadmium. An electrochemical analysis by polarography indicated that the wave properties of the fish MBPs resemble that of rat metallothionein, further contributing to metalloprotein characterization in an ecotoxicology approach (Andersen et al. 1986).

A review on the evolution of environmental metalloproteomics in the last 15 years has been recently published (Hauser-Davis et al. 2017). The authors demonstrate, through bibliometric techniques, that the recent advances in bioanalytical techniques, as discussed previously, have allowed for several applications in the field of environmental metalloproteomics, including the analysis of non-model organisms, since studies in this field have increased over the last two decades, although research interactions in this field still seem to be country- and organization-specific. In addition, they conclude that environmental metalloproteomics now seem to be reaching a more mature stage, in which analytical techniques are now well established and show the potential to be routinely applied in environmentally realistic and relevant scenarios (Hauser-Davis et al. 2017). Thus, the field of metalloproteomics in an aquatic toxicology and public health context may still be considered in its "adolescent stage", since bioanalytical metalloproteome methodologies are already established but their practical applications are still not fully realized.

Concluding Remarks

Proteomics, and especially, metalloproteomics, although still considered in their "adolescent stage" due to several caveats, such as the still limited number of genetically sequenced organisms, limiting protein identification, the lack of basic understanding of the implications of proteome alterations in cellular and metabolic pathways and, finally, differential proteome and metalloproteome expression due to environmental factors, such as temperature and CO_2 levels, are increasingly becoming established as valuable tools in the fields of environmental research. This will surely lead to increased applications in Aquatic Toxicology and Public Health, as seen from the brief discussion conducted herein, as knowledge on the many applications of these areas contributes to further information on the many facets of these fields of investigation.

References

Abdel-Shafy, H.I. and M.S.M. Mansour. 2016. A review on polycyclic aromatic hydrocarbons: Source, environmental impact, effect on human health and remediation. Egypt. J. Pet. 25: 107–123.

Albertsson, E., P. Kling, L. Gunnarsson, D.G. Larsson and L. Förlin. 2007. Proteomic analyses indicate induction of hepatic carbonyl reductase/20 beta-hydroxysteroid dehydrogenase B in rainbow trout exposed to sewage effluent. Ecotoxicol. Environ. Saf. 68: 33–39.

Alexova, R., P.A. Haynes, B.C. Ferrari and B.A. Neilan. 2011. Comparative protein expression in different strains of the bloom-forming cyanobacterium *Microcystis aeruginosa*. Mol. Cell. Proteomics. 10: M110.003749.

Andersen, N.R. 1997. An early warning system for the health of the oceans. Oceanography. 10: 14–23.

Andersen, R., J. Frazier and P.C. Huang. 1986. Transition metal-binding proteins from three Chesapeake Bay fish species. Environ. Health Perspect. 65: 149–156.

Banci, L. 2003. Molecular dynamics simulations of metalloproteins. Curr. Opin. Chem. Biol. 7: 143–149.

Bassil, K.L, C. Vakil, M. Sanborn, D.C. Cole, J.S. Kaur and K.J. Kerr. 2007. Cancer health effects of pesticides: Systematic review. Can. Fam. Physician. 53: 1704–1711.

Bunton, T.E. and J.M. Frazier. 1994. Extrahepatic tissue copper concentrations in white perch with hepatic copper storage. J. Fish Biol. 45: 627–640.

Burkhardt-Holm, P. 2010. Endocrine disruptors and water quality: A state of the art review. Int. J. Water Resour. D. 26: 477–493.

Censi, P. et al. 2006. Heavy metals in coastal water systems. A case study from the northwestern Gulf of Thailand. Chemosphere. 64: 1167–1176.

Cohen, J.E. 1995. Population growth and earth's human carrying capacity. Science. 269: 341–346.

Costanza, R. et al. 1997. The value of the world's ecosystem services and natural capital. Nature. 387: 253–260.

de Souza, K.B., F. Jutfelt, P. Kling, L. Förlin and J. Struve. 2014. Effects of increased CO_2 on fish gill and plasma proteome. PLOS One. 9: e10290.

Dewailly, E. and A. Knap. 2006. Food from the oceans and human health. Balancing risks and benefits. Oceanography. 19: 84–93.

Dhillon, A.S. et al. 2008. Pesticide/environmental exposures and Parkinson's disease in East Texas. J. Agromedicine. 13: 37–48.

Dijkstra, M., R. Havinga, R.J. Vonk and F. Kuipers. 1996. Bile secretion of cadmium, silver, zinc and copper in the rat. Involvement of various transport systems. Life Sci. 59: 1237–1246.

Dineshram, R., K.K. Wong, S. Xiao, Z. Yu, P.Y. Qian and V. Thiyagarajan. 2012. Analysis of Pacific oyster larval proteome and its response to high-CO_2. Marine Poll. Bull. 64: 2160–2167.

Dorts, J., P. Kestemont, M. Dieu, M. Raes and F. Silvestre. 2011. Proteomic response to sublethal cadmium exposure in a sentinel fish species, *Cottus gobio*. J. Proteome Res. 10: 470–478.

Dowling, V.A. and D. Sheehan. 2006. Proteomics as a route to identification of toxicity targets in ecotoxicology. Proteomics. 6: 5597–5604.

Enerstvedt, K.S, M.O. Sydnes and D.M. Pampanin. 2017. Study of the plasma proteome of Atlantic cod (*Gadus morhua*): Effect of exposure to two PAHs and their corresponding diols. Chemosphere. 183: 294–304.

Espino, G.L. 2000. Organismo indicadores de la calidade del agua y de la contaminación (bioindicadores). Plaza y Valdes Editores, Mexico. pp. 17–42.

Fleming, L.E. and E. Laws. 2006. Overview of the oceans and human health. Oceanography. 19: 18–23.

Galgani, F., G. Bocquene, P. Truquet, T. Burgeot, J.-F. Chiffoleau and C. Didier. 1992. Monitoring of pollutant biochemical effects on marine organisms of the French coasts. Oceanol. Acta. 15: 355–364.

Gao, Y., C. Chen and Z. Chai. 2007. Advanced nuclear analytical techniques for metalloproteomics. J. Anal. At. Spectrom. 22: 856–866.

Garcia, J.S., C.S. de Magalhães and M.A.Z. Arruda. 2006. Trends in metal-binding and metalloprotein analysis. Talanta. 69: 1–15.

Gomes, T. et al. 2014. Proteomic response of mussels *Mytilus galloprovincialis* exposed to CuO NPs and Cu^{2+}: An exploratory biomarker discovery. Aquat. Toxicol. 155: 327–366.

Gómez-Ariza, J.L., T. García-Barrera, F. Lorenzo, V. Bernal, M.J. Villegas and V. Oliveira. 2004. Use of mass spectrometry techniques for the characterization of metal bound to proteins (metallomics) in biological systems. Analyt. Chim. Acta. 524: 15–22.

Gulland, F.M.D. and A.J. Hall. 2007. Is marine mammal health deterioring? Trends in the global reporting of marine mammal disease. EcoHealth. 4: 135–150.

Haraguchi, H. 2004a. Metallomics as integrated biometal science. J. Anal. At. Spectrom. 19: 5–14.

Haraguchi, H. 2004b. Metallomics as integrated biometal science. J. Anal. At. Spectrom. 19: 5–14.

Hauser-Davis, R.A., R.A. Gonçalves, R.L. Ziolli and R.C. de Campos. 2012. A novel report of metallothioneins in fish bile: SDS-PAGE analysis, spectrophotometry quantification and metal speciation characterization by liquid chromatography coupled to ICP-MS. Aquat. Toxicol. 116: 54–60.

Hauser-Davis, R.A. et al. 2014. Bile and liver metallothionein behavior in copper-exposed fish. J. Trace Elem. Med. Biol. 28: 70–74.

Hauser-Davis, R.A., R.M. Lopes, F.B. Mota and J.C. Moreira. 2017. The evolution of environmental metalloproteomics over the last 15 years through bibliometric techniques. Ecotoxicol. Environ. Safety. 140: 279–287.

Hogstrand, C., S. Balesaria and C.N. Glover. 2002. Application of genomics and proteomics for study of the integrated response to zinc exposure in a non-model fish species, the rainbow trout. Comp. Biochem. Physiol. B Biochem. Mol. Biol. 133: 523–535.

Jones, K.C. and P. de Voogt. 1999. Persistent organic pollutants (POPs): state of the science. Environmental Pollution. 100: 209–221.

Kanaya, S. et al. 2000. Proteome analysis of Oncorhynchus species during embryogenesis. Electrophoresis. 21: 1907–1913.

Karim, M., S. Puiseux-Dao and M. Edery. 2011. Toxins and stress in fish: Proteomic analyses and response network. Toxicon. 57: 959–969.

Kling, P., A. Norman, P.L. Andersson, L. Norrgren and L. Förlin. 2008. Gender-specific proteomic responses in zebrafish liver following exposure to a selected mixture of brominated flame retardants. Ecotoxicol. Environ. Safety. 71: 319–327.

Kultz, D. and G.N. Somero. 1996. Differences in protein patterns of gill epithelial cells of the fish *Gillichthys mirabilis* after osmotic and thermal acclimation. J. Comp. Physiol. B Biochem. Syst. Environ. Physiol. 166: 88–100.

Lafontaine, A. et al. 2017. Proteomic response of *Macrobrachium rosenbergii* hepatopancreas exposed to chlordecone: Identification of endocrine disruption biomarkers? Ecotoxicol. Environ. Safety. 141: 306–314.

Lavradas, R.T., R.C. Rocha, T.D. Saint' Pierre, J.M. Godoy and R.A. Hauser-Davis. 2016. Investigation of thermostable metalloproteins in *Perna perna* mussels from differentially contaminated areas in Southeastern Brazil by bioanalytical techniques. J. Trace Elem. Med. Biol. 34: 70–78.

Li, L. et al. 2008. Detection of mercury-, arsenic-, and selenium-containing proteins in fish liver from a mercury polluted area of Guizhou Province, China. J. Toxicol. Environ. Health - Part A. 71: 1266–1269.

López-Barea, J. and J.L. Gómez-Ariza. 2006. Environmental proteomics and metallomics. Proteomics. 6: S51–S62.

Lothian, A., D.J. Hare, R. Grimm, T.M. Ryan, C.L. Masters and B.R. Roberts. 2013. Metalloproteomics: principles, challenges and applications to neurodegeneration. Front. Aging Neurosci. 5: 1–7.

MacFarlane, G.R. and M.D. Burchett. 2000. Cellular distribution of copper, lead and zinc in the grey mangrove, *Avicennia marina* (Forsk.) Vierh. Aquat. Bot. 68: 45–59.

Mezhoud, K. et al. 2008. Proteomic and phosphoproteomic analysis of cellular responses in medaka fish (*Oryzias latipes*) following oral gavage with microcystin-LR. Toxicon. 51: 1431–1439.

Mi, J., I. Apraiz and S. Cristobal. 2007. Peroxisomal proteomic approach for protein profiling in blue mussels (*Mytilus edulis*) exposed to crude oil. Biomarkers. 12: 47–60.

Miller, G.G., L.I. Sweet, J.V. Adams, G.M. Omann, D.R. Passino-Reader and P.G. Meier. 2002. *In vitro* toxicity and interactions of environmental contaminants (Arochlor 1254 and mercury) and immunomodulatory agents (lipopolysaccharide and cortisol) on thymocytes from lake trout (*Salvelinus namaycush*). Fish Shellfish Immunol. 13: 11–26.

Miracle, A.L. and G.T. Ankley. 2005. Ecotoxicogenomics: linkages between exposure and effects in assessing risks of aquatic contaminants to fish. Reprod. Toxicol. 19: 321–326.

Monicou, S., J. Szpunar and R. Lobinski. 2009. Metallomics: the concept and methodology. Chem. Soc. Rev. 38: 1119–1138.

Moura, J.F., M. Cardozo, M.S.S.P. Belo, S. Hacon and S. Siciliano. 2011. A interface da saúde pública com a saúde dos oceanos: produção de doenças, impactos socioeconômicos e relações benéficas. Cien. Saude Colet. 16: 3469–3480.

NRC. 1999. From monsoons to microbes: understand the ocean's whole in human health. National Academic Press, Washington.

Oberemm, A., L. Onyon and U. Gundert-Remy. 2005. How can toxicogenomics inform risk assessment? Toxicol. Appl. Pharmacol. 207: 592–598.

Parente, T. and R.A. Hauser-Davis. 2013. The use of fish biomarkers in the evaluation of water pollution. pp. 164–181. *In*: Ribeiro, C.A.O. (ed.). Pollution and Fish Health in Tropical Ecosystems. CRC Press.

PNUMA. 2004. Integração entre o meio ambiente e o desenvolvimento: 1972–2002. Perspectivas do Meio Ambiente Mundial 2002 GEO-3: Passado, presente e futuro. IBAMA/PNUMA. 1–28.

Powers, D.A. 1989. Fish as model systems. Science. 246: 352–358.

Prange, A. and D. Profrock. 2005. Application of CE-ICP-MS and CE-ESI-MS in metalloproteomics: challenges, developments, and limitations. Anal. Bioanal. Chem. 383: 372–389.

Quackenbush, J. 2001. Computational analysis of microarray data. Nature Reviews Genetics. 2: 418–427.

Roesijadi, G. 1986. Mercury-binding proteins from the marine mussel, *Mytilus edulis*. Environ. Health Perspect. 65: 45–48.

Sandifer, P.A., A.F. Holland, T.K. Rowles and G.I. Scott. 2004. The ocean and human health. Environ. Health Perspect. 112: A454–A455.

Santos, A. et al. 2017. Potentially toxic filamentous fungi associated to the economically important *Nodipecten nodosus* (Linnaeus, 1758) scallop farmed in southeastern Rio de Janeiro, Brazil. Marine Poll. Bull. 115: 75–79.

Schunter, C. et al. 2016. Molecular signatures of transgenerational response to ocean acidification in a species of reef fish. Nat. Clim. Change. 6.

Singh, R., N. Gautam, A. Mishra and R. Gupta. 2011. Heavy metals and living systems: An overview. Indian Journal of Pharmacology. 43: 246–253.

Snape, J.R., S.J. Maund, D.B. Pickford and T.H. Hutchinson. 2004. Ecotoxicogenomics: the challenge of integrating genomics into aquatic and terrestrial ecotoxicology. Aquat. Toxicol. 67: 143–154.

Somboonwiwat, K., V. Chaikeeratisak, H.C. Wang, C. Fang Lo and A. Tassanakajon. 2010. Proteomic analysis of differentially expressed proteins in *Penaeus monodon* hemocytes after *Vibrio harveyi* infection. Proteome Sci. 8: 39.

Stentiford, G.D. et al. Zhu. 2005. Liver tumors in wild flatfish: A histopathological, proteomic, and metabolomic study. Omics. 9: 281–299.

Sun, B., Z. Wang, Z. Wang, X. Ma and F. Zhu. 2017. A proteomic study of hemocyte proteins from Mud Crab (*Scylla paramamosain*) infected with White Spot Syndrome Virus or *Vibrio alginolyticus*. Front. Microbiol. 8: 468.

Sveinsdóttir, H., O. Vilhelmsson and A. Gudmundsdóttir. 2008. Proteome analysis of abundant proteins in two age groups of early Atlantic cod (*Gadus morhua*) larvae. Comp. Biochem. Physiol. -D: Genomics & Proteomics. 3: 243–250.

Szökefalvi-Nagy, Z., C. Bagyinka, I. Demeter, K. Hollós-Nagy and I. Kovács. 1999. Speciation of metal ions in proteins by combining PIXE and thin layer electrophoresis. Fresenius J. Anal. Chem. 363: 469–473.

Tay, T.L., Q. Lin, T.K. Seow, K.H. Tan, C.L. Hew and Z. Gong. 2006. Proteomic analysis of protein profiles during early development of the zebrafish, *Danio rerio*. Proteomics. 6: 3176–3188.

Tonietto, A., B.A. Petriz, W.C. Araújo, A. Mehta, B.S. Magalhães and O.L. Franco. 2012. Comparative proteomics between natural *Microcystis isolates* with a focus on microcystin synthesis. Proteome Sci. 10: 38.

Williams, T.D., K. Gensberg, S.D. Minchin and J.K. Chipman. 2003. A DNA expression array to detect toxic stress response in European flounder (*Platichthys flesus*). Aquat. Toxicol. 65: 141–157.

Yadetie, F. et al. 2016. Quantitative analyses of the hepatic proteome of methylmercury-exposed Atlantic cod (*Gadus morhua*) suggest oxidative stress-mediated effects on cellular energy metabolism. BMC Genomics. 17: 554.\

2

Biodiversity and Ecotoxicology

The Case of Loricariidae Fish

IIIIIIIIIIIIIIIIIIIIIIIIIIIIIIIIIIIIIIIIIIIIIIIIIIIIIIIIIIIIIIIIIIIIIIIIIIIIIIIIIIIIIIIIIIIIIIIIIIIIIIIIIIIIIIIIIIIIIIIIIIIIIIIIIIIIIIIIIIIIIIIIIIIIIIIIIIIIIIII

Thiago Estevam Parente

*"The obvious inability of present-day physics and chemistry to account for such events
is no reason at all for doubting that they can be accounted for by those sciences."*
Erwin Schrödinger, 1944

"Nothing in biology makes sense except in the light of evolution."
Theodosius Dobzhansky, 1973

Introduction

In recognising that human health is dependent on ecosystem's health, Ecotoxicology emerged from classical toxicology during the second half of the 20th century to be "concerned with the study of toxic effects, caused by natural and synthetic pollutants, to the constituents of ecosystems, animals (including human), vegetables and microbial, in an integrated context" (Truhaut 1977). Since its inception, the concept of Ecotoxicology has been declared in a variety of other forms reflecting the multidimensional approach of this area of investigation (Newman 2015). In practice, the field has been dominated by environmental chemistry and classical toxicological assays adapted to few non-human species, generally with mild ecological and some economic relevance. The "eco" of Ecotoxicology has always been a great challenge to be addressed effectively. This chapter aims to discuss some of these challenges and to analyze current perspectives to account for the diversity of life in Ecotoxicology.

Instituto Oswaldo Cruz, FIOCRUZ, Avenida Brasil 4036, sala 913, Manguinhos, CEP: 21040-361, Rio de Janeiro, Brasil.
E-mail: parente@ioc.fiocruz.br

The "Eco" in Ecotoxicology

The origin of the challenges to account for the "eco" in Ecotoxicology relies, at least in part, on a distorted comprehension of what it means. At a first glance, the meaning of the "eco" in Ecotoxicology is straight-forward: Ecology. Therefore, Ecotoxicology would be a contraction for Ecological Toxicology. Indeed, this is the most intuitive and routinary interpretation for Ecotoxicology.

However, a more careful look at the published definitions reveal that the word "Ecosystem" is consistently and more often used than "Ecology" or "Ecological" (Newman 2015). In fact, even the original definition by Truhaut (1977) uses the expression "to the constituents of ecosystems" (Truhaut 1977). Therefore, it seems plausible that the "eco" in the original proposition of Ecotoxicology stand for "Ecosystems", instead of "Ecological" as it has been interpreted often. Hence, Ecotoxicology should be regarded as the science investigating the effects of pollutants "to the constituents of ecosystems", including (but not restricted to) the ecological interactions among them.

This latter definition encompasses the three major areas of the field: toxicology (both human and wildlife), analytical chemistry and ecology. While toxicologists investigate the effects of pollutants on the living organisms (animals, including humans, vegetables, and microorganisms), chemists study the transport and fate of natural and synthetic pollutants through the many environmental compartments (either biotic or abiotic), and ecologists integrate these data with their evaluation of the interactions among each component of the system aiming to develop and test predictive models of the ecosystems, which ideally would be capable of anticipating environmental responses to natural or human-induced changes—the ultimate goal of Ecotoxicology.

The inherent multidimensionality of Ecotoxicology is another issue at the origin of the challenges preventing the development of reliable predictive ecosystemic models accounting for the "eco" of Ecotoxicology. Each of the three major areas of Ecotoxicology has different levels of complexity. An exhaustive discussion of these different levels of complexity in a single chapter is unpractical, and goes far beyond the scope of this one. Herein, the great diversity of living organisms will be used as an elucidative example of one of the many complex dimensions (eco)toxicologists must deal with.

Biodiversity

How to investigate the effect of pollutants on living organisms, if not all the living organisms are known? Estimates for the total number of species on Earth vary greatly, but it is generally accepted that the approximate 1.5 million species currently described only correspond to one-third of the total species count (Costello 2015, Costello et al. 2013). Surely, it is, and will continue to be, impossible to test the effects of the increasing number of pollutants on all the living organisms. Even if the necessary technology to perform ecotoxicological assays advances in ways one cannot predict, the task to test the effects of pollutants to all species would still be impractical due to limitations to access most species, in a simple example.

Although several species are not easily accessible to humans, this shall not be the case to pollutants that are carried throughout the globe by particulate matter suspended in the air, dissolved in the water or through the trophic chain. In fact, aside from habitat change, overexploitation, exotic species and climate change, pollution is a major driver of the exacerbated rate of species extinction observed since the beginning of the Anthropocene epoch (Pereira et al. 2012, Seddon et al. 2016, Young et al. 2016, Dirzo et al. 2014, Waters et al. 2016, McGill et al. 2015). However, it has long been known that pollution does not equally affect all living organisms. Truhaut, in his seminal work, called this phenomenon the "Influence of Type Species" (Truhaut 1977). Well ahead of his time, Truhaut in 1977 also recognized the importance of uncovering the molecular mechanisms underlying the susceptibility or resistance to a particular chemical, and that much work remained to be done in this area.

Since then, a lot has been learned about the susceptibility-resistance equilibrium and about the genetic mechanisms underlying such phenotypic differences among metazoan species. Nonetheless, the progress obtained so far is based on an extremely limited number of species (Celander et al. 2011), generally either of biomedical or economical relevance. Most often, these model species have been chosen due to their usability, including availability, but with no or little biological evidence supporting that the obtained results could be extrapolated to an entire group of related species.

Ray-finned fishes as an example

Ray-finned fishes (Actinopterygii) serve as a striking example of the limited number of environmentally relevant model species. Actinopterygii fishes are the most abundant monophyletic group of vertebrates, with more than 30,000 valid species and approximately 400 new species being described each year since 1998 (Eschmeyer et al. 2017). In addition, ray-finned fishes are prominent regarding the diversity of colonized habitats, ecological niches occupied and body shapes and sizes. The taxonomic, ecological and morphological diversities displayed by actinopterygian fishes come along with a myriad of physiological peculiarities, that have long been documented in the scientific literature and that are often subsidized by genetic adaptations. Despite this multidimensional diversity, only a very limited number of fish species have been intensively studied and are currently recommended for use in ecotoxicological tests.

For example, regarding ecotoxicological testing, in the guide for measuring the acute toxicity of effluents and receiving waters to freshwater and marine organisms, the United States Environmental Protection Agency (US EPA) recommends the use of two saltwater, *Cyprinodon variegatus* and *Menidia* spp., and three freshwater species, *Pimephales promelas*, and two trout species belonging to the same family and tribe, *Oncorhynchus mykiss* and *Salvelinus fontinalis*. In addition to these species, US EPA recognizes three other freshwater (*Cyprinella leedsi*, *Lepomis macrochirus*, *Ictalurus punctatus*) and 12 saltwater species from cold (*Parophrys vetulus*, *Citharichys sitigmaeus*, *Pseudopleuronectes americanus*) or warm habitats (*Paralichthys dentatus*, *P. lethostigma*, *Fundulus simillis*, *F. heteroclitus*, *Lagodon rhomboides*, *Orthipristis chrysoptera*, *Leostomus xanthurus*, *Gasterosteus aculeatus*, *Atherinops affinis*) as suitable for toxicity tests (US EPA 2002).

Notably, in the above mentioned guide, the US EPA only recommend the use of species with natural distribution in the US, therefore excluding the zebrafish (*Danio rerio*). Following this same line, this US agency acknowledges the possible existence of species indigenous to few states that might be as sensitive as or more sensitive than the fish species recommended in the above mentioned guideline. In such cases, the US EPA allows the use of these species if there are specific state regulations requiring their use or prohibiting the importation of the recommended fishes and if the indigenous species sensitivity has been experimentally proved to be equal or higher than the sensitivity of one or more of the species listed by the national legislation (US EPA 2002). On the contrary, another and more recent guideline from the US EPA for freshwater and saltwater fish acute toxicity test accepts the use of few non-native fish species (e.g., *Danio rerio, Oryzias latipes, Poecilia reticulata* and *Cyprinus carpio*) (US EPA 2016).

The Organisation for Economic Co-operation and Development (OECD) recommends seven freshwater and three saltwater fish species for ecotoxicological testing (OECD 1992). Among the recommended freshwater species, three belong to the same taxonomic family (*D. rerio, P. promelas* and *Cyprinus carpio*; Cyprinidae), while the others are representative of different orders (*Oryzias latipes*, Beloniformes; *Poecilia reticulata*, Cyprinodontiformes; *Lepomis macrochirus*, Centrarchiformes; and *O. mykiss*, Salmoniformes). Among the three recommended saltwater species, one belongs to an order already represented among the freshwater species (*C. variegatus*, Cyprinodontiformes), while the other two represent distinct taxa (*Menidia* spp., Athèriniformes and *Gasterosteus aculeatus*, Perciformes).

The greatest richness of freshwater fish species is observed in the Neotropical region, with Brazil appearing as the leading country (Buckup et al. 2007). Despite its diverse native and endemic ichthyofauna, the only two freshwater fish species recommended for ecotoxicological tests in Brazil, the zebrafish (*Danio rerio*) and the fathead minnow (*Pimephales promelas*), are not indigenous (ABNT NBR 15088:2016 and ABNT NBR 15499:2015) (ABNT 2016, ABNT 2015).

Dalzochio et al. (2016) recently reviewed the use of biomarkers to assess the health of aquatic ecosystems in Brazil, finding 99 published papers since the year 2000 (Dalzochio et al. 2016). Although not exhaustive, the work from Dalzochio et al. (2016) provides a rather good general panorama of the diversity of aquatic species that have been used in ecotoxicological investigations in Brazil. As for freshwater fishes, these authors encountered papers on 26 native and two widely distributed exotic species, belonging to 12 families and five orders. As demonstrated in Table 1, these numbers are far from being representative of more than 2,500 native freshwater fish species classified in 37 families and seven orders.

The work from Melo et al. (2013) stands out from the others identified by Dalzochio et al. (2016), for being the only one to investigate a biomarker response in an evolutionary context (Melo et al. 2013). These authors established a baseline frequency for micronuclei and other nuclear abnormalities in an order of electric ells (Gymnotiformes), enabling the identification of potentially useful species as models for genotoxicity studies. As the diversity of genera within each of the five Gymnotiformes families is low, only up to three species of each family were used in that study. This low diversity of genera within a taxonomic family, however, is

Table 1. **Representativeness of fish species being used for ecotoxicological studies in Brazil.** The number of fish species used for biomarker research in Brazil was obtained from Dalzochio et al. (2016), while the number of valid fish species per taxonomic family was obtained from Buckup et al. (2007).

Class	Order	Family	Freshwater fish species in Brazil	
			Total	Used for biomarker research
Actinopterygii	Osteoglossiformes	Osteoglossidae	3	–
	Characiformes	Parodontidae	19	–
		Curimatidae	75	–
		Prochilodontidae	12	2
		Anostomidae	92	–
		Chilodontidae	5	–
		Crenuchidae	52	–
		Hemiodontidae	25	–
		Gasteropelecidae	5	–
		Characidae	597	9
		Acestrorhynchidae	14	–
		Cynodontidae	10	–
		Erythrinidae	8	1
		Lebiasinidae	29	–
		Ctenoluciidae	5	–
	Siluriformes	Cetopsidae	16	–
		Aspredinidae	14	–
		Trichomycteridae	144	–
		Callichthyidae	123	–
		Scoloplacidae	4	–
		Loricariidae	418	1
		Pseudopimelodidae	18	–
		Heptapteridae	100	–
		Pimelodidae	83	1
		Doradidae	62	–
		Auchenipteridae	74	–
	Gymnotiformes	Gymnotidae	23	2
		Sternopygidae	21	1
		Rhamphichthyidae	9	1
		Hypopomidae	12	3
		Apteronotidae	30	1
	Cyprinodontiformes	Rivulidae	174	–
		Poeciliidae	54	2
		Anablepidae	11	–
	Synbranchiformes	Synbranchidae	7	–
	Perciformes	Polycentridae	2	–
		Cichlidae	220	4

not the case for several families of Brazilian freshwater fish. While the work from Melo et al. (2013) takes into account the phylogenetic dimension of biodiversity, it evaluated only one kind of biomarker, and thus, did not explore the molecular or genetic dimension of biodiversity.

Accounting for Biodiversity in Ecotoxicology

A much deeper exploration of the genetic and molecular dimension of biodiversity has been made feasible by the current popularization of high-throughput technologies for the study of biomolecules, especially high-throughput DNA and RNA sequencing. However, during the first years of a wider usage of high-throughput sequencing, this new technology has been largely used for phylogenomic and RNA-Seq types of studies (Irisarri et al. 2017, McGettigan 2013). Despite the great progress made in a vast array of research areas in such a short period of time, the recent applications of high-throughput sequencing have been basically the usage of a more powerful tool to answer traditional questions.

For instance, phylogenetics has long been using small pieces of DNA (e.g., microsatellites), while for phylogenomics the great expansion of the number and length of DNA loci used (e.g., ultraconserved elements), as well as the unrequired *a priori* knowledge regarding the genetics of the studied organisms, allowed the investigation and resolution of unsolved or even untested phylogenies for a variety of species. However, most often the biological functions performed by those microsatellites and ultraconserved elements have yet to be elucidated. In contrast, the variety of expressed transcripts once investigated almost one-by-one, mostly protein-coding, are now studied all together in RNA-Seq experiments, but still only in a limited number of species elected to serve as models.

More recently, Phylotranscriptomics and Evolutionary Toxicology have independently emerged as two fast-developing areas of investigation, applying high-throughput RNA sequencing to a group consisting of somehow related species or of individuals from a population. While the utmost goal of Phylotranscriptomics is to achieve a single species tree describing the true evolutionary relationships among the studied organisms, Evolutionary Toxicology aims to understand the evolution of the genetic pathways involved in determining species susceptibility to toxicants. The changes promoted by these two new disciplines exceeds a simple increment in the numbers of loci used in phylogenies and of species used in ecotoxicological tests; for each field it opens a new dimension of biodiversity, significantly increasing the meaning of the genetic data acquired by phylogenetic investigations and considering evolution in attempts to understand the balance between susceptibility and resistance to xenobiotics among the diversity of life. As in many other areas of biological research, high-throughput nucleic acid sequencing is used as a new tool, but unlike most of those areas, Phylotranscriptomics and Evolutionary Toxicology use this more powerful tool in an innovative manner.

As different as these two emerging disciplines may seem, the raw data produced by both is the same. When deposited in public repositories, this data can be analyzed in an interchangeable mode in order to achieve the objectives of both disciplines and more importantly, for the context of this chapter, to cluster species based on the sequence similarity of genes involved in the responses to a particular environmental threat. This information allows an evidence-based selection of a model species, which shall be a true representative of an entire group.

The case of Loricariidae fish

For a number of reasons, loricarids or suckermouth catfishes (Loricariidae, Siluriformes) are an adequate system for both Phylotranscriptomics and Evolutionary Toxicology investigations using high-throughput RNA sequencing. First, summing more than 950 valid species, 232 of those described during the last ten years (2008–2017) (Eschmeyer et al. 2017), suckermouth catfishes are among the most species-rich family of vertebrates. In addition to the abundance of species, these fish species occupy a diverse range of ecological niches, colonize different habitats throughout the Neotropical region, and display large morphological variations in size, shape and color pattern. Furthermore, at least some Loricariidae species are more resistant to the lethal effects of organic pollutants, such as diesel oil, than other fishes frequently used in acute toxicity tests (Nogueira et al. 2011, Felício et al. 2015). Interestingly, these Loricariidae species possesses a unique Cytochrome P450 1A (*CYP1A*) gene, which encodes a protein with altered structure, resulting in a low-to-absent EROD activity, a catalytic reaction toward its most classical substrate (Parente et al. 2009, Parente et al. 2011, Parente et al. 2014, Parente et al. 2015). Altogether, this extreme diversity found in Loricariidae fishes reflect a rather complex evolutionary history, about which many hypotheses remain to be tested, and from which most ecotoxicological consequences are still to be determined.

Recently, we used high-throughput sequencing technology to sequence the liver transcriptome from 34 individual loricariid fish, representing 31 species and 23 genera. As an external group, we also sequenced the liver transcriptomes from six individual Callichthyidae fish, representing three species and two genera. Our major objective is directly related to Ecotoxicology, to identify a representative species of the Loricariidae family to be used as model organism in ecotoxicological tests. Towards this major aim, we deal with Evolutionary Toxicology in order to characterize the diversity of genes coding for enzymes involved in the biotransformation and transport of xenobiotics and their metabolites, with particular emphasis on the Cytochromes P450 super-family. In addition, we are exploring the large amount of newly generated genetic data in order to achieve Phylotranscriptomics goals, including the development of a high-confidence backbone phylogenetic tree for the Loricariidae family. Furthermore, this information-rich dataset has been mined for the development of genetic makers that might be used in Ecotoxicology as well as in Population and Conservation Genetics.

Data mining and phylogenetic inference

The information content in transcriptomic data is so high that patterns are evident even to the naked eye, without the need to use sophisticated data-mining algorithms. This was exactly the case during the very initial processing steps of the recently sequenced liver transcriptomes from Loricariidae and Callichthyidae fishes. The transcripts coding for the Cytochrome Oxidase subunit I (COI) gene were retrieved from each of the assembled transcriptomes after a search using the BLASTn algorithm with the mitochondrial genome of the closest species available as the subject database sequence. Initially, this was done with the sole purpose to test the taxonomic identification of each fish specimen, which had been performed by experienced taxonomists using morphological characters. However, the average length of the transcripts in which the COI gene was encoded corresponded to almost one-third of the complete mitochondrial genome (Moreira et al. 2015).

After the identification of transcripts coding for mitochondrial genes located far from the COI, it was not difficult to resolve this "mitochondrial genome puzzle" only by looking at the BLASTn summary table, which describes the start and end position for each of the transcripts aligned to the reference mitochondrial genome. The transcripts coding for other mitochondrial genes were retrieved and scaffolded by their overlapping sequences at the flanking regions or, whenever there was no overlap, in accordance with the mitochondrial genome from the closest species as a reference. Using this procedure, which was described in detail by Moreira et al. (2015), it was possible from the RNA-Seq data of each of the studied species to assemble their quasi-complete mitochondrial genomes. Generally, only few nucleotides either in the very short tRNA-coding genes or in intergenic regions are missed or show low sequencing depth by this or other similar procedures, which have been recently developed by others (Tian and Smith 2016, Dilly et al. 2015, Fabre et al. 2013, Mercer et al. 2011).

Depth is a key issue in transcriptome sequencing, as it provides another layer of information contained in the assembled transcripts or in the mitochondrial genomes scaffolded from them. Information is also easily extracted from this additional layer. For example, Magalhães et al. (2017) and Parente et al. (2017a) used the information contained in this layer to identify heteroplasmic positions in the mitochondrial genomes from, respectively, *Hypancistrus zebra* (Loricariidae), an endangered species, and *Hoplosternum littorale* (Callichthyidae), a species widely distributed in the Neotropical region that have been causing ecological problems after being introduced in habitats outside its native range. Parente et al. (2017a) demonstrated the remarkable identity between the mitochondrial genomes of *H. littorale* from two populations geographically isolated by more than 5,000 km, which shared even the position of several heteroplasmic sites.

Polymorphic or heteroplasmic sites can be identified from the data simply by mapping the reads obtained from the high-throughput sequencing technology to the assembled mitochondrial genomes. The alignment can be visualized in specific software (e.g., Integrative Genomics Viewer, IGV) and polymorphic positions counted manually or, preferentially, called using algorithms either customized or available in bioinformatics toolkits (e.g., SAMtools). Magalhães et al. (2017) also used this information to identify that the mitochondrial transcription in fish follow the punctuation pattern described for mammals, corroborating the findings of Moreira et al. (2015) with other fish species. Another recent example of information extracted from the large amount of data obtained in transcriptome sequencing was the discovery of a variable number of nucleotides inserted between the ATPase6 and COIII genes in the mitochondrial genomes of Callichthyidae species (Moreira et al. 2016, Parente et al. 2017a).

The mitochondrial genomes and the nuclear orthologs assembled from RNA-Seq data can be used to infer the phylogenetic relationship among the studied organisms. For instance, we have recently provided a high-confidence backbone tree with representative species from six subfamilies of Loricariidae (Fig. 1), using only the mitochondrial genomes assembled from RNA-Seq data (Moreira et al. 2017). While analyzing these data, another evident genetic pattern was observed. A region in the mitochondrial control region (CR), spanning approximately 60 nucleotides, was deleted in a monophyletic clade comprising species belonging to the *Baryancistrus*, *Pterygoplichthys*, *Hypostomus*, *Aphanotorulus*, *Peckoltia*, *Ancistomus* and *Panaqolus* genera. This deletion included part of the 3' end of the conserved sequence block D (CSB-D), which has recently been shown to be conserved among 250 species throughout the diversity of ray-finned fishes (Satoh et al. 2016) and which is also conserved in other vertebrate species (Nilsson 2009, Wang et al. 2011). Although the biological function of the CSB-D is unknown, it is assumed to be relevant due to its evolutionary conservation. Additionally, more than 400 nuclear orthologs sequenced in the liver transcriptomes from all the investigated species were identified. We can anticipate that the retrieved phylogeny using these nuclear orthologs resemble the one obtained using the mitochondrial genes, but with few interesting modifications including a deeper clusterization of Otothyrini among Neoplecostomini species. Among the nuclear orthologs, several genetic patterns are currently under investigation, including the ones presented in the next section with potential implications on the Ecotoxicology of these species.

Exploring the diversity of defensome genes

The term Defensome has been used to refer to the many genes involved in the responses of an organism to the potential harmful effects originating from the exposure to a chemical toxicant (Goldstone et al. 2006). Although these genes participate collectively in the organismal defenses to chemical threats, they often do not share a close phylogenetic origin, being classified in distinct gene families.

Among the species we are currently working on, we have completed the analyses of the defensome genes from a single fish, *Pterygoplicthys anisitsi* (Parente

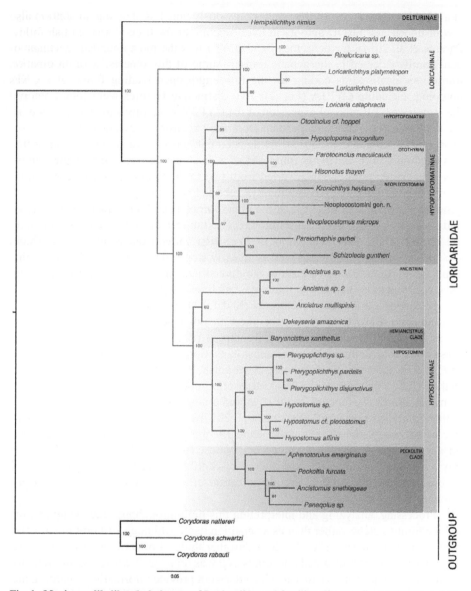

Fig. 1. Maximum likelihood phylogeny of Loricariidae subfamilies. The two ribosomal RNA and 13 protein-coding genes (comprising 14,116 nucleotides) were aligned using MUSCLE. Bootstrap support values are shown on each node and are based on 1,000 replicates. Callichthyidae species were used to root the tree. Loricariidae subfamilies are highlighted in gray scale. The scale bar represents the nucleotide substitution rate, using the GTR + GAMMA + I model. Modified from Moreira et al. (2017).

et al. 2017b). This is one of the species previously noted as showing an abnormally low or undetected EROD activity in liver subcellular fractions (Parente et al. 2011, Parente et al. 2014). Cytochromes P450 (CYP) was the most abundant defensome gene family detected in the hepatic transcriptome of this species, with 43 distinct transcripts identified as coding for the full-length open reading frame of a CYP homolog, including CYP1A (Fig. 2). Two distinctive features were found among the *P. anisitsi* CYP, a novel expansion of the CYP2Y subfamily and an expansion of the CYP2AA subfamily, independent from the expansion previously described for *Danio rerio* (Kubota et al. 2013). While zebrafish possesses a single CYP2Y gene, this subfamily in *P. anisitsi* is composed of at least the 12 transcripts sequenced in this liver transcriptome, which varied from two to 90 amino acids changes among them. As for the CYP2AA subfamily, zebrafish has ten genes identified in its genome and *P. anisitsi* has at least the eight complete coding sequences expressed and sequenced in its liver transcriptome. The number of amino acids changes in the translated CYP2AA transcripts of *P. anisitsi* varies from eight to 201, which include an early start codon, as well as an early stop codon. Curiously, however, the duplication events that gave birth to the diversification in this subfamily appear to have occurred independently in these two fish lineages (Fig. 2).

Following CYP, Sulfotransferases (SULT), Nuclear receptors (NR) and ATP binding cassette (ABC) were the other most abundant defensome gene families with respectively 33, 32 and 21 transcripts coding a complete open reading frame. For these other gene families, however, most transcripts sequenced in the transcriptome of *P. anisitsi* showed a close ortholog in zebrafish, except for another gene expansion in the SULT3 subfamily, which has 13 transcripts coding for a complete open reading frame in *P. anisitsi*, four in *Danio rerio* and a single one in the American channel catfish (*Ictalurus punctatus*) (Parente et al. 2017b). Together, these findings support our earlier suggestion that at least some *Pterygoplichthys* species might display an altered susceptibility to organic compounds. However, the question about the phylogenetic distribution of these altered susceptibility inferred by the genotype of defensome genes, as well as the identification of the best suitable model species, remain.

Processing, analyzing and interpreting this high-throughput sequencing dataset are the limiting steps, rather than its acquisition itself. Although still preliminary, the data from defensome gene families from the other studied Loricariidae species indicate a similar number of sequenced transcripts as it was found in *P. anisitsi*. However, this is only a broad quantitative metric which does not provide information regarding the distribution of these transcripts among subfamilies or about subtle nucleotide changes altering amino acids with potentially important rules in substrate selectivity. Currently, our analyses of transcripts annotated as Cytochromes P450 are more advanced than the analyses of transcripts annotated as other gene families. The number of CYP transcripts coding for a complete coding sequence sequenced in the liver transcriptome of each species varied from 13 (*Loricariichthys castaneus*) to 60 (*Otocinclus* cf. *hoppei*) (Table 2). In terms of transcripts distribution among CYP subfamilies, CYP2AA was the most abundant with more than 100 transcripts coding for a complete open reading frame. As this information is derived from transcriptomes, the actual number of CYP genes encoded in the genomes of these species is expected to be even higher.

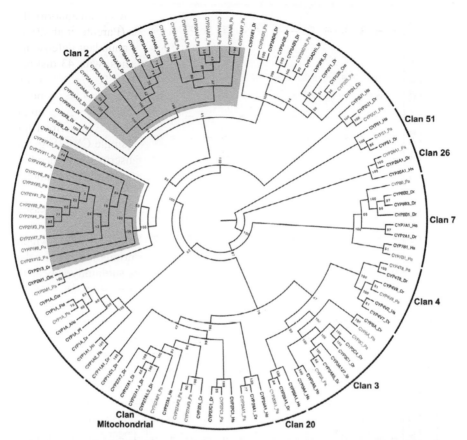

Fig. 2. Maximum-likelihood phylogeny of *Pterygoplichthys anisitsi* cytochromes P450 and homologs. The tree is rooted on CYP51. Sequences of *P. anisitsi* are shown in light gray. Expansions of CYP2Ys and CYP2AAs are highlighted in dark gray. Bootstrap values are shown on each node (1,000 replicates). The translated amino acid sequences were aligned using Muscle and the tree was constructed using RAxML with the LG model for amino acid substitution optimized for invariable sites and across site rate variation. Pa = *Pterygoplichthys anisitsi*; Pte = *Pterygoplichthys* sp.; Anc = *Ancistrus* sp.; Cor = *Corydoras* sp.; Hs = *Homo sapiens*; Dr = *Danio rerio*; Ip = *Ictalurus punctatus*; Pf = *Pelteobagrus fulvidraco*. Modified from Parente et al. (2017b).

Importantly, however, the opposite might also be true as transcripts differing only by few nucleotides may reflect errors during the transcriptome assembly. As a draft genome for the close related Loricariidae species, *Pterygoplichthys pardalis*, was recently released (Liu et al. 2016), we should be able to confirm the actual number of genes and their evolutionary history during these expansion events.

A single isoform coding for the complete coding sequence of CYP1A was sequenced in all but six species (Table 2). In five of these six species, although the complete coding sequence of CYP1A was not sequenced, a partial sequence was obtained in each case. Interestingly, two CYP1A isoforms were sequenced in one of the two specimens of *Hoplosternum littorale* (Callichthyidae) (Fig. 3). The phylogenetic relationships among the CYP1A from each species are different

Table 2. Diversity of Cytochromes P450 (CYP) transcripts identified in the liver transcriptomes of Loricariidae fish species.

Species x CYP	1A	1B	1C	2AA	2AD	2K	2M	2R	2U	2V	2X	2Y	2Z	3A	3C	4F	4T	4V	5A	7A	7B	8A	8B	19A	20A	21A	24A	26A	26B	27A	27B	27C	51A	TOTAL
Corydoras nattereri	1	0	0	2	3	2	3	2	0	2	5	1	1	1	2	0	1	2	1	1	0	0	1	0	1	0	3	0	0	1	1	1	1	39
Corydoras schwartzi	1	0	0	1	0	0	0	0	0	0	1	1	2	1	2	0	0	2	1	1	0	0	0	0	1	1	0	1	1	3	0	3	2	27
Hoplosternum littorale AM	2	0	0	5	1	3	1	1	0	1	5	1	1	1	2	2	2	2	2	0	0	0	1	0	1	0	3	1	0	2	0	1	1	40
Hoplosternum littorale RJ	1	0	0	7	1	6	2	1	0	1	13	1	2	4	1	1	2	1	2	2	0	0	0	0	1	0	1	0	0	4	0	0	1	55
Hemipsilichthys nimius	1	0	0	0	2	1	1	0	1	0	0	1	1	1	1	0	1	1	5	4	1	1	0	0	1	0	1	1	1	1	0	1	1	31
Loricariichthys castaneus	1	0	0	0	0	0	0	0	0	0	1	0	1	1	0	0	0	0	0	1	1	0	0	0	0	0	2	0	1	1	0	1	0	13
Loricariichthys platymetopon	1	1	0	0	0	0	1	1	0	0	0	0	0	1	1	0	1	2	1	1	1	0	0	0	1	0	1	0	0	3	0	1	1	17
Loricaria cataphracta	1	1	0	2	5	1	1	1	0	0	1	1	0	1	0	1	0	2	1	2	4	0	0	0	1	1	1	0	3	3	1	1	1	33
Rineloricaria sp.	1	0	0	11	1	2	2	1	0	2	2	1	1	1	1	0	1	3	1	1	2	0	0	0	1	0	2	0	3	3	1	1	1	42
Rineloricaria cf. *lanceolata*	1	0	0	10	3	1	2	2	0	0	4	1	1	2	2	0	1	3	1	2	0	1	0	1	0	0	2	0	9	1	1	1	1	55
Otocinclus cf. *hoppei*	1	0	0	10	2	3	1	1	0	1	0	4	5	2	2	0	0	2	1	2	1	1	0	0	1	0	7	2	8	1	1	1	1	60
Hypoptopoma incognitum	0	0	0	0	2	0	1	0	0	0	0	3	2	0	1	0	1	2	1	2	1	1	0	0	0	0	1	1	2	1	1	1	1	27
Schizolecis guntheri	1	0	0	0	1	0	0	0	0	0	0	0	1	1	1	0	1	1	1	1	1	1	0	1	0	0	3	0	4	0	1	1	1	24
Pareiorhaphis garbei	1	0	4	4	0	1	1	0	0	0	1	4	1	2	1	0	0	1	2	1	1	0	3	0	0	0	1	0	3	0	2	0	1	33
Hisonotus thayeri	1	0	10	1	1	1	1	0	0	0	0	2	3	3	1	0	4	1	1	1	1	0	2	0	0	0	3	0	6	0	0	1	1	45
Parotocinclus maculicauda	1	0	3	2	0	1	0	2	0	0	0	2	1	1	1	0	1	1	2	1	1	1	0	0	0	0	0	0	4	1	1	1	1	29
Kronichthys heylandi	1	0	0	2	1	1	1	0	0	1	0	1	1	2	0	0	1	3	1	1	0	0	0	0	1	0	1	1	2	2	0	2	1	28
Neoplecostomus microps	1	0	9	1	1	1	1	0	0	0	1	1	1	1	1	0	3	3	1	4	0	4	0	0	3	0	2	0	3	2	2	2	2	49
Neoplecostomini gen. n.	1	0	7	0	1	0	0	0	0	0	0	2	7	1	0	0	0	1	0	1	2	0	0	0	0	0	1	0	2	2	2	0	1	33
Ancistrus multispinis	1	1	0	2	2	1	1	0	1	0	0	2	4	4	1	1	0	2	1	2	1	0	0	1	0	0	2	0	2	2	1	1	1	35
Ancistrus sp. 1	1	0	3	0	3	3	3	0	3	0	1	2	2	1	4	4	0	3	2	1	2	1	0	1	0	0	0	0	3	3	0	1	1	43
Ancistrus sp. 2	1	0	2	2	2	1	1	0	1	0	7	1	2	2	1	0	1	2	1	1	2	0	0	0	1	0	2	0	5	1	0	1	1	39

Species																																		TOTAL
Baryancistrus xanthellus	1	0	0	12	1	0	2	1	1	0	2	2	0	1	2	0	2	3	2	2	1	0	0	0	2	0	2	1	0	2	0	0	1	42
Dekeyseria amazonica	0	0	0	10	3	0	1	0	0	0	0	4	0	1	1	1	2	2	0	1	2	0	1	1	2	0	3	0	0	3	0	0	1	40
Hypostomus sp.	1	0	0	2	2	0	2	1	2	0	4	2	1	2	2	1	1	1	1	0	0	0	0	1	0	1	3	1	0	3	1	1	1	29
Hypostomus cf. plecostomus	0	0	0	2	0	3	0	0	0	0	1	0	2	0	1	1	1	1	1	0	1	0	0	0	1	0	3	0	0	3	1	1	1	24
Hypostomus affinis	1	0	1	0	0	0	0	1	0	0	2	1	0	1	0	1	0	0	0	0	1	0	0	0	1	0	3	0	0	3	0	0	1	15
Pterygoplichthys sp.	1	0	0	9	1	0	2	2	0	0	8	4	2	2	2	1	0	1	2	1	2	0	2	1	2	0	8	2	0	8	2	2	1	58
Pterygoplichthys anisitisi	1	0	0	8	2	0	0	0	1	0	13	1	0	1	1	1	0	1	2	0	2	0	1	1	1	0	6	1	0	6	0	1	1	46
Pterygoplichthys pardalis	1	0	0	0	3	0	1	0	0	0	2	1	0	0	1	1	1	1	2	0	1	0	0	1	0	0	6	1	0	6	0	0	1	26
Aphanotolurus emarginatus	0	0	0	2	2	0	1	0	0	0	0	0	0	1	1	0	1	1	4	0	1	0	0	0	1	0	3	1	0	3	0	1	0	21
Panaqolus sp.	1	0	0	3	2	0	1	1	1	0	4	2	1	0	4	0	0	2	2	1	2	0	0	1	1	0	4	0	0	4	0	1	1	36
Ancistomus snethlageae	1	0	0	2	1	0	1	1	1	0	1	3	0	0	2	0	3	2	1	0	0	0	1	0	1	0	3	1	0	3	0	1	0	30
Peckoltia furcata	0	0	0	5	0	0	0	0	0	0	0	4	1	1	2	1	1	2	2	0	0	0	0	0	1	0	2	1	0	2	0	1	1	25
TOTAL	30	4	1	138	54	28	38	16	28	4	43	76	48	54	39	10	37	63	47	44	25	3	38	1	35	1	54	22	5	120	15	36	32	1189

from the species phylogeny as inferred by the mitochondrial genome (Fig. 1 and Fig. 3); in other words, the gene tree is different from the species tree. The position of *Loricaria cataphracta* changed from the sister taxon of *Loricariichthys* spp. in the species tree (Fig. 1) to the sister taxon of *Rineloricaria* spp. in the CYP1A tree (Fig. 3). Likewise, the position of the two species belonging to the Otothirini tribe (*Parotocinclus maculicauda* and *Hisonotus thayeri*) changed from the sister clade of the five species belonging to the Neoplecostomini tribe to the sister of only three of these Neoplecostomini species, with the other two (*Pareiorhaphis garbei* and *Schizolecis guntheri*) as the external group in the gene tree. All these species are inferred to possess a CYP1A with normal capabilities to catalyze the EROD activity, as they are positioned in-between *Corydoras* spp. (Callichthyidae) and *Ancistrus* spp. (Loricariidae), both in the gene and in the species phylogenetic tree.

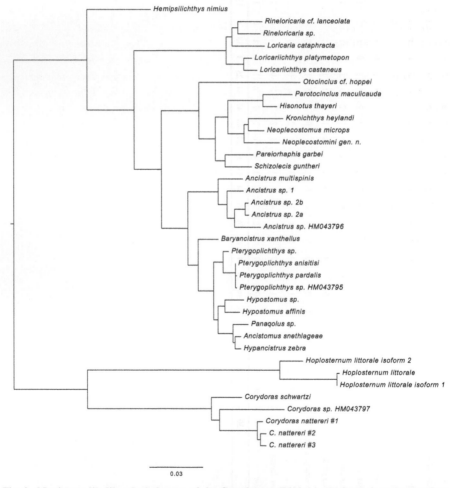

Fig. 3. Maximum likelihood phylogeny of the Cytochrome P450 1A (CYP1A) from Loricariidae species. The CYP1A nucleotide sequence of each species was aligned using MUSCLE. Callichthyidae species were used to root the tree. The scale bar represents the nucleotide substitution rate, using the GTR + GAMMA + I model.

On the contrary, we cannot infer the CYP1A/EROD phenotype for the species belonging to the six tribe-level clades closer to Hypostomini (low-to-absent EROD) than to Ancistrini (normal EROD). The *Peckoltia* and the *Hemiancistrus* clades are two of these six clades that are represented in our CYP1A gene tree. The phylogenetic position of the species belonging to the *Peckoltia*-clade changed from the sister taxon of the Hypostomini tribe (represented here by *Pterygoplichthys* spp. and *Hypostomus* spp.) in the species tree to the sister taxon of *Hypostomus* spp., with *Pterygoplichthys* spp. as the external group in the gene tree (Fig. 3). As the Hypostomini species shows the low-to-absent EROD phenotype, it is now possible to infer that the species belonging to the *Peckoltia*-clade will also share this phenotype.

The same inference cannot be made directly from the gene tree for *Baryancistrus xanthellus* (the representative of *Hemiancistrus* clade). A closer look at the inferred amino acid sequences is also contradictory. In an earlier work, we have identified six exclusive amino acids substitutions in *Pterygoplichthys* sp. in comparison to *Ancistrus* sp., *Corydoras* sp. and a set of 24 other fish species (Parente et al. 2011). Two of these six amino acid substitutions, at the positions 32 and 59, are shared with *Baryancistrus xanthellus* and also with the species belonging to the *Peckoltia*-clade. Other two of these substitutions are shared only with the *Peckoltia*-clade species, at the positions 94 and 98. Another substitution (position 159) is shared with the *Peckoltia*-clade species and paraphyletic with the species from the Hypoptomatinae family, except *Otocinclus* cf. *hoppei*. The sixth amino acid substitution (position 255), previously identified to be exclusive from *Pterygoplichthys* sp., remained exclusive of this genus, but not common to all its species as it was not identified in another unindentified *Pterygoplichthys* species (*Pterygoplichthys* sp.).

So far, the analyses of the Cytochromes P450 system in Loricariidae fish indicate the extension of the current phylogenetic distribution of the low-to-absent EROD phenotype from two genera of the Hypostomini subfamily to all species belonging to this subfamily in addition to at least several (probably all) genera belonging to the *Peckoltia*-clade group. Whether or not the species belonging to the *Hemiancistrus* and the other clades closer to Hypostomini and *Peckoltia* than to Ancistrini (namely, *Pseudancistrus*, *Lithoxus*, another *Pseudancistrus* and *Acanthicus*, according to Lujan et al. (2015)) share the same low-to-absent EROD phenotype is still unclear. Moreover, a number of distinctive features were identified in the Cytochromes P450 system of Loricariidae fish in comparison to the pattern observed in well studied and model fish species, especially the parallel expansion of the CYP2AA subfamily and the novel expansion of CYP2Y subfamily. How these genetic features are linked to a molecular phenotype and to the organism susceptibility to chemical compounds remain an open and intriguing question.

Linking Genotypes to Supraorganismal Effects

Linking genotypes to supraorganismal effects is a goal of Systems Biology, which investigates how the parts of a system sustain its whole, as well as the opposite, how the functioning of the whole influences the parts, their functions and interconnections. In the words of Prof. Hiroaki Kitano, Systems Biology "is a new field in biology that aims at system-level understanding of biological systems"

(Kitano 2001). In his seminal chapter establishing the foundations of Systems Biology, Prof. Kitano recognized that Systems Biology is not the first attempt of the scientific community to gain a systemic understanding of biological and non-biological systems. Following this line, earlier in this chapter, it has been argued that originally the term Ecotoxicology is the contraction of Ecosystem Toxicology. Having distinct areas of scientific investigation independently seeking for a systemic view is possible because the concept of System is abstract, a collection of individual parts assembled in a particular formation, and because the notion that "The whole is more than the sum of its parts", which dates back to the *Metaphysics* by Aristotle. Therefore, each of the many dimensions of the biological diversity can be defined as a unique biological system to be investigated, in parts or as a whole, from a single molecule embedded in its biological matrix interacting with a chemical ligand to the interactions among biotic (e.g., distinct species) and abiotic (e.g., naturally occurring chemicals or anthropogenic contaminants) elements of a given ecosystem.

The crucial difference between Systems Biology and the previous attempts to a holistic view in many fields, including Ecotoxicology, was also noted by Prof. Kitano: "It is the first time that we may be able to understand biological systems grounded in the molecular level as a consistent framework of knowledge". Genes are the fundamental unit carrying the information underlying the diversity of life, while the encoded proteins sustain the cellular metabolism as well as organismal homeostasis by interacting in a myriad of ways with an astonishing diversity of chemical compounds. The advancements in high-throughput technologies are allowing a continuously greater capacity to identify and quantify these molecules in distinct biological matrixes, making possible the development not only of Phylotranscriptomics and Evolutionary Toxicology, as mentioned earlier, but also of Systems Biology, Predictive Ecotoxicology and other approaches with broad potential such as the Adverse Outcome Pathway (AOP) (Ankley et al. 2010, Vinken 2013, Villeneuve and Garcia-Reyero 2011, Hartung et al. 2017). Nonetheless, it is still striving to generate a consistent and reliable AOP or a whole cell model, either prokaryotic or eukaryotic, which can be considered the simplest biological system (Karr et al. 2012, Kramer et al. 2011).

The reason why it is still complicated to develop reliable predictive models even for a simple biological system is straightforward: the whole is more than the sum of its parts. As Systems Biology develops, our capacity to predict the system behavior from the collection of its constituents will increase. Likewise, our ability to link suborganismal responses to population-level effects and population-level effects to alterations in the whole ecosystem is increasing as the system approach has been applied to Toxicology and Ecotoxicology (Garcia-Reyero and Perkins 2011, Hartung et al. 2017, Ideker et al. 2001, Ananthasubramaniam et al. 2015, Amiard-Triquet 2009, Forbes et al. 2017). Eventually, but still in a not so near future, the goals of Ecotoxicology and Systems Biology will merge and be achieved by resolving the broadest of all biological systems, the ecosystem, under homeostatic or stress conditions at the molecular level, the finest biological scale resolution. Until then, the system approach can be applied to narrower systems (e.g., the biotransformation of xenobiotics) in order to inform the selection of candidate species to serve as models of toxic responses of larger taxa.

Concluding Remarks

Despite the advancements in the field of Ecotoxicology since its formal establishment by Truhaut four decades ago, it is still challenging to evaluate, in an integrated context, the toxic effects of natural and synthetic pollutants to the constituents of ecosystems. Technological improvements have always marked the progress of Ecotoxicology, allowing more precise and accurate measurements of pollutants in a progressively wider array of biological and environmental matrixes, as well as the development of newer and more reliable biomarkers. Nonetheless, the currently available tools do not provide enough power to face all the obstacles imposed by the complexity of ecosystems, from which the diversity of life forms stands out.

The development and the current dissemination of high-throughput technologies, especially for DNA and RNA sequencing, increase our ability to produce data in such a way that actually offers a real opportunity to cope with biodiversity in the context of Ecotoxicology. Without any need for previous knowledge about the genetics of a given species, it is now possible to access genotypes in a relatively easy and fast way from species never investigated before. This information shall allow the grouping of species according to their infered phenotypes regarding a specific ecotoxicological endpoint. Although data acquisition is not (or, at least, is about not to be) a limiting step any longer, the computational processing, the biological interpretation and the linking of suborganismal endpoints to supraorganismal (including ecosystemic) responses remain to be challenging limiting steps.

These current limiting steps of Ecotoxicology, however, are shared by the newer fields of Phylotranscriptomics, Evolutionary Toxicology and Systems Biology. It is remarkable how the forty years old eco(system)toxicology and the young Systems Biology share the same fundamental objective of understanding biological systems, at any level of complexity, grounded in the molecular level. Towards this end, the words of Truhaut in 1977 continue to be valid: "Much work remains to be done in this area particularly in regard to uncovering the biochemical mechanisms which underlies the susceptibility or resistance of this or that constituent to this or that toxic effect of terrestrial or aquatic ecosystems". The availability of high-throughput technologies, as well as the development of the correlated fields of Phylotranscriptomics and Evolutionary Toxicology, make this an exciting time to face the vast array of anthropogenic impacts on natural ecosystems.

Acknowledgments

I am deeply in debt to my students, namely: Daniel Moreira, Maithê Magalhães and Paula Andrade. The continuous support from the scientists and staff from the Laboratório de Toxicologia Ambiental (ENSP, FIOCRUZ) has been indispensable. I also want to acknowledge the financial support from the United States Agency for International Development (USAID) through its Partnerships for Enhanced Engagement in Research (PEER) (PGA-2000003446 and PGA-2000004790) and from the Brazilian federal government agency Coordenação de Aperfeiçoamento de Pessoal de Nível Superior (CAPES) for a fellowship from the National Postdoctoral Program (PNPD).

References

ABNT, Associação Brasileira de Normas Técnicas, 2015. NBR 15499:2015—Ecotoxicologia aquática–Toxicidade crônica de curta duração–Método de ensaio com peixes.

ABNT, Associação Brasileira de Normas Técnicas, 2016. NBR 15088:2016—Ecotoxicologia aquática–Toxicidade aguda–Método de ensaio com peixes (Cyprinidae).

Amiard-Triquet, C. 2009. Behavioral disturbances: The missing link between sub-organismal and supra-organismal responses to stress? Prospects based on aquatic research. Hum. Ecol. Risk Assess. 15: 87–110.

Ananthasubramaniam, B., E. McCauley, K.A. Gust, A.J. Kennedy, E.B. Muller, E.J. Perkins et al. 2015. Relating suborganismal processes to ecotoxicological and population level endpoints using a bioenergetic model. Ecol. Appl. 25: 1691–1710.

Ankley, G.T., R.S. Bennett, R.J. Erickson, D.J. Hoff, M.W. Hornung, R.D. Johnson et al. 2010. Adverse outcome pathways: A conceptual framework to support ecotoxicology research and risk assessment. Environmental Toxicology and Chemistry. 29(3): 730–41.

Buckup, P.A., N.A. Menezes and M.S. Ghazzi. 2007. Catálogo das Espécies de Peixes de Água Doce do Brasil. Museu Nacional, Rio de Janeiro.

Celander, M.C., J.V. Goldstone, N.D. Denslow, T. Iguchi, P. Kille, R.D. Meyerhoff et al. 2011. Species extrapolation for the 21st Century. Environmental Toxicology and Chemistry. 30(1): 52–63.

Costello, M.J., R.M. May and N.E. Stork. 2013. Can we name earth's species before they go extinct? Science. (80)339: 413–416.

Costello, M.J. 2015. Biodiversity: The known, unknown, and rates of extinction. Curr. Biol. 25: R368–R371.

Dalzochio, T., G.Z.P. Rodrigues, I.E. Petry, G. Gehlen and L.B. da Silva. 2016. The use of biomarkers to assess the health of aquatic ecosystems in Brazil: A review. Int. Aquat. Res. 8: 283–298.

Dilly, G.F., J.D. Gaitán-Espitia and G.E. Hofmann. 2015. Characterization of the Antarctic sea urchin (*Sterechinus neumayeri*) transcriptome and mitogenome: a molecular resource for phylogenetics, ecophysiology and global change biology. Mol. Ecol. Resour. 15: 425–436.

Dirzo, R., H.S. Young, M. Galetti, G. Ceballos, N.J.B. Isaac and B. Collen. 2014. Defaunation in the Anthropocene. Science. (80)345: 401–406.

Eschmeyer, W.N., R. Fricke and R. van der, Laan. 2017. Catalog of fishes: genera, species, references. http://researcharchive.calacademy.org/research/ichthyology/catalog/SpeciesByFamily.asp. Accessed on 29 August 2017.

Fabre, P.H., K.a. Jønsson and E.J.P. Douzery. 2013. Jumping and gliding rodents: Mitogenomic affinities of pedetidae and anomaluridae deduced from an RNA-Seq approach. Gene. 531: 388–397.

Felício, A.A., T.E.M. Parente, L.R. Maschio, L. Nogueira, L.P.R. Venancio, M.D.F. Rebelo et al. 2015. Biochemical responses, morphometric changes, genotoxic effects and CYP1A expression in the armored catfish *Pterygoplichthys anisitsi* after 15 days of exposure to mineral diesel and biodiesel. Ecotoxicol. Environ. Saf. 115: 26–32.

Forbes, V.E., C.J. Salice, B. Birnir, R.J.F. Bruins, P. Calow, V. Ducrot et al. 2017. A framework for predicting impacts on ecosystem services from (sub)organismal responses to chemicals. Environ. Toxicol. Chem. 36: 845–859.

Garcia-Reyero, N. and E.J. Perkins. 2011. Systems biology: Leading the revolution in ecotoxicology. Environ. Toxicol. Chem. 30: 265–273.

Goldstone, J.V., A. Hamdoun, B.J. Cole, M. Howard-Ashby, D.W. Nebert, M. Scally et al. 2006. The chemical defensome: Environmental sensing and response genes in the *Strongylocentrotus purpuratus* genome. Dev. Biol. 300: 366–384.

Hartung, T., R.E. FitzGerald, P. Jennings, G.R. Mirams, M.C. Peitsch, A. Rostami-Hodjegan et al. 2017. Systems toxicology: Real world applications and opportunities. Chem. Res. Toxicol. 30: 870–882.

Ideker, T., T. Galitski and L. Hood. 2001. A new approach to decoding life: Systems biology. Annu. Rev. Genomics Hum. Genet. 2: 343–372.

Irisarri, I., D. Baurain, H. Brinkmann, F. Delsuc, J. Sire, A. Kupfer et al. 2017. Phylotranscriptomic consolidation of the jawed vertebrate timetree. Nature Ecology & Evolution. (1): 1370–1378.

Karr, J.R., J.C. Sanghvi, D.N. MacKlin, M.V. Gutschow, J.M. Jacobs, B. Bolival et al. 2012. A whole-cell computational model predicts phenotype from genotype. Cell. 150: 389–401.

Kitano, H. 2001. Systems biology: Toward system-level understanding of biological systems. *In*: Kitano, H. (ed.). Foundations of Systems Biology. Massachusetts Institute of Technology.

Kramer, V.J., M.A. Etterson, M. Hecker, C.A. Murphy, G. Roesijadi, D.J. Spade et al. 2011. Adverse outcome pathways and ecological risk assessment: Bridging to population-level effects. Environ. Toxicol. Chem. 30(1): 64–76.

Kubota, A., A.C.D. Bainy, B.R. Woodin, J.V. Goldstone and J.J. Stegeman. 2013. The cytochrome P450 2AA gene cluster in zebrafish (*Danio rerio*): Expression of CYP2AA1 and CYP2AA2 and response to phenobarbital-type inducers. Toxicol. Appl. Pharmacol. 272: 172–179.

Liu, Z., S. Liu, J. Yao, L. Bao, J. Zhang, Y. Li et al. 2016. The channel catfish genome sequence provides insights into the evolution of scale formation in teleosts. Nat. Commun. 7: 11757.

Lujan, N.K., J.W. Armbruster, N. Lovejoy and H. López-fernández. 2015. Multilocus molecular phylogeny of the suckermouth armored catfishes (Siluriformes: Loricariidae) with a focus on subfamily Hypostominae. Mol. Phylogenet. Evol. 82: 269–288.

Magalhães, M.G.P., D.A. Moreira, C. Furtado and T.E. Parente. 2017. The mitochondrial genome of *Hypancistrus zebra* (Isbrücker & Nijssen, 1991) (Siluriformes: Loricariidae), an endangered ornamental fish from the Brazilian Amazon. Conserv. Genet. Resour. 9(2): 319–324.

McGettigan, Paul A. 2013. Transcriptomics in the RNA-Seq Era. Curr. Opin. Chem. Biol. 17(1): 4–11.

McGill, B.J., M. Dornelas, N.J. Gotelli and A.E. Magurran. 2015. Fifteen forms of biodiversity trend in the anthropocene. Trends Ecol. Evol. 30: 104.

Melo, K.M., I.R. Alves, J.C. Pieczarka, J.A. de O. David, C.Y. Nagamachi and C.K. Grisolia. 2013. Profile of micronucleus frequencies and nuclear abnormalities in different species of electric fishes (Gymnotiformes) from the Eastern Amazon. Genet. Mol. Biol. 36: 425–429.

Mercer, T.R., S. Neph, M.E. Dinger, J. Crawford, M.A. Smith, A.M.J. Shearwood et al. 2011. The human mitochondrial transcriptome. Cell. 146: 645–658.

Moreira, D.A., C. Furtado and T.E. Parente. 2015. The use of transcriptomic next-generation sequencing data to assemble mitochondrial genomes of *Ancistrus* spp. (Loricariidae). Gene. 573: 171–175.

Moreira, D.A., P.A. Buckup, P.C.C. Andrade, M.G.P. Magalhães, M. Brito, C. Furtado et al. 2016. The complete mitochondrial genome of *Corydoras nattereri* (Callichthyidae: Corydoradinae). Neotrop. Ichthyol. 14: e150167.

Moreira, D.A., P.A. Buckup, C. Furtado, A.L. Val, R. Schama and T.E. Parente. 2017. Reducing the information gap on Loricarioidei (Siluriformes) mitochondrial genomics. BMC Genomics. 18: 345.

Newman, M.C. 2015. Fundamentals of Ecotoxicology: The Science of Pollution, Fourth. ed. CRC Press Taylor & Francis Group, Boca Raton, FL.

Nilsson, M.A. 2009. The structure of the Australian and South American marsupial mitochondrial control region. Mitochondrial DNA. 20: 126–138.

Nogueira, L., A.C.F. Rodrigues, C.P. Trídico, C.E. Fossa and E.A. De Almeida. 2011. Oxidative stress in Nile tilapia (*Oreochromis niloticus*) and armored catfish (*Pterygoplichthys anisitsi*) exposed to diesel oil. Environ. Monit. Assess. 180: 243–255.

OECD. Organisation for Economic Co-operation and Development, 1992. OECD guideline for testing of chemicals.

Parente, T.E., D.A. Moreira, P.A. Buckup, P.C.C. de, Andrade, M.G.P. Magalhães, C. Furtado et al. 2017a. Remarkable genetic homogeneity supports a single widespread species of *Hoplosternum littorale* (Siluriformes, Callichthyidae) in South America. Conserv. Genet. Resour., 1-7, DOI 10.1007/ s12686-017-0831-0.

Parente, T.E., D.A. Moreira, M.G.P. Magalhães, P.C.C. De, Andrade, C. Furtado, B.J. Haas et al. 2017b. The liver transcriptome of suckermouth armoured catfish (*Pterygoplichthys anisitsi*, Loricariidae): Identification of expansions in defensome gene families. Mar. Pollut. Bull. 115: 352–361.

Parente, T.E.M., A.C.A.X. De-Oliveira, D.G. Beghini, D.A. Chapeaurouge, J. Perales and F.J.R. Paumgartten. 2009. Lack of constitutive and inducible ethoxyresorufin-O-deethylase activity in the liver of suckermouth armored catfish (*Hypostomus affinis* and *Hypostomus auroguttatus*, Loricariidae). Comp. Biochem. Physiol. -C Toxicol. Pharmacol. 150: 252–260.

Parente, T.E.M., M.F. Rebelo, M.L. Da-Silva, B.R. Woodin, J.V. Goldstone, P.M. Bisch et al. 2011. Structural features of cytochrome P450 1A associated with the absence of EROD activity in liver of the loricariid catfish *Pterygoplichthys* sp. Gene. 489: 111–118.

Parente, T.E.M., P. Urban, D. Pompon and M.F. Rebelo. 2014. Altered substrate specificity of the *Pterygoplichthys* sp. (Loricariidae) CYP1A enzyme. Aquat. Toxicol. 154: 193–199.

Parente, T.E.M., L.M.F. Santos, A.C.A.X. de Oliveira, J.P. de M. Torres, F.G. Araújo, I.F. Delgado et al. 2015. The concentrations of heavy metals and the incidence of micronucleated erythrocytes and liver EROD activity in two edible fish from the Paraíba do Sul river basin in Brazil. Vigilância Sanitária em Debate. 1: 88–92.

Pereira, H.M., L.M. Navarro and I.S. Martins. 2012. Global biodiversity change: the bad, the good, and the unknown. Annu. Rev. Environ. Resour. 37: 25–50.

Satoh, T.P., M. Miya, K. Mabuchi and M. Nishida. 2016. Structure and variation of the mitochondrial genome of fishes. BMC Genomics. 17: 719.

Seddon, N., G. Mace, S. Naeem, A. Pigot, D. Mouillot, R.D. Cavanagh et al. 2016. Biodiversity in the anthropocene: prospects and policy. Proc. R. Soc. B Biol. Sci. 1–9.

Tian, Y. and D.R. Smith. 2016. Recovering complete mitochondrial genome sequences from RNA-Seq: A case study of *Polytomella* non-photosynthetic green algae. Mol. Phylogenet. Evol. 98: 57–62.

Truhaut, R. 1977. Ecotoxicology: Objectives, principles and perspectives. Ecotoxicol. Environ. Saf. 1: 151–173.

U.S. EPA, United States Environmental Protection Agency, 2002. Methods for Measuring the Acute Toxicity of Effluents and Receiving Waters to Freshwater and Marine Organisms.

U.S. EPA, United States Environmental Protection Agency, 2016. OCSPP 850.1075: Freshwater and Saltwater Fish Acute Toxicity Test.

Villeneuve, Daniel L. and Natàlia Garcia-Reyero. 2011. Predictive Ecotoxicology in the 21st Century. Environ. Toxicol. Chem. 30(1): 1–8.

Vinken, Mathieu. 2013. The adverse outcome pathway concept: A pragmatic tool in toxicology. Toxicology. 312(1): 158–65.

Wang, L., X. Zhou and L. Nie. 2011. Organization and variation of mitochondrial DNA control region in pleurodiran turtles. Zoologia. 28: 495–504.

Waters, C.N., J. Zalasiewicz, C. Summerhayes, A.D. Barnosky, C. Poirier, A. Gauszka et al. 2016. The anthropocene is functionally and stratigraphically distinct from the Holocene. Science. (80)351: 137–148.

Young, H.S., D.J. McCauley, M. Galetti and R. Dirzo. 2016. Patterns, causes, and consequences of anthropocene defaunation. Annu. Rev. Ecol. Evol. Syst. 47: 333–358.

3

Ecophysiological Implications of Climate Change Applied to Aquatic Ecotoxicology

IIIIIIIIIIIIIIIIIIIIIIIIIIIIIIIIIIIIIIIIIIIIIIIIIIIIIIIIIIIIIIIIIIIIIIIIIIIIIIIIIIIIIIIIIIIIIIIIIIIIIIIIIIIIIIIIIIIIIIIIIIIIIIIIIIIIIIIIIIIIIIIIIII

Tiago Gabriel Correia[1] and *Adalberto Luis Val*[2,]*

Introduction

Life on earth depends on a delicate and complex interrelationship between the biotope and biocenosis, resulting in the multiplicity of well-known ecosystems encompassing an intricate biodiversity. In this context, the ecological and evolutionary success of a species depends on the relative stability of the abiotic factors that operate within a given ecosystem, as well as the trophic relationships (Quince et al. 2002). It is also of note that abiotic factors influence the dynamics (Gerwing et al. 2016) and the distribution of the population in a given ecosystem (Lewis et al. 2017).

The abiotic factors influence the biological processes within organisms (e.g., growth, reproduction), thereby contributing to the genetic variability (Foll and Gaggiotti 2006, Paulls et al. 2013) observed in the ecological dynamics of a given population (Lovejoy and Hannah 2005). Such abiotic factors include temperature, oxygen saturation, carbon dioxide, water pH, rainfall and light intensity. Changes in environmental factors are often seasonal, with the adaptive processes of organisms then reflecting this seasonality. However, unexpected environmental changes can constitute a significant ecophysiological challenge, thereby providing stress driven selective pressures on organisms (Crozier et al. 2008, Turcotte et al. 2012).

[1] Federal University of Amapá (UNIFAP), Rod. Juscelino Kubitscheck, km 02 - Jd Marco Zero, 68903-419, Macapá, AP, Brazil.
   E-mail: tiago.correia@unifap.br
[2] Brazilian National Institute for Research of the Amazon (INPA), Av. André Araújo, 2936 – Petrópolis, 69067-375, Manaus, AM, Brazil.
* Corresponding author: dalval@inpa.gov.br

For ecophysiologists and ecotoxicologists, knowing the physiological effects that environmental stressors can promote in organisms is of fundamental importance. In this context, the influence of polluting or relevant abiotic factors arising from climate change is important to determine, allowing a modelling of predictions on environmental impact and changes in the ecological structure.

Physiological stress arising from environmental stressors has a very broad operational definition (McEwen 2005, Goodnite 2014). More practically, it refers to the responses that an organism makes in order to prevent large variations in its steady state (Hochachka and Somero 2002), which can be considered a fundamental organizing paradigm within the discipline of ecophysiology (Bradshaw 2007). The classical physiological response to stress, Selye's general adaptation syndrome (Selye 1950), encompasses endocrine responses and metabolic effects, including changes in catecholaminergic hormones and corticosteroids, which promotes a series of metabolic adjustments and the mobilization of energetic substrates (Guerriero and Ciarcia 2006).

Although classical conceptualizations of stress may be broad, and perhaps even ambiguous, it is important to mention allostasis, which provides a model for the regulation and maintenance of homeostasis through physiological and/or behavioral change (McEwen 2005). This model advocates that efficient regulation requires anticipation of the needs of the organism, preparing it even before these needs arise, providing a predictive physiological regulation, through anticipatory adjustments and positive feedbacks (Sterling 2012).

Allostatic responses have metabolic cost for the organism preparing the physiological systems capable of sustaining homeostasis when imposed by different stressors (McEwen and Wingfield 2003). This is complicated by the proposed synergistic interaction between environmental contaminants and climate change, which has consequences for biodiversity that are primarily driven by impacts on the trophic structure of ecosystems, including species distribution and richness. This links to the 'metabolic theory of ecology' (MTE) (Brown 2004), which will be briefly discussed next.

Although much criticized, MTE can be considered as an organizing principle of ecology supported by the tripod: biology, physics and chemistry, through an allometric and thermodynamic approach, which suggests, in a predictive way, how climatic effects, more precisely, the environmental temperature, considered as the most important abiotic factor, influences the patterns of abundance, richness and geographical distribution of species (Brown 2004). In the scope of MTE, the metabolic rate of an animal, especially ectothermic, is influenced by the variation of the environmental temperature, though the increase in temperature implies elevation of metabolic rate (Hochachka and Somero 2002).

Subsequently, as a thermodynamic result of this process, predicted climate change will therefore require greater energy expenditure. However, the toxicity of many chemical compounds will also be potentiated, further increasing the energy cost for maintenance of basal metabolism (Derelanko and Auletta 2014). Environmental temperature influences the metabolic balance of ecosystems (Durocher et al. 2010), thereby modifying its trophic structure by influencing all levels of organization, from single organisms to communities (Brown 2004).

Climatic, especially temperature, variations will therefore be an important determinant of alterations in metabolism and thereby with consequences for the allostatic adjustments following environmental stress, which underpin homoeostasis and are indispensable to the understanding and prediction of possible impacts on biodiversity. Figure 1 shows an entity-relationship diagram (ER), which gives a simple model of MTE in this context.

The imminent projections for climate change, and those having already occurred, indicate dramatic impacts on biodiversity, with a prognosis suggesting possible collapse of some ecosystems (Morris 2010). Ecosystem collapses are often not avoided because predictive ecology lacks extensive evidence of events and the association between forces that promote ecological impacts, with unexpected combinations and unpredictable changes (Montoya and Raffaelli 2010, Connel et al. 2013).

The notoriety of this scenario is exacerbated by the disastrous perspective attributed to the expected increase in toxicity, promoted by chemical compounds from predominantly anthropogenic sources that pollute ecosystems (Moe et al. 2013), since one of the premises that permeate the ecophysiological assumptions applicable to ecotoxicology is that the occurrence and permanence of any species in a given ecosystem is partly due to the ability to reproduce and face the environmental factors (Correia et al. 2010).

Walther (2010) argues that the effects of climate change on biodiversity are virtually undeniable, with ample ecological evidences to date. This author also highlights the role of changes in abiotic factors that trigger unfavorable environmental conditions, due, in part, to the break in the synchronized seasonal rhythms of many ecological processes. Such temporal asynchronies alter species composition and disorganize trophic chains to the point of being perceptible, including plant

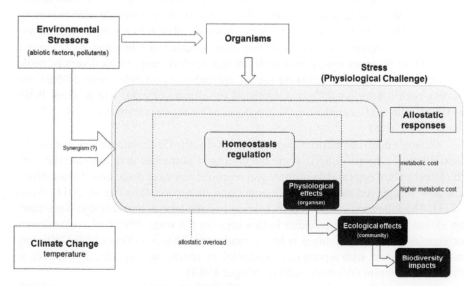

Fig. 1. Entity-relationship conceptual diagram. Association between environmental stressors, homoeostasis and ecological effects.

phenology and interspecific biotic relationships, such as insect-plant and parasite-host (Walther 2010).

For Woodward and co-authors (2010), climate change is such a diverse and complex combination of factors that when associated with anthropogenic chemical compounds, will result not only in already apparent abiotic effects, such as habitat fragmentation and increased eutrophication rates, but also in barely perceptible biotic effects, such as species invasion and even extinction processes.

However, Bellard et al. (2012) argue that there is still little evidence of species extinction as a result of climate change, although they admit that habitat destruction arising from abiotic factors, such as rainfall, photoperiod and temperature, can impact biodiversity due to a failure in acclimatizing to new rhythms. These authors also suggest that the resilience of an ecosystem is dependent upon the capacity of different populations to physiologically adjust, and thus to tolerate the new abiotic conditions (Bellard et al. 2012).

This indicates that in ecosystems impacted by sublethal pollutants, biocenosis should have sufficient plasticity and energy resources to maintain basal metabolism and homeostasis, as well as for detoxification against the effects imposed by the stressors. In this sense, the processes of acclimatization and adaptation of the species are decisive in the resilience of certain ecosystems (Huey et al. 2012). The following is a brief overview of this interrelationship between climate change and the contamination of aquatic ecosystems and the physiological and ecological effects on organisms and biodiversity.

The Future Challenge is Already the Present Challenge

Following the publication of Rachel Carson's book *Silent Spring* in 1962, the world was alerted to the dangers of persistent organic pollutants (POPs) to human health, as well as to wildlife and the flora. This inspired the worldwide environmental movement (Vail 2015). In spite of Carson's positive influence on new environmental paradigms, the reduction in pesticide use only occurred in a few nations (Pimentel 2012). Over 50 years ago, it was realized that such damage to biodiversity could be irreversible, with the increased use of agricultural pesticides now evident and having their deleterious effects potentiated by climate change, which alters POPs bioavailability and exacerbating the processes of bioaccumulation (Borgå et al. 2010, Nadal et al. 2015).

Carson's main contribution occurred in 1968 at the Conference of Environmental Toxicity in Rochester (USA), where the effects of pesticides in decreasing the shell thickness of bird eggs and their impact on reproduction were discussed. These effects are now recognized as arising from endocrine disruption (Mnif et al. 2011, Weiss 2011). The following year, René Truhaut coined the term ecotoxicology; since then, an extensive subsequent research in this area on the toxic effects of contaminants or xenobiotics on living things is being conducted. This is an area of long-standing historical interest, with reports of contamination, specifically aquatic, dating back to the Roman Empire (Wijibenga and Hutzinger 1984).

The interaction of climate change with environmental pollutants is currently an area of extensive research. However, much is still to be learned in this area, especially with regard to future consequences, although the World Meteorological Organization's Global Climate Impact Program (WICP) has existed since the 1970s. According to Kates and co-authors (1985), the WICP program should have 5 main objectives:

1. Improvement of our knowledge of the impact of climatic variability and change in terms of the specific primary responses to natural and human systems.

2. Development of our knowledge and awareness of the interactive relations between climate variability and socio-economic activities.

3. Improvement of the methodology employed so as to deepen the understanding and improve the simulation of the interactions among climatic, environmental and socio-economic factors.

4. Determining the characteristics of human societies at different levels of development and in different natural environments which make them especially resilient to climatic variability and change and which also permit them to take advantage of the opportunities posed by such changes.

5. Application of this new knowledge of techniques to practical problems of concern to developing countries or which are related to a common need for all mankind.

These objectives are still pertinent. However, a series of new metrics have been proposed which draws on the cause-and-effect relationships (Levasseur et al. 2016), thereby constructing a new conceptual model for the main agents of changing climatic conditions and how these can negatively influence aquatic ecosystems, including temperature, rainfall and salinity (Ward et al. 2016), as well as ocean acidification (Speers et al. 2016), dissolved CO_2 and depletion of O_2, resulting in hypoxic conditions (Altieri and Gedan 2015).

Climate change is affecting humanity, both directly and indirectly (Hooper et al. 2013). Among the many systems that can be impacted is the agricultural sector, which is one of the most vulnerable to the effects of climate change (Cai et al. 2016). Reductions in fish stocks (Belhabib et al. 2016) are also worrisome, increasing the demand for food production (Ogier et al. 2016). In addition, threats to public health should also be noted (Vardoulakis et al. 2015).

Schiedek and co-authors (2007) suggest that there is an approximation between research involving climate change and ecotoxicology in such a way that a better basis can be provided to assist in understanding and predicting future changes. According to authors, different types of contaminants or abiotic factors can interact synergistically, making it difficult to identify the various environmental threats present in an ecosystem under pressure from such environmental changes (Schiedek et al. 2007).

Interactions between Climate Change and Chemical Contaminants

An important aspect of ecotoxicology is the prediction of the possible harmful effects of pollutants in order to protect ecosystems and living creatures. This may require the utilization of valid biomarkers in order to assess the sublethal effects of exposure to chemical, physical or biological agents (Oost et al. 2003, Connon et al. 2012).

However, considering the interaction of these responses with the effects of climate change on organisms (biomarkers), the task becomes much more complex because there are many factors that are subject to several variables that often overlap, making it difficult to interpret the results since many ecotoxicological protocols are still limited (Hook et al. 2014). The interpretation of this interaction can sometimes be dichotomous (Hooper et al. 2013) and to be relevant, requires consideration in an ecological context where experimental designs are complex (Noyes and Lema 2015).

Consequently, experiments in microcosms or mesocosms are indispensable, given that multiple stressors can be considered simultaneously. Physiological biomarkers can indicate health status, physiological integrity, and species susceptibility to specific environmental threats (Connon et al. 2012), while ecological indicators show the consequences of impacts at a population or community level (Bartell 2006).

Table 1 summarizes some of the isolated effects and the synchronous associations between climate changes and some chemical contaminants, together with their physiological responses and ecological consequences. Several taxa are highlighted in this context, providing a global view for different biomes subject to specific combinations of stressors, which indicate the following physiological effects: endocrine dysregulation (Jenssen 2006, Gustavson et al. 2015), metabolic impairment, decrease in growth, reproduction and biomass (Sogard and Spencer 2004, Eissa and Zaki 2011, Hallinger and Cristol 2011, Ainsworth et al. 2011), osmoregulation disturbances (Fortin et al. 2008, Adeyami et al. 2012), oxidative stress (Greco et al. 2011), changes in biotransformation enzymes (Buckman et al. 2007), and respiratory allergy (D'Amato et al. 2016). In addition, ecological impacts on phenology (Scaven and Rafferty 2013, Lötters et al. 2014), abundance (Khasnis and Nettleman 2005, Russell et al. 2009, Falkenberg et al. 2012) and migratory behavior (Carey 2009) should also be considered.

In this sense, it is imperative to consider that chemical contaminants may be considered as being comprised of two classes: organic compounds, including petroleum derived substances, such as polycyclic aromatic hydrocarbons (HPAs), bisphenols, pesticides and other POPs, and inorganic compounds, generally comprising the heavy metals. Some of the most relevant abiotic factors, in the context of climate change interactions with chemical contaminants in aquatic ecosystems, include pH, temperature, gas saturation (O_2 and CO_2) and salinity.

It is important to emphasize that Noyes and co-authors (2009) as well as Noyes and Lema (2015) have proposed that the interaction between climate change and chemical toxicity may result in non-linear effects. Such proposed non-linearity links to Ludwig von Bertalanffy's General Theory of Systems (1951).

By not starting with the supposition from a pre-deterministic premise but rather to be a presupposition of complex systems, multiple possibilities arise from the resultant interactions. Therefore, given that future outcomes (prognostics) are directly dependent on the present reality, any intervention in the present may lead to radical future changes. Therefore, an epistemological approach, utilizing holistic-

Table 1. Interactive effects between climate change and contaminants on biomarkers.

Outcome biomarkers	Environmental threats & Anthropogenic contaminants	Ref.
Endocrine disruption (polar bears)	OH-PCBs + Climate change	Gustavson et al. 2015
Endocrine disruption causes interference on adaptation capacity to environmental stress in Artic marine mammals and seabirds	EDCs + Climate change	Jenssen 2006
Changes in sexual proportions (vertebrates) Skeletal deformities (fishes)	Thermal stress	Eissa and Zaki 2011 Guidini et al. (under review)
Impairment in somatic and reproductive fish growth (deficit in metabolic requirements)		Sogard and Spencer 2004
Increase in mosquito population vectors of diseases and agricultural pests	Thermal stress	reviewed by Delorenzo 2015 Tadei et al. 2016
Loss of osmoregulatory function (fishes)	Atrazine + salinity	reviewed by Delorenzo 2015
Inhibit antioxidant defenses (bivalve mussel)	Herbicide + Temperature	reviewed by Delorenzo 2015
Changes on migratory behavior and breeding (birds)	Climate Change	Carey 2009
Human respiratory allergy	Urbanization (CO_2 vehicle) + Diverse Climate Change Factors	D'Amato et al. 2016
Osmoregulation effects (fishes)	Cu + Salinity	Adeyami et al. 2012
Reproductive effects (birds)	Environmental temperature + Hg	Hallinger and Cristol 2011
Effects on enzymes of biotransformation process (fishes)	Temperature + OH-PCBs	Buckman et al. 2007
Changes in phenology (amphibian)	Glyphosate + Climate Change	Lötters et al. 2014
Changes in the relative abundance of algae species	CO_2 + nutrients	Russell et al. 2009, Falkenberg et al. 2012
Physiological effects on flowering plants and pollinating insects	Climate warming	Scaven and Rafferty 2013
Decline fisheries biomass	Climate effects	Ainsworth et al. 2011

multidisciplinary and non-reductionist perspectives, is required for the proposals of studies in this thematic.

It is important to point out in this context that ecotoxicological experiments in the laboratory (bioassays) are, as a rule, reductionist and, consequently, may impede or limit the interpretation of more complex approaches (Hook et al. 2014). Figure 2, in a general way, shows the relationship between environmental stressors and some response mechanisms (biomarkers) for fish.

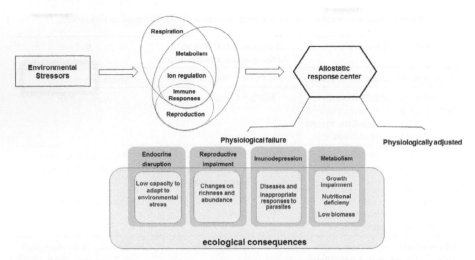

Fig. 2. Schematic representation of the main physiological responses and their ecological consequences in the case of homeostatic adjustment failure.

Increased Environmental Temperature

Few ecological factors have a greater influence on animal energy metabolism than temperature (Bícego et al. 2007). For ectothermal aquatic organisms, temperature is the main abiotic factor that modulates most of its physiological processes, including endocrine function (Norris 2007), metabolic rate (Donelson et al. 2014), cell membrane fluidity (Murata and Los 1997) and, consequently, the homeoviscous adaptation (Ernst et al. 2016).

Obviously, modifications in the fatty acid structure of the cell membrane will influence the entry and deposition of compounds, mostly organic, within the cell (Noyes and Lema 2015). This process must be considered simultaneously with diffusion rates, given that molecular kinetics are influenced by temperature arise, which will also modulate the chemical structure of contaminants, their bioavailability and their toxicity (Nikinmaa 2014).

Relevant toxicological aspects of contaminants released into aquatic ecosystems that are influenced by increased temperature include changes in toxicokinetics (absorption, distribution, metabolism and excretion) and toxicodynamics (molecular interaction, cellular response and body toxic effects), given the possible synergistic interaction between temperature and contaminants (Hooper et al. 2013).

Generally, all chemical reactions are affected by temperature variation, with consequences for behavioral and physiological processes, including O_2 consumption and basal metabolic rate (Schmidt-Nielsen 2002). Importantly, the expected temperature increase of 0.2°C for the coming decades and 1.4–5.8°C by 2100 are attributed to increased greenhouse gas emissions, including CO_2, CH_4, and N_2O, which are the main drivers of climate change (IPCC 2014).

Both vertebrates and invertebrates have limited tolerance to environmental thermal variation. Although these limits are not fixed, animals need time to acclimatize (Schmidt-Nielsen 2002). However, the expected synergistic effect of increasing temperature with chemical contaminants may occur at a very rapid rate and greatly diminish the thermal tolerance of many organisms (Cahill et al. 2012), resulting in significant ecological impacts.

In spite of being a worldwide phenomenon, only recent studies have explored the effects of climate change beyond the borders of Europe and the USA (Noyes et al. 2009). As Neotropical regions are relatively under-explored, many of these effects and their interactions are unknown, including for Amazonian species. Because the interaction between climate changes (e.g., temperature) and pollutants is very complex, it is often difficult to identify effects separately. This exacerbates the situation for species living at the limit of their physiological tolerance, particularly as chemical compounds may impair the organism's ability to acclimatize adequately (Stahl et al. 2013). It is important to emphasize that being an abiotic factor that significantly modulates some key vital processes for life, as well the toxicity of chemical agents, temperature is important for both physiological (metabolism) and toxicological (toxicodynamics) processes (Noyes et al. 2009).

In the case of teleost fish, the main physiological processes impacted by changes in environmental temperature are aerobic metabolism (rate of O_2 consumption), cardiac output, opercular ventilation, excretion and reproduction, which are well documented (Reid et al. 1997, Pörtner and Peck 2010). However, the interaction with chemical contaminants still requires clarification.

The bioenergetic implications of climate change, as indicated above, highlight their ecophysiological relevance, especially for high-energy processes such as growth and reproduction. An important aspect of these processes may be the conversion of food to energy (Bostock et al. 2010). In a chronic microcosm experiment, Oliveira and Val (2017) investigated the effects of different climate scenarios on the growth and physiology of juveniles of the Amazonian teleost species, *Colossoma macropomum*. The results showed that the expected climatic changes for year 2100 led to a mass gain and increased food conversion, with no significant effect on growth. These authors concluded that the increased temperature above the optimum for this species caused a displacement of energy to meet the increased metabolic demand. In a natural environment, these characteristics would result in ecological imbalances in the food chain.

According to Noyes and Lema (2015), the relationship between thermal tolerance, chemical contaminants and bioenergetics must be analysed simultaneously. This allows consideration of not only the thermal performance of a species, but also its ability to deal with multiple stressors and, therefore, better predict ecological impacts. This suggests that indirect physiological measures, such as O_2 consumption, behavioral analysis and swimming capacity, will provide data with more ecological relevance. In our laboratory, a swimming tunnel was used to evaluate the maximum velocity a fish can maintain in a stream before it becomes fatigued (Ucrit) (Farrell 2008) under different conditions.

At the same time, it is possible to obtain data on O_2 consumption, indicative of aerobic metabolism, CO_2 excretion, nitrogen (NH_3) and to evaluate the swimming performance. This type of approach is non-invasive, of low cost and clarifies the metabolic profile of species with different swimming characteristics, and readily

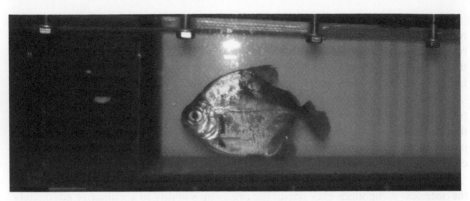

Fig. 3. A specimen of *Myloplus asterias* in a closed swimming tunnel to evaluate swimming performance and to determine the Ucrit. Coupled to a respirometer, the tunnel allows control of temperature, oxygen levels and especially water velocity.

allows the investigation of environmental variables and/or contaminants. Much still needs to be investigated, including the effects of climate change on migratory *versus* non-migratory species. Figure 3 illustrates the exposure of an Amazonian species, *Myloplus asterias*, submitted to the Ucrit test.

Unpublished data from our laboratory analysed the effect of heavy metal exposure in a simulated climate change environment on the ovoviparous teleost species, *Xiphophorus helleri*, during the embryonic period. Results showed that in an extreme climatic scenario, there was a remodelling in the fatty acid profile of embryos during the final stage of development as well metabolic disturbance. Results also showed a synergism between metals and climate changes that is lethal for both males and females of this species.

Endocrine Disruption

Endocrine-disrupting compounds (EDCs) are defined by the US Environmental Protection Agency as any exogenous agent that interferes with the synthesis, transport, secretion, and metabolism of natural hormones, and which are transported by blood to their respective receptors on target organs. EDCs can have impacts on reproduction, homeostasis and development (Kandarakis et al. 2009). Both organic compounds and metals can be considered as EDCs, with studies of their effects on the endocrine system primarily investigating the hypothalamic-pituitary-gland axis, especially the thyroid gland, gonads and adrenals or homologous structures, with consequences for metabolism, reproduction and environmental stress responses, respectively. The interaction between EDCs and abiotic factors related to climate change is an important area of investigation (Jenssen 2006b, Keller et al. 2015).

Although there are no published results on these interactions in the Amazonian teleosts, unpublished data from our laboratory shows that acute copper exposure, in a microcosm simulating climate change, altered energy metabolism and led to the depletion of thyroid hormones in the teleost, *Colossoma macropomum* (TGC, unpublished data).

As indicated above, reviews of literature led to the proposal that physiological responses, arising from the interaction of chemical contaminants and abiotic factors related to climate change, are non-linear. Matthiessen and Johnson (2007) point out that EDCs can trigger non-linear and monotonic hormonal effects, which are neither increasing, decreasing or constant, but rather are biphasic effects.

This response profile is related to different biochemical pathways of interaction, regardless of whether EDCs are in high or low doses. Moreover, these authors affirm that this non-linearity has contributed to the acceptance of the idea of the hormesis phenomenon, suggesting the possibility that the non-linear hormetic dose-response curve for EDCs is a standard, and not a linear curve (Matthiessen and Johnson 2007).

Unpublished data obtained in our laboratory from experiments in which the interaction between metals and climate change was investigated indicates a counterproductive hormonal response pattern compared with many reported effects in the literature. This leads us to suspect a biphasic response. Hormonal responses are often considered to be biphasic (Schrek 2010), reinforcing the idea of a hormesis phenomenon occurring in the interactions of EDCs with climate change.

Perhaps one of the most striking examples of deleterious effects of climate change and EDCs is in amphibians. Although little is known about the interaction between these stressors and climate change for this group, there is a consensus that compounds, mainly organic, impair the metamorphosis of these animals because they affect the thyroid gland hormones, as well as the adaptive responses to the selective pressures promoted by climate change (Urban et al. 2013).

Ecophysiological Perspectives of Ocean Acidification

Coral reefs are perhaps one of the most striking examples of the biomes that have suffered the deleterious effects of climate change. Until very recently, it was thought that these formations were exclusively oceanic, but recent discoveries of the existence of biogenic reefs in the mouth of the Amazon River (Moura et al. 2016) have changed perceptions about this biome. Oceanic coral reefs are one of the planet's most important ecosystems and harbor fragile biodiversity (Ruppert and Barnes 1996).

Oceanic coral reef integrity depends on a narrow range of temperature variation, depth, luminosity and other physical and chemical characteristics of water (Speers et al. 2016). The main threats of climate change are not limited to coral reefs; other oceanic environments are vulnerable to rising temperatures, rising sea levels and water acidification, as a consequence of the deposition and solubilization of atmospheric anthropogenic CO_2 (Keller et al. 2009). As for freshwater corals, it is unknown as to which abiotic factors have most direct relevance to their continued functioning, including as to the effects of climate change on this.

For centuries, due to human activity, atmospheric CO_2 concentration has been gradually increasing, and it is forecasted to increase further from its current 400 parts per million (ppm) to 1250 ppm by 2100, which is dependent on projected human activity (IPCC 2014). However, the increased CO_2 concentration is already so high that some of the effects would be irreversible for about 1000 years after the end of emissions (Solomon et al. 2009).

In oceans, CO_2 depositions promote a series of changes in water's physicochemical characteristics, including a reduction in $CaCO_3$ and changes in the chemical balance between organic and inorganic carbon species (Coelho et al. 2013). However, the main stressor is the decrease in pH, leading to acidification of the oceans (Connel et al. 2013), which is often referred to as "the other problem" (Doney et al. 2009).

Acidification of the oceans is affecting all marine ecosystems globally (Kroeker et al. 2013), primarily by the solubilization of calcium carbonate from carapace or invertebrate shells, changes in the trophic chain (Godbold and Calosi 2013), the population structure of species, including phytoplankton, the rate of photosynthesis, and changes in the biogeochemical cycle of micronutrients, with a consequent increase in eutrophication and proliferation of red tides (Moore et al. 2008).

When considering the effects of ocean acidification, several environmental stressors and abiotic factors have a heightened likelihood of interaction, with resultant consequences being unpredictable. The physico-chemical variables of the water are of note in this context. Dissolved oxygen, temperature and salinity may modulate the toxicity, biotransformation and bioaccumulation of organic compounds, but mainly on the speciation and bioavailability of heavy metals (Lewis et al. 2016). There is general agreement that ocean acidification will act synergistically with heavy metal ions potentiating these toxic effects on aquatic biota, mainly by directly interfering with speciation and bioavailability (Nikinmaa 2014, Zeng et al. 2015).

However, in spite of this agreement, Roberts and co-authors (2013) showed a counter-claim that the toxicity resulting from this interaction cannot be explained by the processes of metal speciation and that the physiological effects will be additive and not synergistic, as previously proposed. It is clear that future mechanistic research will be required to clarify the nature of such interactions that underpin heightened toxicity.

The application of physiological biomarkers to access the effects of oceanic acidification on marine organisms is an arduous task because the interpretation of the results is multifactorial and ambiguous, especially when it comes to metals. For example, although reducing the pH of water promotes an increase in copper concentration from the sediment to the water, other metals, such as cadmium, may have their concentration reduced or unaffected (Roberts et al. 2013). It is important to note that the toxicological relevance of complex mixtures (where more than one contaminant is involved) may result in interactions that are difficult to predict, including synergistic, additive, potentiating and antagonistic effects (Zagatto and Bertoletti 2006).

In an experiment conducted by Lewis and co-authors (2016) investigating the relationship of ocean acidification and Cu, there was still ambiguity as to whether the results arose from additive or synergistic interactions, due to limitations in the experimental design. However, the authors emphasized that a number of meta-analyzes indicate that synergistic effects more commonly arise from the interactions between multiple abiotic factors. Environmental stressors for the marine environment are much more common than additive effects. It is clear that future investigations and appropriate experimental protocols are required to clarify the nature of the interactions of climate change factors and environmental contaminants. These will be important to investigate as it is clear that the available current data acts to limit the predictability of ecological effects.

Marine invertebrate species can be considered as promising ecophysiological models for the study of ocean acidification interacting with other environmental stressors. This may be especially true for sessile or less mobile species, since they meet specific ecotoxicological premises of representativeness, local relevance and constancy of exposure to environmental factors. For example, in a study by Lewis and co-authors (2006) using the mussel, *Mytilus edulis*, and purple sea urchin, *Paracentrotus lividus*, copper exposure under ocean acidification resulted in DNA damage, which was more pronounced in mussels. In the same study, oxidative stress and lipoperoxidation were evaluated, with the antioxidant enzyme, superoxide dismutase, suppressed only in *Mytilus edulis*, whilst lipoperoxidation only occurred in *Paracentrotus lividus*. This demonstrates that the use of different species with different physiological sensitivities is fundamental until a species that can be considered an ideal model for this type of study is found because the physiological peculiarities of each species denote the need for the application of different biomarkers.

In addition to the impacts of ocean acidification on metal toxicity, acidification slows the degradation of organic pollutants, thereby increasing bioavailability (Zeng et al. 2015). An example to show how these pollutants will be affected will be by reducing bioavailability of the metal, Fe (III), which is an important cofactor of many enzymes involved in the degradation of organic compounds, and at the same time may lead to a reduction in the availability of oxygen and nitrogen, thereby impairing the metabolism and microbial degradation of organic compounds (Zeng et al. 2015).

As indicated above, ocean acidification will affect the oceanic trophic structure as well as interfere with the physicochemical processes of organic compounds. Alava and co-authors (2017) provide, in a general way, how climatic changes can generate serious ecological problems, highlighting changes in the composition of species and several inter-specific relations, for example, predator-prey. These authors have traced the relationship between inorganic and organic pollutants, Hg and PCBs respectively, coupled with increased CO_2 concentration in the marine trophic chain, with physiological effects involving endocrine components, energetic substrates (lipids) and bioaccumulation (Alava et al. 2017).

Alava and co-authors (2017) illustrate this scenario when presenting the combined actions of the above stressors in the resultant high metabolic cost for the chinook salmon (*Oncorhynchus tshawytscha*), which accumulates environmental mercury and PCBs. In order to maintain their basal metabolism in face of the imposed physiological challenge, these animals use a large part of their energy substrates (lipids), and consequently, individuals have gradually lost biomass, whilst offspring numbers have decreased. This resulted in their predator, *Orcinus orca*, having to consume a much larger number of salmon, highlighting the biomagnification of pollutants that have intensified in the food chain from interaction with climate change (Alava et al. 2017).

Finally, the crisis in coral reefs arising from 'coral bleaching syndrome' and the extermination of their constituent organisms related with oxidative stress has well documented (Downs et al. 2002). The need for wider physiological biomarkers appropriate to the particular species and context is clearly needed. This is highlighted in the recent disruption of the Samarco mining dam in Mariana—Brazil, which led to the release of large quantities of iron ore tailings, containing different heavy metals, directly into the Doce River (Fernandes et al. 2016). The Coral Vivo project was set up to study the interaction of climate change with heavy metal pollution in Brazilian coral reefs using a novel marine mesocosm facility and was tasked with the elaboration of the physiological biomarkers and ecological indicators to enable protection against such ecological disasters (Duarte et al. 2015).

Brief Comments on Pollutants Interactions with Hypoxia

The solubility of oxygen is directly influenced by temperature in virtually all aquatic environments, including oceanic and continental (Nikinmaa 2002). Under natural conditions, the dissolved oxygen concentration in the water can vary to become hypoxic, and even anoxic, with both daily and seasonal rhythms. These variations are more pronounced in the rivers and lakes of tropical environments and in shallow and eutrophic coastal areas (Childress and Seibel 1998, Rowe 2001). The threat of climate change in interaction with anthropogenic compounds is responsible for coastal 'dead zones' arising from oxygen depletion, and exacerbated by climate change (Altieri and Gedan 2015).

Tropical rivers, such as those composing the Amazon Basin, naturally present extreme environmental conditions, such as acidic and ion-poor waters, high concentrations of dissolved hydrogen sulfide and CO_2, high temperatures and often hypoxic and even anoxic conditions. However, these adverse environmental conditions may be even more challenging in the context of climate change, resulting in the expansion of deeper hypoxic areas and more acidic environments (Val et al. 2015). Such hypoxia has become a worldwide environmental concern due to the enrichment of aquatic ecosystems by anthropogenic compounds rich in nitrogen and other nutrients (Breitburg et al. 2009). Chronic exposure to hypoxia results in impaired reproduction, immune response and teleost growth, as well as changes in interspecific interactions in the trophic chain (Breitburg et al. 2009).

Clearly, climate change exacerbates the expansion of hypoxic areas and 'dead zones' by increasing factors such as temperature, ocean acidification, rising sea levels, and storms, which can synergistically interact with pollutants (Altieri and Gedan 2015). The most important pollutants include the agricultural run-off residues containing high NO_3^- concentrations (Keller et al. 2009), resulting in sites with high eutrophication rates.

The increase in oceanic pCO_2 is directly related to hypoxia and oceanic acidification. In a study conducted by Labarthe and co-authors (2012), increased caesium bioaccumulation was associated with decreased pH under high CO_2 concentration in the eggs of the cuttlefish species, *Sepia officinalis*. This study illustrates how metal toxicity can be increased under the influence of these abiotic factors.

Nikinmaa (2013), in a very general way, proposed that any type of chemical stressor can result in the formation of reactive oxygen species, leading to the oxidative stress that can contribute to hypoxia. Hypoxia-inducible factors (HIFs) are transcriptional factors that respond to the decrease in cellular oxygen. HIFs are bHLH-PAS proteins that are heterodimeric transcription factors that respond to environmental signals, including anthropogenic chemical compounds, physiological signals, hypoxia, and circadian rhythms (Bernsten et al. 2013).

Among the bHLH-PAS transcription factor families is the aryl hydrocarbon receptor (AhR), which is a binding-dependent transcription factor that binds to xenobiotics and regulates the expression of the response genes required by the metabolic detoxification machinery of these compounds (Wu et al. 2013). In this sense, according to Nikinmaa (2013), HIFs and AhR share biochemical pathways and, therefore, a possible activation of the AhR may occur, either stimulated by xenobiotics that induce their own metabolism, or by abiotic factors of climate change in response to the hypoxia.

Marine aquatic animals, such as fish, which are confronted by hypoxia environments/situations, require an adequate physiological response in order to maintain metabolism and adjustments in the respiratory system. However, fish in the Amazon basin are regularly confronted with hypoxia on a physiological and environmental basis (Val and Almeida-Val 1995). Some Amazonian teleosts have morphological, behavioral and biochemical adjustments against hypoxia, whereas for other species, it is only biochemical (Val et al. 2015) and/or physiological adjustments (Ferreira et al. 2010). However, although hypoxia can be a common phenomenon for Amazonian fish, it is likely that under the additional onus of climate change, hypoxia will become a major ecophysiological challenge for the continuity of many tropical species in the Amazon (Val et al. 2015).

The tambaqui, *Colossoma macropomum*, is one of the most important species of Amazonian teleosts and is used in many ecophysiological studies, given that it is adaptive and highly tolerant to changes in pH, temperature and oxygenation among the different rivers that inhabit the Amazon Basin (Val and Almeida-Val 1995). In the context of climate change, the tambaqui may be an important physiological model for the study of molecular mechanisms, underpinning resilience to the environmental challenges posed by climate change and its interactions with abiotic factors (Lima and Val 2016).

The transcriptomic characterization of the tambaqui, when exposed to a microcosm scenario simulating climate change, shows a complex cellular response, involving the expression of several genes that can be controlled by different mechanisms of transcription and translation (Lima and Val 2016). This study demonstrates that even for species already adapted and subjected to a great abiotic variation, climate change imposes challenges to survival that can be seen as an attempt to drive the acclimatization of the species to the new environmental conditions. Further research is required in order to clarify the relevant biological underpinnings that determine survival under the interactive challenge of climate change and abiotic factors, perhaps being especially fruitful to investigate in Amazonian species.

Closing Remarks and Future Directions

It is clear that aquatic ecotoxicology needs both physiological and ecological approaches for the investigation of the interactions between climate change and chemical contaminants on biocenosis. More realistic and ecologically relevant experimental designs in microcosm or mesocosm should help to prioritize the multifactorial factors underpinning the effects of different stressors and their interactions while at the same time, given the limitation of many biomarkers, omics technologies may provide important information facing new challenges and current needs.

References

Adeyami, J.A., L.W. Deaton, T.C. Pesacreta and P.L. Klerks. 2012. Effects of copper on osmoregulation in sheepshead minnow, *Cyprinodon variegatus* acclimated to different salinities. Aquat. Toxicol. 109: 111–117.

Ainsworth, C.H., J.F. Samhouri, D.S. Busch, W.W.L. Cheung, J. Dunne and T.A. Okey. 2011. Potential impacts of climate change on Northeast Pacific marine food webs and fisheries. J. Mar. Sci. 68(6): 1217–1229.

Alava, J.J., W.W.L. Cheung, P.S. Ross and U.R. Sumaila. 2017. Climate change–contaminant interactions in marine food webs: Toward a conceptual framework. Global Change Biol. 00: 1–18.

Altieri, A.H. and K.B. Gedan. 2015. Climate change and dead zones. Global Change Biol. 21: 1395–1406.

Bartell, S.M. 2006. Biomarkers, bioindicators, and ecological risk assessment—a brief review and evaluation. Environ. Bioind. 1: 60–73.

Belhabib, D., V.W.Y. Lam and W.W.L. Cheung. 2016. Overview of West African fisheries under climate change: Impacts, vulnerabilities and adaptive responses of the artisanal and industrial sectors. Mar. Policy. 71: 15–28.

Bellard, C., C. Bertelsmeier, P. Leadley, W. Thuiller and F. Courchamp. 2012. Impacts of climate change on the future of biodiversity. Ecol. Lett. 15(4): 365–377.

Bersten, D.C., A.E. Sullivan, D.J. Peet and M.L. Whitelaw. 2013. Nature Rev. 13: 827–841.

Bertalanffy, L.V. 1951. General system theory: A new approach to unity of science—toward a physical theory of organic teleology—feedback and dynamics. Hum. Biol. 23: 346–361.

Bícego, K.C., R.C.H. Barros and L.G.S. Branco. 2007. Physiology of temperature regulation: Comparative aspects. Comp. Biochem. Physiol. A Mol. Integr. Physiol. 147: 616–639.

Borgå, K., T.M. Saloranta and A. Ruus. 2010. Simulating climate change-induced alterations in bioaccumulation of organic contaminants in an Arctic marine food web. Environ. Toxicol. Chem. 29(6): 1349–1357.

Bostock, J., B. McAndrew, R. Richards, K. Jauncey, T. Telfer, K. Lorenzen, D. Little et al. 2010. Aquaculture: global status and trends. Philosophical Transactions of the Royal Society B. 365: 2897–2912.

Bradshaw, D. 2007. Ecofisiologia dos Vertebrados. Uma Introdução aos Seus Princípios e Aplicações. Santos Press, BR.

Breitburg, D.L., D.W. Hondorp, L.A. Davias and R.J. Diaz. 2009. Hypoxia, nitrogen, and fisheries: Integrating effects across local and global landscapes. Annu. Rev. Mar. Sci. 1: 329–349.

Brown, J.H. 2004. Toward a metabolic theory of ecology. Ecology. 85(7): 1771–1789.

Buckman, A.H., S.B. Brown, J. Small, D.C.G. Muir, J. Parrott, K.R. Solomon et al. 2007. Role of temperature and enzyme induction in the biotransformation of polychlorinated biphenyls and bioformation of hydroxylated polychlorinated biphenyls by rainbow trout (*Oncorhynchus mykiss*). Environ. Sci. Technol. 41(11): 3856–3863.

Cai, Y., J.S. Bandara and D. Newth. 2016. A framework for integrated assessment of food production economics in South Asia under climate change. Environ. Model. Softw. 75: 459–497.

Cahill, A.E., M.E.A. Lammens, M.C.F. Reid, X. Hua, C.J. Karanewsky, H.Y. Ryu et al. 2013. How does climate change cause extinction? Proc. R Soc. Lond. [Biol]. 280(1750): 1–9.

Carey, C. 2009. The impacts of climate change on the annual cycles of birds. Philos. Trans. Royal Soc. B. 364: 3321–3330.

Childress, J.J. and B.A. Seibel. 1998. Life at stable low oxygen levels: adaptations of animals to oceanic oxygen minimum layers. J. Exp. Biol. 201(8): 1223–1232.

Coelho, F.J.R.C., A.L. Santos, J. Coimbra, A. Almeida, A. Cunha, D.F.R. Cleary et al. 2013. Interactive effects of global climate change and pollution on marine microbes: the way ahead. Ecol. Evol. 3(6): 1808–1818.

Connell, S.D., K.J. Kroeker, K.E. Fabricius, D.I. Kline and B.D. Russell. 2013. The other ocean acidification problem: CO_2 as a resource among competitors for ecosystem dominance. Philos. Trans. Royal Soc. B. 368: 1–9.

Connon, R.E., J. Geist and I. Werner. 2012. Effect-based tools for monitoring and predicting the ecotoxicological effects of chemicals in the aquatic environment. Sensors. 12: 12741–12771.

Correia, T.G., A.M. Narcizo, A. Bianchini and R.G. Moreira. 2010. Aluminum as an endocrine disruptor in female Nile tilapia (*Oreochromis niloticus*). Comp. Biochem. Physiol. C Toxicol. Pharmacol. 151: 461–466.

Crozier, L.G., A.P. Hendry, P.W. Lawson, T.P. Quinn, N.J. Mantua, J. Battin et al. 2008. Potential responses to climate change in organisms with complex life histories: evolution and plasticity in Pacific salmon. Evol. Appl. 1: 252–270.

D´Amato, G., R. Pawankar, C. Vitale, M. Lanza, A. Molino, A. Stanziola et al. 2016. Climate change and air pollution: Effects on respiratory allergy. Allergy Asthma Immunol. Res. 8(5): 391–395.

Delorenzo, M.E. 2015. Impacts of climate change on the ecotoxicology of chemical contaminants in estuarine organisms. Curr. Zool. 61(4): 641–652.

Derelanko, M.J. and C.S. Auletta. 2014. Handbook of Toxicology. 3th edition. CRC Press.

Donelson, J.M., M.I. McCormick, D.J. Booth and P.L. Munday. 2014. Reproductive acclimation to an increased water temperature in a tropical reef fish. Plos One. 9(5): e97223.

Doney, S.C., V.J. Fabry, R.A. Feely and J.A. Kleypas. 2009. Ocean acidification: The other CO_2 problem. Annu. Rev. Mar. Sci. 1: 169–192.

Downs, C.A., J.E. Fauth, J.C. Halas, P. Dustan, J. Bemiss and C.M. Woodley. 2002. Oxidative stress and seasonal coral bleaching. Free Radic. Biol. Med. 33(4): 533–543.

Duarte, G., E.N. Calderon, C.M. Pereira, L.F.B. Marangoni, H.F. Santos, R.S. Peixoto et al. 2015. Novel marine mesocosm facility to study global warming, water quality, and ocean acidification. Ecol. Evol. 5(20): 4555–4566.

Durocher, G.Y., J.I. Jones, M. Trimmer, G. Woodward and J.M. Montoya. 2010. Warming alters the metabolic balance of ecosystems. Philos. Trans. Royal Soc. B. 365: 2117–2126.

Eissa, A.E. and M.M. Zaki. 2011. The impact of global climatic changes on the aquatic environment. Procedia Environ. Sci. 4: 251–259.

Ernst, R., C.S. Ejsing and B. Antonny. 2016. Homeoviscous adaptation and the regulation of membrane lipids. J. Mol. Biol. 428(24): 4776–4791.

Falkenberg, L.J., B.D. Russell and S.D. Connell. 2012. Stability of strong species interactions resist the synergistic effects of local and global pollution in kelp forests. Plos One. 7(3): 1–7.

Farrell, A.P. 2008. Comparisons of swimming performance in rainbow trout using constant acceleration and critical swimming speed tests. J. Fish Biol. 72: 693–710.

Fernandes, G.W., F.F. Goulart, B.D. Ranieri, M.S. Coelho, K. Dales, N. Boesche et al. 2016. Deep into the mud: ecological and socio-economic impacts of the dam breach in Mariana, Brazil. Natureza e Conservação. 14: 35–45.

Ferreira, M.S., A.M. Oliveira and A.L. Val. 2010. Velocidade crítica de natação (Ucrit) de matrinxã (*Brycon amazonicus*) após exposição à hipóxia. Acta Amaz. 40: 699–704.

Fool, M. and O. Gaggiotti. 2006. Identifying the environmental factors that determine the genetic structure of populations. Genetics. 174: 875–891.

Gerwing, T.G., D. Drolet, D.J. Hamilton and M.A. Barbeau. 2016. Relative importance of biotic and abiotic forces on the composition and dynamics of a soft-sediment intertidal community. Plos One. 20: 1–15.

Godbold, J.A. and P. Calosi. 2013. Ocean acidification and climate change: advances in ecology and evolution. Philos. Trans. Royal Soc. B. 368(1627): 1–5.

Goodnite, P.M. 2014. Stress: A concept analysis. Nurs. Forum. 49: 71–74.

Guerriero, G. and G. Ciarcia. 2006. Stress biomarkers and reproduction in fish. pp. 665–692. *In*: Reinecke, M., G. Zaccone and B.G. Kapoor (eds.). Fish Endocrinology. Vol 2. Science Publishers Press, Enfield, NH, USA.

Guidini, I., A.L. Val, J.T. Kojima, T. Silva-Dairiki and M.C. Portella. (under review). Predicted 2100 climate scenario affects growth and skeletal development of tambaqui (*Colossoma macropomum*) larvae. Global Change Biol.

Gustavson, L., T.M. Ciesielski, J. Bytingsvik, B. Styrishave, M. Hansen, E. Lie et al. 2015. Hydroxylated polychlorinated biphenyls decrease circulating steroids in female polar bears (*Ursus maritimus*). Environ. Res. 138: 191–201.

Hallinger, K.K., K.I. Cornell, R.I. Brasso and D.A. Cristol. 2011. Mercury exposure and survival in free-living tree swallows (*Tachycineta bicolor*). Ecotoxicol. 20: 39–46.

Hochachka, P.W. and G.N. Somero. 2002. Biochemical Adaptation: Mechanism and Process in Physiological Evolution. Oxford University Press.

Hook, S.E., E.P. Gallagher and G.E. Batley. 2014. The role of biomarkers in the assessment of aquatic ecosystem health. Integr. Environ. Assess. Manag. 10(3): 327–341.

Hooper, M.J., G.T. Ankley, D.A. Crystol, L.A. Maryoung, P.D. Noyes and K.T. Pinkerton. 2013. Interactions between chemical and climate stressors: a role for mechanistic toxicology in assessing climate change risks. Environ. Toxicol. Chem. 32(1): 32–48.

Huey, R.B., M.R. Kearney, A. Krochenberger, J.A.M. Holtum, M. Jess and S.E. Willians. 2012. Philos. Trans. Royal Soc. B. 367: 1665–1679.

IPCC (Intergovernmental Panel on Climate Change). Climate change 2014: synthesis report. Contribution of working groups I, II and III to the fifth assessment report of the Intergovernmental Panel on Climate Change. Cambridge University Press.

Jenssen, B.M. 2006. Endocrine-disrupting chemicals and climate change: A worst-case combination for arctic marine mammals and seabirds? Environ. Health Perspect. 114: 76–80.

Jenssen, B.M. 2006b. Effects of anthropogenic endocrine disrupters on responses and adaptations to climate change. *In*: Grotmol, T., A. Bernhoft, G.S. Eriksen and T.P. Flaten (eds.). Endocrine Disrupters. Oslo: The Norwegian Academy of Science and Letters.

Kandarakis, E.D., J.P. Bourguignon, L.C. Giudice, R. Hauser, G.S. Prins, A.M. Soto et al. 2009. Endocrine-disrupting chemicals: An endocrine society scientific statement. Endocr. Rev. 30(4): 293–342.

Kates, R.W. 1985. The interactions of climate and society. pp. 3–36. *In*: Kates, R.W., J.H. Ausubel and M. Berberian (eds.). Climate Impact Assessment: Studies of the Interaction of Climate and Society. ICSU/SCOPE Report Nº 27, John Wiley.

Keller, B.D., D.F. Gleason, E. McLeod, C.M. Woodley, S. Airamé, B.D. Causey et al. 2009. Climate change, coral reef ecosystems, and management options for marine protected areas. Environ. Manage. 44: 1069–1088.

Keller, V.D.J., P. Lloyd, J.A. Terry and R.J. Williams. 2015. Impact of climate change and population growth on a risk assessment for endocrine disruption in fish due to steroid estrogens in England and Wales. Environ. Pollut. 197: 262–268.

Kroeker, K.J., R.L. Kordas, R. Crim, I.E. Hendriks, L. Ramajo, G.S. Singh et al. 2013. Impacts of ocean acidification on marine organisms: quantifying sensitivities and interaction with warming. Global Change Biol. 19: 1884–1896.

Labarthe, T.L., S. Martin, F. Oberhänsli, J.L. Teyssié, R. Jeffree, J.P. Gattuso et al. 2012. Temperature and pCO_2 effect on the bioaccumulation of radionuclides and trace elements in the eggs of the common cuttlefish, *Sepia officinalis*. J. Exp. Mar. Biol. Ecol. 413: 45–49.

Levasseur, A., O. Cavalett, J.S. Fuglesvedt, T. Gasser, D.J.A. Johansson, S.V. Jørgensen et al. 2016. Enhancing life cycle impact assessment from climate science: Review of recent findings and recommendations for application to LCA. Ecol. Indic. 71: 163–174.

Lewis, C., R.P. Ellis, E. Vernon, K. Elliot, S. Newbatt and R.W. Wilson. 2016. Ocean acidification increases copper toxicity differentially in two key marine invertebrates with distinct acid-base responses. Sci. Rep. 6(21554): 1–10.

Lewis, J.S., L.M. Farnsworth, L.C. Burdett, D.M. Theobald, M. Gray and R.S. Miller. 2017. Biotic and abiotic factors predicting the global distribution and population density of an invasive large mammal. Sci. Rep. 7(44152): 1–12.

Lima, M.P. and A.L. Val. 2016. Transcriptomic characterization of tambaqui (*Colossoma macropomum*, Cuvier, 1818) exposed to three climate change scenarios. Plos One. 11(3): 1–21.

Lötters, S., K.J. Filz, N. Wagner, B.R. Schmidt, C. Emmerling and M. Veith. 2014. Hypothesizing if responses to climate change affect herbicide exposure risk for amphibians. Environ. Sci. Eur. 26–31.

Lovejoy, T.E. and L.J. Hannah. 2005. Climate Change and Biodiversity. Yale University Press, USA.

Matthiessen, P. and I. Johnson. 2007. Implications of research on endocrine disruption for the environmental risk assessment, regulation and monitoring of chemicals in the European Union. Environ. Pollut. 146: 9–18.

McEwen, B.S. and J.C. Wingfield. 2003. The concept of allostasis in biology and biomedicine. Horm. Behav. 43(1): 2–15.

McEwen, B.S. 2005. Stressed or stressed out: What is the difference? J. Psychiatry Neurosci. 30(5): 315–318.

Mnif, W., A.I.H. Hassine, A. Bouaziz, A. Bartegi, O. Thomas and B. Roig. 2011. Effect of endocrine disruptor pesticides: A review. Int. J. Environ. Res. Publ. Health. 8: 2265–2303.

Moe, S.J., K.D. Schamphelaere, W.H. Clements, M.T. Sorensen, P.J.V. Brink and M. Liess. 2013. Combined and interactive effects of global climate change and toxicants on populations and communities. Environ. Toxicol. Chem. 32: 49–61.

Montoya, J.M. and D. Raffaelli. 2010. Climate change, biotic interactions and ecosystems services. Philos. Trans. Royal Soc. B. 365: 2013–2018.

Moore, S.K., V.L. Trainer, N.J. Mantua, M.S. Parker, E.A. Laws, L.C. Baker et al. 2008. Impacts of climate variability and future climate change on harmful algal blooms and human health. Environ. Health. 7(2): 1–12.

Morris, R.J. 2010. Anthropogenic impacts on tropical forest biodiversity: a network structure and ecosystem functioning perspective. Philos. Trans. Royal Soc. B. 365: 3709–3718.

Moura, R.L., G.M.A. Filho, F.C. Moraes, P.S. Brasileiro, P.S. Salomon, M.M. Mahiques et al. 2016. An extensive reef system at the Amazon River mouth. Sci. Adv. 2(4): e1501252–e1501252.

Murata, N. and D.A. Los. 1997. Membrane fluidity and temperature perception. Plant Physiol. 11(5): 875–879.

Nadal, M., M. Marquès, M. Mari and J.L. Domingo. 2015. Climate change and environmental concentrations of pops: A review. Environ. Res. 143: 177–185.

Nikinmaa, M. 2002. Oxygen-dependent cellular functions—why fishes and their aquatic environment are a prime choice of study. Comp. Biochem. Physiol. A Mol. Integr. Physiol. 133: 1–16.

Nikinmaa, M. 2013. Climate change and ocean acidification—Interactions with aquatic toxicology. Aquatic Toxicology. 126: 365–372.

Nikinmaa, M. 2014. An Introduction to Aquatic Toxicology. Academic Press.

Norris, D.O. 2007. Vertebrate Endocrinology. Elsevier Academic Press.

Noyes, P.D., M.K. McElwee, H.D. Miller, B.W. Clark, L.A.V. Tiem, K.C. Walcott et al. 2009. The toxicology of climate change: Environmental contaminants in a warming world. Environ. Int. 35: 971–986.

Noyes, P.D. and S.C. Lema. 2015. Forecasting the impacts of chemical pollution and climate change interactions on the health of wildlife. Curr. Zool. 61(4): 669–689.

Ogier, E.M., J. Davidson, P. Fidelman, M. Haward, A.J. Hobday, N.J. Holbrook et al. 2016. Fisheries management approaches as platforms for climate change adaptation: Comparing theory and practice in Australian fisheries. Mar. Policy. 71: 82–93.

Oliveira, A.M. and A.L. Val. 2017. Effects of climate scenarios on the growth and physiology of the Amazonian fish tambaqui (*Colossoma macropomum*) (Characiformes: Serrasalmidae). Hydrobiologia. 789: 167–178.

Oost, R.V., J. Beyer and N.P.E. Vermeulen. 2003. Fish bioaccumulation and biomarkers in environmental risk assessment: a review. Environ. Toxicol. Pharmacol. 13: 57–149.

Pauls, S.U., C. Nowak, M. Bálint and M. Pfenninger. 2013. The impact of global climate change on genetic diversity within populations and species. Mol. Ecol. 22: 925–946.

Pimentel, D. 2012. Silent spring, the 50th anniversary of Rachel Carson's book. BMC Ecology. 12–20.

Pörtner, H.O. and M.A. Peck. 2010. Climate change effects on fishes and fisheries: towards a cause-and-effect understanding. J. Fish Biol. 77(8): 1745–1779.

Quince, C., P.G. Higgs and A.J. McKane. 2002. Food web structure and the evolution of ecological communities. pp. 281–298. *In*: Lässig, M. and A. Valleriani (eds.). Biological Evolution and Statistical Physics. Springer-Verlag, Press, Berlin, DE.

Reid, S.D., J.J. Dockray, T.K. Linton, D.G. McDonald and C.M. Wood. 1997. Effects of chronic environmental acidification and a summer global warming scenario: protein synthesis in juvenile rainbow trout (*Oncorhynchus mykiss*). Can. J. Fish. Aquat. Sci. 54: 2014–2024.

Roberts, D.A., S.N.R. Birchenough, C. Lewis, M.B. Sanders, T. Bolam and D. Sheahan. 2013. Ocean acidification increases the toxicity of contaminated sediments. Global Change Biol. 19: 340–351.

Rowe, G.T. 2001. Seasonal hypoxia in the bottom water off the Mississippi River delta. J. Environ. Qual. 30(2): 281–290.

Ruppert, E.E. and R.D. Barnes. 1996. Zoologia dos Invertebrados. 6ª ed. Roca, Press. São Paulo-BR.

Russell, B., J.A.I. Thompson, L.J. Falkenberg and S.D. Connell. 2009. Synergistic effects of climate change and local stressors: CO_2 and nutrient-driven change in subtidal rocky habitats. Global Change Biol. 15: 2153–2162.

Scaven, V.L. and N.E. Rafferty. 2013. Physiological effects of climate warming on flowering plants and insect pollinators and potential consequences for their interactions. Curr. Zool. 59(3): 418–426.

Schiedek, D., B. Sundelin, J.M. Readman and R.W. Macdonald. 2007. Interactions between climate change and contaminants. Mar. Poll. Bull. 54: 1845–1856.

Schmidt-Nielsen, K. 2002. Fisiologia Animal Adaptação e Meio Ambiente. Santos, Press, BR.

Schreck, C.B. 2010. Stress and fish reproduction: The roles of allostasis and hormesis. Gen. Comp. Endocrinol. 165: 54–556.

Selye, H. 1950. Stress and the general adaptation syndrome. BMJ. 1(4667): 1383–1392.

Sogard, S.M. and M.L. Spencer. 2004. Energy allocation in juvenile sablefish: effects of temperature, ration and body size. J. Fish Biol. 64: 726–738.

Solomon, S., G.K. Plattner, R. Knutti and P. Friedlingstein. 2009. Irreversible climate change due to carbono dioxide emissions. PNAS. 106(6): 1704–1709.

Speers, A.E., E.Y. Besedin, J.E. Palardy and C. Moore. 2016. Impacts of climate change and ocean acidification on coral reef fisheries: An integrated ecological–economic model. Ecol. Econ. 128: 33–43.

Stahl, R.G.J., M.J. Hooper, J.M. Balbus, W. Clementes, A. Fritz, T. Gouin et al. 2013. The influence of global climate change on the scientific foundations and applications of environmental toxicology and chemistry: Introduction to a SETAC International Workshop. Environ. Toxicol. Chem. 32(1): 13–19.

Sterling, P. 2012. Allostasis: A model of predictive regulation. Physiol. Behav. 106: 5–15.

Tadei, W.P., I.B. Rodrigues, M.S. Rafael, R.T.M. Sampaio, H.G. Mesquita, V.C.S. Pinheiro et al. 2017. Adaptative processes, control measures, genetic background, and resilience of malaria vectors and environmental changes in the Amazon region. Hydrobiologia. 789: 179–196.

Turcotte, M.M., M.S.C. Corrin and M.T.J. Johnson. 2012. Adaptive evolution in ecological communities. Plos Biol. 10(5): 1–6.

Urban, M.C., J.L. Richardson and N.A. Freindenfelds. 2013. Plasticity and genetic adaptation mediate amphibian and reptile responses to climate change. Evol. Appl. 7(1): 88–103.

Vail, D.D. 2015. Toxicity abounds: New histories on pesticides, environmentalism, and silent spring. Stud. Hist. Philos. Sci. C. 53: 118–121.

Val, A.L. and V.M.F. Almeida-Val. 1995. Fishes of the amazon and their environment. Physiological and Biochemistry Features. Springer-Verlag, Press, Berlin, DE.

Val, A.L., K.R.M. Gomes and V.M.F.A. Val. 2015. Rapid regulation of blood parameters under acute hypoxia in the Amazonian fish *Prochilodus nigricans*. Comp. Biochem. Physiol. A Mol. Integr. Physiol. 184: 125–131.

Vardoulakis, S., C. Dimitroulopoulou, J. Thornes, K.M. Lai, J. Taylor, I. Myers et al. 2015. Impact of climate change on the domestic indoor environment and associated health risks in the UK. Environ. Int. 85: 299–313.

Walther, G.R. 2010. Community and ecosystem responses to recent climate change. Philos. Trans. Royal Soc. B. 365: 2019–2024.

Ward, R.D., D.A. Friess, R.H. Day and R.A. Mackenzie. 2016. Impacts of climate change on mangrove ecosystems: a region by region overview. Ecosyst. Health Sustainability. 2(4): 1–25.

Weiss, B. 2011. Endocrine disruptors as a threat to neurological function. J. Neurol. Sci. 305: 1–17.
Wijbenga, A. and O. Hutzinger. 1984. Chemicals, man and the environment: a historic perspective of pollution and related topics. Sci. Nat. 71(5): 239–246.
Woodward, G., D.M. Perkins and L.E. Brown. 2010. Climate change and freshwater ecosystems: impacts across multiple levels of organization. Philos. Trans. Royal Soc. B. 365: 2093–2106.
Wu, D., N. Ploturi, Y. Kim and F. Rastinejad. 2013. Structure and dimerization properties of the Aryl hydrocarbon receptor PAS-A domain. Mol. Cell. Biol. 33(21): 4346–4356.
Zagatto, P.A. and E. Bertoletti. 2008. Ecotoxicologia Aquática Princípios e Aplicações. Rima, Press, BR.
Zeng, X., X. Chen and J. Zhuang. 2015. The positive relationship between ocean acidification and pollution. Mar. Pollut. Bull. 91: 14–21.

4

Marine Mammals as Environmental Sentinels Focusing on Mercury Contamination

Helena do Amaral Kehrig,[1,]* *Ana Paula Madeira Di Beneditto*[1] and *Tércia Guedes Seixas*[2]

Introduction

Most marine mammals are top predators that accumulate pollutants in their tissues through bioaccumulation and biomagnification processes. The effects of pollutants on marine mammals include immunosuppression, cancer, skin lesions, secondary infections, diseases, and reduced reproductive success. By determining the health status of marine mammals, it is possible to identify anthropogenic influences on the marine environmental health itself, and on the well-being of these animals. In this chapter, a brief description of marine mammals and a discussion on their role as sentinel species shall be made. Subsequently, emphasis shall be given to mercury contamination in these animals, since environmental exposure to Hg, particularly for higher trophic level consumers, is significantly higher that other the elements, as this metal presents high toxicity and the ability to undergo biomagnification along trophic chains.

[1] Universidade Estadual do Norte Fluminense; Laboratório de Ciências Ambientais, Av. Alberto Lamego, 2000 - Parque California, Campos dos Goytacazes - RJ, CEP: 28035-200, Brazil.
E-mail: anapaula@uenf.br
[2] Fundação Oswaldo Cruz; Escola Nacional de Saúde Pública Sergio Arouca, Rua Leopoldo Bulhões, 1480, Bonsucesso, Rio de Janeiro, RJ, CEP"21041-210, Brazil.
E-mail: terciaguedes@gmail.com
* Corresponding author: helena.kehrig@pq.cnpq.br

Marine Mammals

Most information discussed in this section was compiled from Geraci and Lounsbury (1993) and Jefferson et al. (1993), with other additional information sources. In mammal evolution, a variety of forms began to explore marine waters as an alternative to living on land. Mammalian species that have a strong relationship with the marine environment, spending the whole life cycle in this environment or depending on it to obtain feeding resources, are known as marine mammals. Sea otters, polar bear and pinnipeds (sea lions, fur seals, walruses and true seals) are marine mammals partially adapted to this environment, while still preserving vital ties to the land, especially for reproduction and parental care. On the other hand, cetaceans (whales and dolphins) and sirenians (manatees and dugongs) complete their entire life cycle in the marine environment.

Marine mammals are not randomly distributed around the world. Some species are found exclusively or primarily in waters of a particular depth, temperature range, and/or oceanographic conditions. One major factor affecting productivity, and thus, indirectly influencing the distribution of marine mammals, is the pattern of ocean currents, and the presence of marine mammals in an area is related primarily to prey, and secondarily to the water conditions supporting that productivity (Pompa et al. 2011).

Adjusting to an aquatic environment required certain adaptations in mammal bodies, both anatomical and physiological (Newell 2013). For thermal protection, otters, some pinnipeds, such as seals, and the polar bear depend on a blanket of thick fur. Cetaceans and other pinnipeds, as sea lions and walruses, rely instead on blubber, a fatty tissue. Besides providing thermal protection, blubber is buoyant and enables marine mammals to remain at the surface to breathe and rest without much effort. Additionally, by regulating blood circulation, marine mammals are able to deal with extreme variations in temperature when swimming from the surface to the bottom. Pinnipeds and cetaceans display adaptations for efficiently acquiring, storing and utilizing oxygen, allowing long and deep dives.

Most carnivores are terrestrial mammals, and besides pinnipeds, only two Carnivora families contain marine mammal representatives: Mustelidae (sea otters) and Ursidae (polar bear). Considering mustelids, only two species are truly marine (*Enhydra lutris* and *Lutra felina*). There are seven species of bears in the world, and the single marine species, the polar bear (*Ursus maritimus*), is qualified as the least aquatic of all marine mammals.

Pinnipeds are distributed in three families with more than 30 species (Otariidae, Phocidae and Odobenidae). They are highly specialized aquatic carnivores, but all must return to a solid substrate, such as land or ice, to raise their pups. In this sense, all species are amphibious. Their cardiovascular system is specialized for diving, with an immense hepatic sinus, an enlargement of the vena cava that acts as a reservoir of oxygenated blood during a dive (Riedman 1990). Females of most pinniped species become sexually mature by about four to six years of age and give birth to a single offspring per reproductive effort after 11 to 12-month pregnancy period. Males reach sexual maturity at about the same age or older, but may not breed successfully until several years later. Females of most species remain with their pups continuously until weaning, and the maternal care can spend for a few months to a year or more. The preferred preys of pinnipeds are fish and squids, but the diet may also include invertebrates, mammals (including other pinnipeds) and birds. They are top predators, and most species have distinct preferences in their choice of prey, determined by temporal or spatial abundance. Some species feed in coastal waters, and often enter rivers, while others forage in deep water, offshore. Depending on their prey, certain pinniped species may be more exposed to environmental contaminants through their diet, since certain prey, such as squid, are known do accumulate high levels of Cd for example (Dorneles et al. 2007).

Regarding cetaceans, currently, around 80 living species exist, classified as Mysticeti, baleen whales, or Odontoceti, toothed whales. Cetacea is the oldest and most diverse group of marine mammals, with fossil evidence dating back at least 40 to 50 million years. This groups shows a body well-adapted to a fully aquatic life: streamlined spindle shaped torso, flattened paddle-like fore flippers, telescoped skull, nasal openings on top of the head, well-developed blubber layer, internal reproductive organs, newly derived boneless structures in the form of tail flukes and a dorsal fin (not present in some species), and loss of such aquatic hindrances as hind limbs, external ear flaps and fur. The internal anatomy of cetaceans is like that of land mammals, with adaptations regarding with its aquatic life. The cardiovascular system has a unique adaptation of arteries and veins, which helps cetacean regulate body temperature.

External conditions, such as population density and food availability, influence age at sexual maturity, lactation period and calving interval of cetacean species. The smaller odontocetes have shorter life spans compared with the larger species (e.g., seven to 30 *vs* 60 or more years). Besides, the reproductive cycles of smaller species are more accelerated than larger species (e.g., sexually mature at age three to six *vs* eight to 10 years; gestation period of 10 to 12 months *vs* 14 to 16 months; and six to eight months of nursing *vs* two years or more). The baleen whales evolved reproductive cycles synchronized with their annual migrations between low latitude (calving grounds) and high latitude (feeding grounds). These cetaceans mature relatively young (four to 10 years), have a gestation period for 10 to 12 months, nurse for four to 10 months, and can reach ages of 50 to 80 years or more.

Most toothed whales feed primarily on fish and squids, and may include shrimps and crabs in their diets. The killer whale is an exception, because it can include other marine mammals in its diet. The baleen whales are adapted to foraging on prey that can be engulfed and strained from the water, as patches of euphausiid (krill) and copepod crustaceans, and small schooling fishes. The gray whale has a diverse feeding behavior, scour the bottom in search of benthic invertebrates. Environmental contaminants levels in cetaceans increase with the trophic position and top predators, like most toothed whales, present higher levels than baleen whales (Nomiyama et al. 2010, Law et al. 2012).

Another group of marine mammals comprises the sirenians, with currently four living species, three of which are considered marine mammals: two manatees (*Trichechus manatus* and *T. senegalensis*) and the one dugong (*Dugong dugon*). Sirenians, like cetaceans, are totally aquatic. They are restricted to coastal waters of tropical and subtropical habitat. Both females and males may reach sexual maturity as early as three to four years old, but they may not breed successfully until they are five to eight years old. They breed primarily during the non-winter months, and most calves are born during warmer weather, after a gestation period of about 12–13 months. The nursing period normally ranges from one year to a year and a half, and the interval between births is at least two to three years. The life span of these marine mammals is long—the oldest known animal was estimated to be more than 50 years old. Manatees and the dugong are the only herbivorous marine mammals, consuming a wide variety of aquatic and semi-aquatic plants, which may be a route for the ingestion of environmental contaminants, since some aquatic plant species are known to accumulate high amounts of pollutants (Haynes et al. 2005, Zhou et al. 2008). While showing some preference for submerged succulent forms, they will feed on floating seaweed, and even algae, detritus, and salt-marsh grasses. To compensate for the low energy content of their diet and low digestive efficiency, they must feed from 6 to 8 hours per day.

Marine Mammals as Environmental Sentinels

Chemical contamination in the aquatic environment has increased substantially over the last decades and it is imperative to investigate the relationship between xenobiotics, environment and exposed organisms (Gadzala-Kopciuch et al. 2004, Jakimska et al. 2011).

Marine mammals occupy a mid to high trophic level that makes them accumulate high amounts of xenobiotics, in different tissues and organs, causing several adverse effects on their metabolism (Arellano-Peralta and Medrano-González 2015). Most marine mammals are distributed in large geographic ranges within which they travel long distances and are, thus, affected by many human activities with complex effects on their feeding, reproduction and/or traveling. Therefore, marine mammals, in general, appear as highly vulnerable to the ongoing processes of environmental deterioration (Acevedo-Whitehouse and Duffus 2009, Aguirre and Tabor 2004, Harwood 2001, Moore 2008, Ross 2000, Smith et al. 2009). For these reasons, research on these vertebrates is currently largely focused on inferring ecosystem modifications and functionality under the concept of sentinel species (Aguirre and Tabor 2004, Moore 2008, Ross 2000).

For example, the health effects from the complexed biomagnified mixture of long-range transported industrial organochlorines (OCs), polybrominated diphenyl ethers (PBDEs), perfluorinated compounds (PFCs) and mercury (Hg) on polar bear (*Ursus maritimus*) have provided information from long-range transported contaminants in Arctic top predators. These environmental stressors can impact exposure and biological responses to toxic and infectious agents (Aguirre and Tabor 2004). According to Sonne (2010), data indicated that hormone and vitamin concentrations, liver, kidney and thyroid gland morphology, as well as reproductive and immune systems of polar bears, are likely to be influenced by environmental stressors. Furthermore, exclusively based on polar bear contaminant studies, bone density reduction and neurochemical disruption and DNA hypomethylation of the brain stem seemed to occur. Mercury concentrations in hair above 5.4 $\mu g.g^{-1}$ dry wt.

cause neurologic damage to polar bears in the Arctic, and correspond to decreased levels of NMDA (N-methyl-D-aspartate) receptors in the brain stem of polar bears sampled in East Greenland in ~ 2000 (Basu et al. 2009, Dietz et al. 2013).

It is worth noting that, specifically in East Greenland where Inuits rely on the same prey species as polar bears as well as polar bears themselves, an extrapolation of contaminant-driven wildlife health effects towards human health is possible. Thus, polar bears may be a useful tool for conventional work as sentinel and species conservation (Sonne 2010). Dietz et al. (2006) demonstrated that approximately 93% of the Hg in East Greenland polar bear hair was of anthropogenic origin and that the concentrations are increasing in West Greenland polar bears.

Arctic pinnipeds and cetaceans are also useful integrators and sentinels of Hg in the Arctic. A comparison of Hg concentrations in ringed seals (*Pusa hispida*) and beluga whales (*Delphinapterus leucas*) from locations across the Arctic and Hudson Bay indicated that this metal was generally present in higher concentrations in marine mammals from the western compared to the eastern Arctic, indicating a possible influence of the different geological settings in the eastern and western Arctic (Wagemann et al. 1995). This was attributed to different Hg natural background concentrations in the western and eastern Canadian Arctic, dictated by different geological formations in the two regions (Wagemann et al. 1995, 1996). Likewise, extrapolation from seal and belugas to Inuit people is possible as they prey on the same species, indicating that these species also show potential in identifying environmental contamination. Arctic beluga, for instance, exhibited brain Hg concentrations one order of magnitude greater than those found in polar bears and seals (Lemes et al. 2011).

In the North Pacific Ocean, Steller sea lions (*Eumetopias jubatus*) are broadly distributed apex predators and, as such, integrate complex food webs and the associated exposure and possible adverse effects of toxic and infectious agents (Aguirre and Tabor 2004). In Alaska, declining Steller sea lion populations accompanied by declines in other marine mammal and bird populations (National Research Council 1996) have signaled major shifts in ecosystem structure and health that may have roots in a number of factors, both natural and anthropogenic (Castellini et al. 2012). Hair, including lanugo, of Alaskan Steller sea lions was examined using regional to assess Hg concentrations. Regionally, higher concentrations of Hg were observed in the endangered western population of Steller sea lions and mirrored patterns were observed in human biomonitoring studies of Alaskan coastal communities (State of Alaska Epidemiology Bulletin 2010). These data have broader implications with respect to human and ecosystem health, as Steller sea lions rely on similar prey species and foraging areas as those targeted by commercial fisheries and subsistence users and are, therefore, valuable sentinels of marine ecosystem health. Alaskan Steller sea lions are an important sentinel species in Alaska and have undergone drastic population changes as a result of a changing environment (Castellini et al. 2012).

Evidence of increasing Hg concentrations in Arctic animals is therefore a concern with respect to ecosystem health. Hg concentrations in Arctic mammals have increased over the past 150 years, resulting in over 92% of Hg body burdens in higher trophic level species, such as marine mammals (Dietz et al. 2009). This indicates that Arctic species, including the human Inuit population, are exposed to higher Hg concentrations today compared to historic times (Dietz et al. 2013).

For centuries, the pilot whale (*Globicephala melas*) has been an important part of Faroese life, both in regard to food and culture. Some studies dating back to 1977 have shown an increase in contamination of the meat, blubber, liver and kidneys of pilot whales. Hg and OC content in the pilot whale tissues and organs were extremely high, since this marine mammal is a long-lived apex predator (Weihe and Joensen 2012). Pilot whales are thus also useful sentinel of environmental health (Bossart 2006).

Several birth cohorts of newborns from Faroe Islands have been established in order to discover the health effects related to Hg and OC exposure *via* human consumption of pilot whale meat and blubber. In short, results have so far shown that Hg from pilot whale meat adversely affects the fetal development of the nervous system, that Hg effects are still detectable during adolescence, that Hg from the maternal diet affects the blood pressure of the children, that contaminants from blubber adversely affect the immune system so that the children react more poorly to immunizations, that contaminants in pilot whales appear to increase the risk of developing Parkinson's disease in populations who have this species as a staple diet, that the risk of hypertension and arteriosclerosis of the carotid arteries increases in adults who have an increased exposure to Hg and, finally, that septuagenarians with type 2 diabetes or impaired fasting glycaemia tend to have higher PCB concentrations and higher past intake of traditional foods, especially during childhood and adolescence (Weihe and Joensen 2012).

Bottlenose dolphins (*Tursiops truncatus*), the apex predator in Florida-USA, are an important sentinel species for ecosystem and public health hazard. These dolphins from the Indian River Lagoon (IRL), Florida, bioaccumulate high concentrations of Hg in their blood, skin and internal organs that are among the highest reported worldwide (Reif et al. 2015). These high Hg concentrations showed association with markers for endocrine, renal, hepatic, hematologic and immune system dysfunction. The IRL occupies 40 percent of the east coast of Florida and is bordered by counties with approximately 2.5 million human inhabitants. Therefore, the local inhabitants in communities bordering the IRL could be at risk of exposure to Hg due to the same consumption of fish and shellfish as this dolphin (Reif et al. 2015).

A comparative study of Hg accumulation in striped dolphin (*Stenella coeruleoalba*) from the French Atlantic and Mediterranean coast showed that the levels observed in the Mediterranean specimens are among the highest observed worldwide. These differences provide additional confirmation for the highest Hg concentrations observed previously in other pelagic species (tuna, sardine anchovy, etc.) from the Mediterranean Sea. Taking into consideration the pelagic habits of the dolphin species and also, the local influence of anthropogenic Hg sources, it seems reasonable to assume that the main source of the high Hg concentrations observed in Mediterranean biota is from the natural Hg deposits located in many regions of the Mediterranean basin (Andre et al. 1991).

Marine mammals have also been shown to be useful sentinels of global environmental changes that are expected to alter selection pressures in many biological systems. Climate change has the potential to have a considerable impact on marine mammals through indirect or direct effects (such as loss of habitats, temperature stress, and exposure to severe weather) on ecosystems or their health (Frouin et al. 2012). Indirect effects could result from changes in host-pathogen associations due to altered pathogen transmission or host resistance, changes in body condition due to alterations in predator-prey relationships or changes in exposure to contaminations (Frouin et al. 2012). For instance, the investigation about the relationship between individual heterozygosity and demographic response to climate change was conducted for three decades of biometric, life history and genetic data from a population of Antarctic fur seals (*Arctocephalus gazella*) on the island of South Georgia, in an area of the southwest Atlantic strongly affected by climate change (Forcada and Hoffman 2014). The local fur seal population showed significant demographic fluctuation linked to modes of climate variation that impacted the local ecosystem, modulating the availability of Antarctic krill (*Euphausia superba*), a keystone species and staple food of these fur seals. Climate change has reduced prey availability and caused a significant decline in seal birth weight, selecting for heterozygosity in a declining fur seal population (Forcada and Hoffman 2014).

A comparative study of Hg and cadmium (Cd) accumulation in Franciscana dolphins (*Pontoporia blainvillei*) showed significant differences in hepatic concentrations of these metals in individuals from the southern and southeastern Brazilian coast (Seixas et al. 2007). This difference can be attributed partly to the distinct populations, the prevalent environmental conditions (water temperature and primary production) and also, to other factors, such as the level of food contamination. The main metal intake in Franciscana is *via* food (Kehrig et al. 2016). Probably, the preys available for individuals from the southern Brazilian coast are richer in Hg and Cd than those available for individuals from the southeastern coast. The low metal concentrations observed in the animals from the southeastern coast may also be related to the low bioavailability of metals in the southeastern environment. It is worth noting that throughout the Brazilian coast, a decline in the density of all Franciscana dolphin populations has been observed due to high mortality rates (Danilewicz et al. 2010). Being one of the most coastal and vulnerable small cetaceans mainly to anthropogenic activities, especially fisheries, this dolphin species is considered the most threatened cetacean in the South-western Atlantic Ocean (Seixas et al. 2007). Since coastal Brazilian human populations rely on the same prey species, fish, cephalopods and crustaceans as Franciscana, an extrapolation of contaminant-driven wildlife health effects towards human health is possible. Thus, Franciscana dolphins may also be useful tools for conventional work as sentinel and species conservation.

Plastic debris contamination has one of the most human impacts on the marine environment, causing impacted degradation. Marine mammals are susceptible to ingesting the plastic materials available, directly to the aquatic environment, or through similarities with the prey consumption (Ferreira et al. 2016). In this sense, the Franciscana dolphins and the Guiana dolphin (*Sotalia guianensis*) are coastal species that are sympatric in southwestern Atlantic Ocean, and used as sentinel of marine debris ingestion. Di Beneditto and Ramos (2014) verified that 15.7% stomach contents samples of Franciscana contained plastic material composed of nylon yarns and flexible plastics. Meanwhile, for Guiana dolphin, only one stomach content sample (1.30%) contained marine debris. Differences in feeding habits between the coastal dolphins were found to drive their differences regarding marine debris ingestion. Guiana dolphin has a near-surface feeding habit. In contrast, the feeding activity of Franciscana is mainly near the sea bottom, which increases its chances of ingesting debris deposited on the seabed. The seabed is the main zone of accumulation of debris, and species with some degree of association with the sea bottom may be local sentinels of marine debris pollution (Di Beneditto and Ramos 2014).

Mercury: Bioconcentration, Bioaccumulation and Biomagnification

A wide range of xenobiotics, including metals, has become widely recognized as the source of adverse effects to the marine environments and organisms. During the past few decades, increasing concern about environmental pollution has led to many investigations on metals and their distribution in the marine ecosystem (Kehrig et al. 2016).

Metals can bioaccumulate over time to reach sub lethal, or even lethal, levels in organisms, unless they are excreted or detoxified. Bioaccumulation of xenobiotics is a process defined as their uptake by an organism from the abiotic (water, sediment) and/or biotic (food) environment, occurring from all sources (Gray 2002).

Metals are capable of interacting with nuclear proteins and DNA, causing oxidative deterioration of biological macromolecules (Flora et al. 2008). This problem is particularly severe for metals in long-lived organisms, such as marine mammals (Lahaye et al. 2007).

In this section, emphasis will be given on Hg and its possible effects on marine mammals. Mercury is a metal of environmental interest that shows naturally high concentrations in several regions, occurring in different chemical and physical forms. The most abundant forms are elemental Hg (Hg^{o}), divalent mercury (Hg^{+2}), methylmercury (MeHg, CH_3Hg^+), dimethylmercury (DMHg, CH_3HgCH_3), and ethylmercury (EtHg, $CH_3CH_2Hg^+$), each of which is unique regarding exposure pattern, metabolism, and toxic effects.

Elemental and particulate-bound ionic forms of Hg are released into the environment from multiple industrial processes such as metal production, waste incineration, mining and the burning of coal for energy as well as natural phenomena such as volcanic eruptions. Inorganic Hg enters the atmosphere, and may be transported globally and re-deposited onto the earth's surface. Much of the re-deposited Hg enters the marine environment, primarily the oceans. However, dry deposition is an unimportant source of Hg to the open ocean but might account for about one third of the total deposition to terrestrial systems (Mason et al. 1994). As ionic Hg species are particle reactive and soluble, they would be readily removed from the atmosphere by precipitation and by dry deposition, accounting for the "short-circuiting" predicted from the wet deposition estimates (Mason and Sheu 2002).

Inorganic Hg is converted to MeHg in aquatic sediments by the action of multiple anaerobic species of sulfate-reducing bacteria. Thus, the sulfate concentration and composition of bacterial communities in marine sediments are important predictors of Hg methylation rates (King et al. 1999). Methylmercury, in turn, is taken up from sediments by phytoplankton and biomagnified through fish species within trophic chain, reaching the highest levels in the apex predators within an ecosystem (Reif et al. 2015). Biomagnification, the process where Hg is transferred from food to an organism resulting in higher concentrations compared with the source (Gray 2002), occurs through at least two trophic positions in a trophic chain (Barwick and Maher 2003). Methylmercury is biomagnified (10^3–10^4) between trophic levels from phytoplankton to top-predators (2–4 trophic levels), and the initial bioconcentration, i.e., uptake from the environment, of MeHg by phytoplankton represents the greatest single contribution to the food chain (Kehrig 2011), leading to higher Hg concentrations in these organisms (Gray 2002). In this sense, there is a consensus that Hg enters the food chain *via* phytoplankton (Mason et al. 1996, Kehrig 2011), and then is magnified in the other links in the chain *via* trophic transfer (Kehrig et al. 2011).

Mercury, in its more toxic organic form MeHg, is biomagnified up to a million times over the aquatic trophic chain from its base (plankton) by adsorption to the body surface to organisms at the top of the food chain (predatory fish and mammals) by food ingestion. Uptake of dissolved MeHg by phytoplankton establishes a pool of bioavailable contaminant that can be taken up by heterotrophic organism (zooplankton, fish), since phytoplankton organisms play a significant role in nutrient cycling, water quality and energy flow (Watras et al. 1998). However, the factors influencing MeHg bioconcentration by phytoplankton in marine ecosystems and, by extension higher trophic levels, are not well elucidated, although, bioavailability and chemical species (especially free ions) are known to influence Hg toxicity and its bioaccumulation by organisms in the marine environment (Wang and Rainbow 2005).

The study of the microbial food chain can be considered essential in the understanding of the energy flow and nutrient cycling loading in coastal ecosystems (Burford et al. 2008). The term "microbial loop" was originally coined by Azam et al. (1983), and includes several trophic levels of the microbial food chain and a large fraction of the organic carbon particulate. These processes can influence the bioaccumulation of Hg by microorganisms. The total amount of this metal accumulated by prokaryotes (microplankton) will affect the quantity of it transferred trophically along the food chain, due to the fact that mesoplankton (microcrustaceans) grazed on microplankton and both of these plankton fractions served as food source for small fish (Fenchel 2008). The nature of metal binding in microplankton also possesses the potential to significantly affect trophic transfer (Ng et al. 2005). The microbial loop is supposed to be an especially important feature in the ecology of tropical waters, where temperature, dissolved organic carbon contents (DOC) and solar radiation are permanently abundant. Both autotrophic and heterotrophic organism in the microbial loop are key components in the transfer of carbon and elements, including Hg, through marine food chains (Fenchel 2008), influencing the biogeochemical cycling of the aquatic ecosystem, as well as being major contributors to vertical fluxes (Fisher et al. 2000).

The main effect of the microbial loop on Hg cycling in the water column is the acceleration of organic matter mineralization and thus regenerates the nutrients for primary production (Fenchel 2008). A large fraction of the organic matter that is synthesized by primary producers becomes dissolved organic matter (DOM) and is taken up almost exclusively by bacteria. Most of the DOM is respired to carbon dioxide and a fraction is assimilated and re-introduced into the classical food chain (phytoplankton to zooplankton to fish to marine mammal) (Fenchel 2008). Therefore, the dynamics of Hg through the base food chain is influenced by the microbial loop. A simplified scheme of the microbial loop and trophic transfer of Hg, as MeHg, through a marine aquatic food chain is presented in Fig. 1.

The assimilation of dissolved Hg in the water column is an important route for the bioaccumulation of this metal by aquatic organisms that have small body size and greater relative surface area, such as microplankton (Reinfelder et al. 1998). However, with the increase in body size of aquatic organisms, as in the case of mesoplankton, a decrease in the contribution of dissolved Hg in the water is observed, and consequently, the trophic transfer becomes more efficient means for assimilation and accumulation of Hg in the form of MeHg (Mason et al. 2000).

Dissolved MeHg, which is the most biologically available organic form of Hg, is bioaccumulated up to a million times in microscopic particles, including phytoplankton and bacteria, at the base of aquatic trophic chain by adsorption to their body surface in the water column (Mason et al. 1996, Miles et al. 2001). These MeHg-enriched particles are then consumed by zooplankton, which in turn are a primary food source of larval, juvenile, and some adult fish (Hall et al. 1997). Zooplanktonic organisms such as copepods assimilate MeHg much more efficiently than Hg_{inorg},

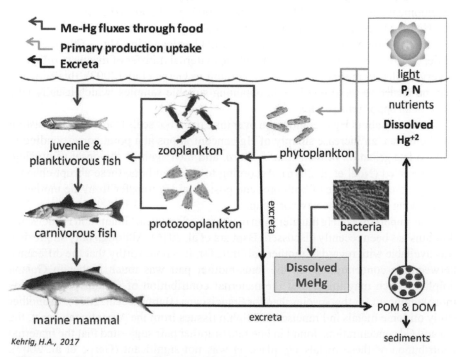

Fig. 1. Microbial loop and trophic transfer of methylmercury (MeHg) through a marine food chain.

presenting the relative assimilation efficiency of MeHg to Hg_{inorg} of 2.0 (Lawson and Mason 1998). Kainz and Mazumder (2005) demonstrated that a bacterial diet could be better at predicting variations of MeHg concentrations in zooplankton (copepods) than essential algal (phytoplankton) diet.

Mercury and marine mammals

Mercury has no known normal metabolic function, being an exogenous and harmful metal that accumulates in marine organisms. Environmental exposure to Hg *via* food chain, particularly for higher trophic level consumers, including marine mammals and humans, is significantly higher compared to other elements since this metal presents high toxicity and the ability to undergo biomagnification along the trophic chains (Agusa et al. 2007).

In general, in long-lived marine mammals, Hg concentrations increase with length or age due to these animals accumulating this metal in tissues throughout their life (Ikemoto et al. 2004), probably related to the continuous accumulation of Hg through diet combined with a much slower turnover rate in the body and also, the rather long biological half-life of this element in these animals (Neathery and Miller 1975), since it shows a strong affinity with the sulfhydryl groups (SH) present in cysteine (Kunito et al. 2004).

Mercury could be transferred *via* placental or lactational transfer from mother to fetus and suckling calves, affecting them during their most sensitive periods of development (Gerpe et al. 2002, Lahaye et al. 2007, Noël et al. 2016). It is noteworthy that Hg, as MeHg, passes through the placental barrier and accumulates in dolphin fetal tissues, whereas the placenta is an important barrier against Hg_{inorg} (Neathery and Miller 1975). However, knowledge about the maternal transfer of metals to offspring is very limited in marine mammals. According to Gerpe et al. (2002), this situation may be related to the difficulties in obtaining suitable samples, which usually take place in an opportunistic way.

In a study about Hg accumulation over time in harbor seals from the Northeastern Pacific Ocean, an increase sharply of Hg concentrations at a point corresponding to mid- to late gestation of their time *in utero*, and then again at the onset of nursing, was presented (Noël et al. 2016). According to these authors, these abrupt changes highlight the importance of both pre- and post-natal Hg transfer from the mother to the growing fetus and the newborn pup.

The importance of Hg transfer from mother to offspring in Guiana and Franciscana dolphins has been recently discussed (Baptista et al. 2016). Although only single data was available with regard to mother-calf transfer, it is noteworthy that the difference between Hg concentrations in the fetus-mother pair was much higher in Guiana dolphin, which may imply that the maternal contribution of Hg *via* placenta was more significant for this species than for Franciscana (Baptista et al. 2016). In another study on some metals in Franciscana dolphin tissues from the Argentinean coast, the Hg and Cd concentrations found in one fetus-mother pair suggested that the maternal contribution of these metals *via* placenta was not significant (Gerpe et al. 2002). Meanwhile, a study with trace element levels in fetus-mother pairs of short-beaked common dolphins (*Delphinus delphis*) from the French coast indicated a limited maternal transfer of Hg during pregnancy, since concentrations in the tissues of fetus were below 1 $\mu g.g^{-1}$ wet wt. (Lahaye et al. 2007). Yang et al. (2004) reported that Hg, Cd and Ag concentrations in the liver of a fetus were apparently lower than those of Dall's porpoise (*Phocoenoides dalli*) mother. Results of blood dynamics of Hg and Se in northern elephant seals (*Mirounga angustirostris*) suggested that maternal Se transfer was prominent during lactation, whereas Hg transfer was higher during gestation (Habran et al. 2011).

Significant Hg concentrations have been associated to potential neurotoxicity and immunotoxicity in marine mammals and human (Basu et al. 2009, Frouin et al. 2011, Krey et al. 2012), and this is of major concern, especially for female of childbearing age and the developing fetus (Weihe and Joensen 2012). However, other effects have also been reported for Hg in marine mammals, including immune-suppression (Kakuschke et al. 2009) and endocrine disruption (Schaeler et al. 2011, Bechshoft et al. 2015).

Thus, exposure to Hg is thought to be a problem for marine mammals because this contaminant is highly hormone-like and cellular toxic substance that negatively affects neuro-endocrine, reproductive, developmental and immune function in mammals. Therefore, osteoid tissue, internal organs, endocrine glands, liver enzymes, hormone and vitamin homeostasis are also negatively influenced by Hg, increasing stress in the mammalian organism (Sonne 2010).

Mercury is known to be toxic in all forms but some forms are more toxic than others, depending on the chemistry of Hg containing molecule, which determines its absorption, distribution, and excretion pattern in the body (Winship 1985). The inorganic and organic form of Hg are, therefore, preferably accumulated in the protein rich tissues of liver, kidneys, hair and blood, while significantly lower concentrations are found in muscle, urine, feces and brain (Sonne 2010).

Alkyl mercuries, especially MeHg, are more toxic than inorganic Hg compounds due to their ability to cross cell membranes, resulting in higher absorption, propensity for nervous system, a disregard for the placental barrier and longer retention within the body (Neathery and Miller 1975). Characteristic outcomes of MeHg poisoning in both humans and mammalian wildlife include structural degeneration of the occipital cortex and the cerebellum, which leads to paresthesia (numbness, tingling), ataxia (incoordination), sensory impairment, and memory loss (Weihe and Joensen 2012). Moreover, MeHg has a much slower turnover rate in the body, i.e., the biological half-life of MeHg for striped dolphin (*Stenella coeruleoalba*) was estimated to be 1000 days (Itano and Kawai 1981) and Tillander et al. (1972) observed a half-life of ~ 500 days in harp seals (*Pagophilus groenlandicus*).

Methylmercury exposure is of particular concern. Chronic exposure at low concentrations can cause subtle adverse effects, particularly on the developing brain (Basu et al. 2009). Methylmercury can also have deleterious effects on many organ systems and laboratory studies have suggested synergistic effects among Hg and other contaminants known to occur in Steller sea lion (Castellini et al. 2012). Methylmercury is readily absorbed and transported across the blood brain barrier and transplacentally (Wagemann et al. 1988). Therefore, the central nervous system of fetuses and neonates is of concern with respect to MeHg toxicity. In this sense, fetuses encounter significant exposure to Hg *in utero*, a critical developmental period (Castellini et al. 2012).

Laboratory trials with mink (*Mustela vison*) inhabiting North America have demonstrated that neuronal lesions, behavioral deficits, and even death are likely outcomes when concentrations of Hg in the brain are between 4 and 5 $\mu g.g^{-1}$ wet wt. (Basu et al. 2007). Furthermore, significant changes in neurochemistry may be apparent for concentrations of Hg in the brain as low as 1 $\mu g.g^{-1}$ wet wt. (Basu et al. 2006).

Polar bears that accumulate low concentrations of Hg in their brain stem region (mean = 0.36 ± 0.12 $\mu g.g^{-1}$ dry wt.) showed significant negative correlations between both Hg and MeHg concentrations and synaptic NMDA (*N*-methyl-D-aspartate) glutamate receptors. These decreased levels of NMDA receptors could be one of the most sensitive indicators of mercury's subclinical and early effects (Basu et al. 2009). It is worth noting that in this same brain region, MeHg comprised 83% of the Hg present. These results suggest that Hg at ecologically relevant levels may exert subtle, sub-clinical neurological changes in the 3 to 5 $\mu g.g^{-1}$ dry wt. concentration in brain of several fish-eating wildlife species (Dietz et al. 2013).

Organic Hg compounds such as ethylmercury and phenylmercury are biotransformed to the inorganic Hg more rapidly than is MeHg. Another factor contributing to longer biological half-life of MeHg is the rapid resorption following excretion into the intestine. Methylmercury endogenously excreted into the gut is combined with cysteine or glutathione and rapidly resorbed, whereas most inorganic Hg excreted into the gut goes out with the feces (Neathery and Miller 1975). In this instance, MeHg is the chemical Hg form preferentially assimilated by living organisms and for that reason, it is the dominant form found in fish, squids and crustaceans consumed by marine mammals.

Hg detoxification in marine mammals

Marine mammals use a variety of homeostasis processes to limit the accumulation of metals that could cause toxic effects. These mammals may be partially protected against the negative effects of Hg through a number of mechanisms, including demethylation (Wintle et al. 2011), excretion (e.g., urine, feces, hair) (Nigro et al. 2002, Correa et al. 2014), interactions with proteins, such as metallothioneins (Das et al. 2000) and elements such as selenium (Se) (Khan and Wang 2009).

Some studies have demonstrated that Se, a micronutrient, may decrease Hg bioavailability, in the form of MeHg, since it blocks Hg in insoluble compounds in liver and kidneys (Feroci et al. 2005), consequently decreasing MeHg toxicity. Like Sulphur (S), Se readily complexes with Hg, and both elements tend to bind to the S groupings present in proteins. Thus, it is reasonable to expect that both Se and Hg bioaccumulate alongside each other in tissues of marine mammals (Ganther et al. 1972). In fact, Se concentrations are usually in molar excess of Hg in almost all marine mammals, indicating that substantial Se is available in enough amounts to counter Hg toxicity, and some studies have demonstrated that Se:Hg molar ratios in excess of 1:1 neutralize the adverse effects of Hg (Ganther et al. 1972, Leonzio et al.

1992, Ralston et al. 2007, Kehrig et al. 2013). Strong positive correlations between Hg and Se concentrations in tissues (e.g., liver, kidney) of many fish-eating wildlife species, especially predatory marine mammals, are well documented (Seixas et al. 2007, Baptista et al. 2016, Kehrig et al. 2016, Romero et al. 2016, Koeman et al. 1973). The Hg–Se relationship is a toxicant–nutrient interaction that has relevance for both basic biology and environmental risk assessment, although important physiological details of the relationship are still unclear. It is worth noting that the differences in the metabolism of certain marine mammals can also influence the accumulation of Hg and Se, as reflected in the Se:Hg molar ratios (Seixas et al. 2007).

A coping mechanism for Hg toxicity in marine mammals is the formation of mercuric selenide (HgSe), the final product of the Hg demethylation process (Kehrig et al. 2016, Romero et al. 2016). For example, HgSe has been observed in the liver of Guiana and Franciscana dolphins, identified as amorphous crystals in Kupffer cells (macrophages) by ultra-structural analysis (Lailson-Brito et al. 2012, Romero et al. 2016). This has also been observed in northern fur seals (*Callorhinus ursinus*), where Hg was demonstrated as preferentially accumulated in liver, mainly as Hg_{inorg} and HgSe (Ikemoto et al. 2004, Arai et al. 2004), the lattes in nuclear and lysosomal mitochondrial liver fractions (Arai et al. 2004), as well as in ringed seals from the Canadian Arctic (Wagemann et al. 2000).

On the other hand, almost the entire Hg content found in marine mammals' muscle tissue is in its methylated form, which is intimately associated with high affinity to Se. MeHg covalently binds to Se present in selenoenzymes, forming a highly stable organic compound, methylmercury-selenocysteine (MeHg-SeCys) in organisms exposed to Hg, resulting in adverse effects associated with Hg toxicity (Ralston 2008).

Metallothionein (MT) concentrations in marine mammals are an important tool that assists in the evaluation of water contamination by metals. Mammalian MTs are cysteine-rich low-molecular-weight proteins that bind with high affinity to metals and whose synthesis is mainly induced in response to the presence of certain elements, such as Cd, zinc (Zn), copper (Cu), as well as Hg_{inorg} (Jakimska et al. 2011). MT induction has been considered one of the most important detoxification processes against metal toxicity (Cáceres-Saez et al. 2016). MT concentrations in marine mammal tissues have been used as a biomarker of exposure to metals, since MT concentrations have been shown to correlate well with mammal metal exposure in biomonitoring programs (Kehrig et al. 2016). However, MT regulation may be influenced by local environmental metal concentrations and differences in prey preference (Cáceres-Saez et al. 2016).

Conflicting data in the literature regarding MT Hg detoxification in marine mammals is available. For example, MT concentrations in Franciscana and Guiana dolphin liver from the Brazilian coast have been implicated as playing an important role in the detoxification process of total Hg and Hg_{inorg}, although not of MeHg (Kehrig et al. 2016). On the other hand, MT appears to play a minor role in the binding and detoxification of hepatic Hg, in contrast to the detoxification of Cd, Zn and Cu in northern fur seals and harbor porpoises (*Phocoena phocoena*) (Ikemoto et al. 2004, Das et al. 2006, Romero et al. 2016). This may be due to the fact that despite a strong affinity for MT, only a small part of Hg_{inorg} in the liver of marine mammals is bound to these proteins (Das et al. 2000). In stranded striped dolphins and bottlenose dolphins from the Mediterranean Sea, hepatic Hg was present mainly in the insoluble subcellular fraction, indicating that MT seemed to play no role in Hg detoxification in these species (Decataldo et al. 2004). It has been postulated that Hg concentrations below the tolerance limit (100–400 $\mu g.g^{-1}$ wet wt., Wagemann and Muir 1984) in marine mammal livers are likely not high enough to induce MT synthesis (Romero et al. 2016). More recently, a new analytical procedure for the identification of Hg complexes with MT was applied in a white-sided dolphin (*Lagenorhynchus acutus*) liver sample, and the presence of Hg-MT binding in this tissue was detected. This demonstrates the probable potential role of MT in Hg detoxification mechanism in the hepatic tissues of marine mammals (Pedrero et al. 2012), contrasting with other studies.

Hepatic and renal MT concentrations in Commerson's dolphins (*Cephalorhynchus commersonii*) from Tierra del Fuego, South Atlantic Ocean did not present significant correlation with Hg, possibly due to their values corresponding to the physiological background levels of the evaluated marine mammal specimens (Cáceres-Saez et al. 2016).

Conclusions

Marine mammals are a diverse group of mid to high trophic level predators that show the potential to be applied as environmental sentinels for several pollutants, since they may accumulate high amounts of xenobiotics, in different tissues and organs. In this sense, extrapolation from marine mammals to humans is possible as they prey on the same species, indicating that these species also show potential in identifying environmental contamination. Marine mammals present several interesting features for the study of xenobiotics accumulation and transfers within marine systems from an ecotoxicological point of view. A wide range of xenobiotics has become widely recognized as the source of adverse effects to the marine environments and organisms, and Hg in particular, has been the subject of many studies due to its highly toxic effects. Lastly, marine mammals have the highest Hg concentrations recorded for any marine species. Environmental exposure to Hg, particularly for higher trophic level consumers, including marine mammals and humans, is significantly higher than other elements, since this metal presents high toxicity and the ability to undergo biomagnification along trophic chains. Significant correlations have been reported between brain stem Hg concentrations and changes in Hg-neurochemical biomarkers for top consumers as marine mammals. Hg concentrations in Arctic marine mammal brain tissue are in the range previously demonstrated as associated to neurochemical effects. Metal detoxification mechanisms, such as Se:Hg interactions and MT-Hg complexes, have been proven to be important for marine mammals, although they are not yet fully elucidated. Further studies are needed, especially on the chemical form in which Hg is accumulated and other regions of the brain with known sensitivity to Hg should also be examined, such as the cerebellum and occipital cortex.

Acknowledgments

The authors would like to thank the Brazilian National Research Council (CNPq), Fundação de Amparo à Pesquisa do Estado do Rio de Janeiro (FAPERJ) and Coordenação de Aperfeiçoamento de Pessoal de Nível Superior (CAPES) for financial support.

References

Acevedo-Whitehouse, K. and A.L. Duffus. 2009. Effects of environmental change on wildlife health. Philos. Trans. R Soc. Lond. B Biol. Sci. 364: 3429–3438.

Aguirre, A.A. and G.M. Tabor. 2004. Introduction: marine vertebrates as sentinels of marine ecosystem health. EcoHealth. 1: 236–238.

Agusa, T., T. Kunito, A. Sudaryanto, I. Monirith, S. Kan-Atireklap, H. Iwata et al. 2007. Exposure assessment for trace elements from consumption of marine fish in Southeast Asia. Environ. Pollut. 145: 766–777.

Anandraj, A., R. Perissinotto, C. Nozais and D. Stretch. 2008. The recovery of microalgal production and biomass in a South African temporarily open/closed estuary, following mouth breaching. Estuar. Coast. Shelf Sci. 79: 599–606.

Andre, J., A. Boudou, F. Ribeyre and M. Bernhard. 1991. Comparative study of mercury accumulation in dolphins (*Stenella coeruleoalba*) from French Atlantic and Mediterranean coasts. Sci. Total Environ. 104: 191–209.

Arai, T., T. Ikemoto, A. Hokura, Y. Terada, T. unito, S. Tanabe et al. 2004. Chemical forms of mercury and cadmium accumulated in marine mammals and seabirds as determined by XAFS analysis. Environ. Sci. Technol. 38: 6468–6474.

Arellano-Peralta, V.A. and L. Medrano-González. 2015. Ecology, conservation and human history of marine mammals in the Gulf of California and Pacific coast of Baja California, Mexico. Ocean Coast Manage. 104: 90–105.

Azam, F., T. Fenchel, J.G. Field, J.S. Gray, L.A. Meyer-Reil and F. Thingstad. 1983. The ecological role of water-column microbes in the sea. Mar. Ecol. Prog. Ser. 10: 257–263.

Baptista, G., H.A. Kehrig, A.P.M. Di Beneditto, R.A. Hauser-Davis, M.G. Almeida, C.E. Rezende et al. 2016. Mercury, selenium and stable isotopes in four small cetaceans from the Southeastern Brazilian coast: Influence of feeding strategy. Environ. Pollut. 218: 1298–1307.

Barwick, M. and W. Maher. 2003. Biotransference and biomagnification of selenium copper, cadmium, zinc, arsenic and lead in a temperate seagrass ecosystem from Lake Macquarie Estuary, NSW, Australia. Mar. Environ. Res. 56: 471–502.

Basu, N., A.M. Scheuhammer, K. Rouvinen-Watt, N. Grochowina, K. Klenavic, R.D. Evans et al. 2006. Methylmercury impairs components of the cholinergic system in captive mink (*Mustela vison*). Toxicol. Sci. 91: 202–209.

Basu, N., A.M. Scheuhammer, S.J. Bursian, J. Elliott, K. Rouvinen-Watt and H.M. Chan. 2007. Mink as a sentinel species in environmental health. Environ. Res. 103: 130–144.

Basu, N., A.M. Scheuhammer, C. Sonne, R.J. Letcher, E.W. Born and R. Dietz. 2009. Is dietary mercury of neurotoxicological concern to wild polar bears (*Ursus maritimus*)? Environ. Toxicol. Chem. 28: 133–140.

Bechshoft, T., A.E. Derocher, E. Richardson, P. Mislan, N.J. Lunn, C. Sonne et al. 2015. Mercury and cortisol in Western Hudson Bay polar bear hair. Ecotoxicology. 24: 1315–1321.

Bossart, G.D. 2006. Marine mammals as sentinel species for oceans and human health. Oceanogr. 19: 133–137.

Burford, M.A., D.M. Alongi, A.D. McKinnon and L.A. Trott. 2008. Primary production and nutrients in a tropical macrotidal estuary, Darwin Harbour, Australia. Estuar. Coast. Shelf Sci. 79: 440–448.

Cáceres-Saez, I., P. Polizzi, B. Romero, N.A. Dellabianca, S.R. Guevara, R.N.P. Goodall et al. 2016. Hepatic and renal metallothionein concentrations in Commerson's dolphins (*Cephalorhynchus commersonii*) from Tierra del Fuego, South Atlantic Ocean. Mar. Pollut. Bull. 108: 263–267.

Castellini, J.M., L.D. Rea, C.L. Lieske, K.B. Beckmen, B.S. Fadely, J.M. Maniscalco et al. 2012. Mercury concentrations in hair from neonatal and juvenile Steller sea lions (*Eumetopias jubatus*): Implications based on age and region in this Northern Pacific marine sentinel piscivore. EcoHealth. 9: 267–277.

Correa, L., L. Rea, R. Bentzen and T. O'Hara. 2014. Assessment of mercury and selenium tissular concentrations and total mercury body burden in 6 Steller sea lion pups from the Aleutian Islands. Mar. Pollut. Bull. 82: 175–182.

Danilewicz, D., I.B. Moreno, P.H. Ott, M. Tavares, A.F. Azevedo, E.R. Secchi et al. 2010. Abundance estimate for a threatened population of franciscana dolphins in southern coastal Brazil: uncertainties and management implications. J. Mar. Biol. Assoc. UK. 90(8): 1649–1657.

Das, K., V. Debacker and J. Bouquegneau. 2000. Metallothioneins in marine mammals. Cell. Mol. Biol. 46: 283–294.

Das, K., A. De Groof, T. Jauniaux and J.M. Bouquegneau. 2006. Zn, Cu, Cd and Hg binding to metallothioneins in harbour porpoises *Phocoena phocoena* from the southern North Sea. BioMed. Cent. Ecol. 6: 1–7.

de Moura, J.F., R.A. Hauser-Davis, L. Lemos, R. Emin-Lina and S. Siciliano. 2014. Guiana dolphins (*Sotalia guianensis*) as marine ecosystem sentinels: Ecotoxicology and emerging diseases. Rev. Environ. Contam. Toxicol. 228: 1–29.

Decataldo, A., A. Di Leo, S. Giandomenico and N. Cardellicchio. 2004. Association of metals (mercury, cadmium and zinc) with metallothionein-like proteins in storage organs of stranded dolphins from the Mediterranean sea (Southern Italy). J. Environ. Monit. 6: 361–367.

Di Beneditto, A.P.M. and R.M.A. Ramos. 2014. Marine debris ingestion by coastal dolphins: What drives differences between sympatric species? Mar. Pollut. Bull. 83: 298–301.

Dietz, R., F. Riget, E.W. Born, C. Sonne, P. Grandjean, M. Kirkegaard et al. 2006. Trends in mercury in hair of Greenlandic polar bears (*Ursus maritimus*) during 1892–2001. Environ. Sci. Technol. 40: 1120–1125.

Dietz, R., P.M. Outridge and K.A. Hobson. 2009. Anthropogenic contribution to mercury levels in present-day Arctic animals—a review. Sci. Total Environ. 407: 6120–6131.

Dietz, R., E.W. Born, F. Riget, A. Aubail, C. Sonne, R. Drimmie et al. 2011. Temporal trends and future predictions of mercury concentrations in Northwest Greenland polar bear (*Ursus maritimus*) hair. Environ. Sci. Technol. 45: 1458–1465.

Dietz, R., C. Sonne, N. Basu, B. Braune, T. O'Hara, R.J. Letcher et al. 2013. What are the toxicological effects of mercury in Arctic biota? Sci. Total Environ. 443: 775–790.

Dorneles, P.R., J. Lailson-Brito, R.A. Santos, P.A.S. Costa, O. Malm, A.F. Azevedo et al. 2007. Cephalopods and cetaceans as indicators of offshore bioavailability of cadmium off Central South Brazil Bight. Environ. Pollut. 148: 352–359.

Endo, T., K. Haraguchi and M. Sakata. 2002. Mercury and selenium concentrations in the internal organs of toothed whales and dolphins marketed for human consumption in Japan. Sci. Total Environ. 300: 15–22.

Fenchel, T. 2008. The microbial loop–25 years later. J. Exp. Mar. Biol. Ecol. 366: 99–103.

Feroci, G., R. Badiello and A. Fini. 2005. Interactions between different selenium compounds and zinc, cadmium and mercury. J. Trace Elem. Med. Biol. 18: 227–234.

Ferreira, G.V., M. Barletta, A.R. Lima, D.V. Dantas, A.K. Justino and M.F. Costa. 2016. Plastic debris contamination in the life cycle of Acoupa weakfish (*Cynoscion acoupa*) in a tropical estuary. ICES J. Mar. Sci. 73: 1–13.

Fisher, N.S., I. Stupakoff, S. Sañudo-Wilhelmy, W.X. Wang, J.L. Teyssié, S.W. Fowler et al. 2000. Trace metals in marine copepods: a field test of a bioaccumulation model coupled to laboratory uptake kinetics data. Mar. Ecol. Prog. Ser. 194: 211–218.

Flora, S.J.S., M. Mittal and A. Mehta. 2008. Heavy metal induced oxidative stress & its possible reversal by chelation therapy. Indian J. Med. Res. 128: 501–523.

Forcada, J. and J.I. Hoffman. 2014. Climate change selects for heterozygosity in a declining fur seal population. Nature. 511: 462–465.

Frouin, H., L.L. Loseto, G.A. Stern, M. Haulena and P.S. Ross. 2012. Mercury toxicity in beluga whale lymphocytes: limited effects of selenium protection. Aquat. Toxicol. 109: 185–193.

Gadzała-Kopciuch, R., B. Berecka, J. Bartoszewicz and B. Buszewski. 2004. Some considerations about bioindicators in environmental monitoring. Pol. J. Environ. Stud. 13: 453–462.

Ganther, H.E., C. Goudie, M.L. Sunde, M.J. Kopecky, P. Wagner, S.-H. Oh et al. 1972. Selenium: relation to decreased toxicity of methylmercury added to diets containing tuna. Science. 175: 1122–1124.

Geraci, J.R. and V.J. Lounsbury. 2005. Decisions on the beach. *In*: Geraci, J.R. and V.J. Lounsbury (eds.). Marine Mammals Ashore: A Field Guide for Strandings. National Aquarium in Baltimore, Baltimore, Maryland, USA.

Gerpe, M., D. Rodríguez, V.J. Moreno, R.O. Bastida and J.D. Moreno. 2002. Accumulation of heavy metals in the franciscana (*Pontoporia blainvillei*) from Buenos Aires Province, Argentina. Lat. Am. J. Aquat. Mamm. 1: 95–106.

Gibičar, D., M. Logar, N. Horvat, A. Marn-Pernat, R. Ponikvar and M. Horvat. 2007. Simultaneous determination of trace levels of ethylmercury and methylmercury in biological samples and vaccines using sodium tetra (n-propyl) borate as derivatizing agent. Anal. Bioanal. Chem. 388: 329–340.

Gray, J.S. 2002. Biomagnification in marine systems: the perspective of an ecologist. Mar. Pollut. Bull. 45: 46–52.

Habran, S., C. Debier, D.E. Crocker, D.S. Houser and K. Das. 2011. Blood dynamics of mercury and selenium in northern elephant seals during the lactation period. Environ. Pollut. 159: 2523–2529.

Hall, B.D., R.A. Bodaly, R.J.P. Fudge, J.W.M. Rudd and D.M. Rosenberg. 1997. Food as the dominant pathway of methylmercury uptake by fish. Water Air Soil Poll. 100: 13–24.

Harwood, J. 2001. Marine mammals and their environment in the twenty-first century. J. Mammal. 82: 630–640.

Haynes, D., S. Carter, C. Gaus, J. Müller and W. Dennison. 2005. Organochlorine and heavy metal concentrations in blubber and liver tissue collected from Queensland (Australia) dugong (*Dugong dugon*). Mar. Pollut. Bull. 51: 361–369.

Ikemoto, T., T. Kunito, I. Watanabe, G. Yasunaga, N. Baba, N. Miyazaki et al. 2004. Comparison of trace element accumulation in Baikal seals (*Pusa sibirica*), Caspian seals (*Pusa caspica*) and northern fur seals (*Callorhinus ursinus*). Environ. Pollut. 127: 83–97.

Itano, K. and S. Kawai. 1981. Changes of mercury contents and biological half-life of mercury in the striped dolphins. Studies on the levels and organochorine compounds and heavy metals in the marine organisms. University of the Ryukyus, Nishihara, Okinawa.

Jakimska, A., P. Konieczka, K. Skóra and J. Namiesnik. 2011. Bioaccumulation of metals in tissues of marine animals, Part I: the role and impact of heavy metals on organisms. Pol. J. Environ. Stud. 20: 1117–1125.

Jefferson, T.A., S. Leatherwood and M.A. Webber. 1993. FAO species identification guide. Marine Mammals of the World. FAO, Rome, Italy.

Kainz, M. and A. Mazumder. 2005. Effect of algal and bacterial diet on methyl mercury concentrations in zooplankton. Environ. Sci. Technol. 39: 1666–1672.

Kakuschke, A., E. Valentine-Thon, S. Fonfara, K. Kramer and A. Prange. 2009. Effects of methyl-, phenyl-, ethylmercury and mercurychlorid on immune cells of harbor seals (*Phoca vitulina*). J. Environ. Sci. 21: 1716–1721.

Kehrig, H.A., T.G. Seixas, E. Palermo, A.P.M. Di Beneditto, C. Souza and O. Malm. 2008. Different species of mercury in the livers of tropical dolphins. Anal. Lett. 41: 1691–1699.

Kehrig, H.A. 2011. Mercury and plankton in tropical marine ecosystems: a review. Oecologia Australis. 15: 869–880.

Kehrig, H.A., T.G. Siexas, E.A. Palermo, A.P. Baêta, O. Malm and I. Moreira. 2011. Bioconcentration and biomagnification of methylmercury in Guanabara Bay, Rio de Janeiro. Quím Nova. 34: 377–384.

Kehrig, H.A., T.G. Siexas, A.P.M. Di Beneditto and O. Malm. 2013. Selenium and mercury in widely consumed seafood from South Atlantic Ocean. Ecotox. Environ. Safe. 93: 156–162.

Kehrig, H.A., R.A. Hauser-Davis, T.G. Seixas, A.B. Pinheiro and A.P.M. Di Beneditto. 2016. Mercury species, selenium, metallothioneins and glutathione in two dolphins from the southeastern Brazilian coast: Mercury detoxification and physiological differences in diving capacity. Environ. Pollut. 213: 785–792.

King, J.K., F.M. Saunders, R.F. Lee and R.A. Jahnke. 1999. Coupling mercury methylation rates to sulfate reduction rates in marine sediments. Environ. Toxicol. Chem. 18: 1362–1369.

Khan, M.A. and F. Wang. 2009. Mercury-selenium compounds and their toxicological significance: toward a molecular understanding of the mercury-selenium antagonism. Environ. Toxicol. Chem. 28: 1567–1577.

Koeman, J., W. Peeters, C. Koudstaal-Hol, P. Tjioe and J. De Goeij. 1973. Mercury-selenium correlations in marine mammals. Nature. 245: 385–386.

Krey, A., S.K. Ostertag and H.M. Chan. 2015. Assessment of neurotoxic effects of mercury in beluga whales (*Delphinapterus leucas*), ringed seals (*Pusa hispida*) and polar bears (*Ursus maritimus*) from the Canadian Arctic. Sci. Total Environ. 509: 237–247.

Kunito, T., S. Nakamura, T. Ikemoto, Y. Anan, R. Kubota, S. Tanabe et al. 2004. Concentration and subcellular distribution of trace elements in liver of small cetaceans incidentally caught along the Brazilian coast. Mar. Pollut. Bull. 49: 574–587.

Lahaye, V., P. Bustamante, R.J. Law, J.A. Learmonth, M.B. Santos, J.P. Boon et al. 2007. Biological and ecological factors related to trace element levels in harbour porpoises (*Phocoena phocoena*) from European waters. Mar. Environ. Res. 64: 247–266.

Lailson-Brito, J., R. Cruz, P.R. Dorneles, L. Andrade, A.F. Azevedo, A.B. Fragoso et al. 2012. Mercury-selenium relationships in liver of Guiana dolphin: the possible role of Kupffer cells in the detoxification process by tiemannite formation. PloS ONE. 7: 42162.

Law, R., J. Barry, J.L. Barber, P. Bersuder, R. Deaville, R.J. Reid et al. 2012. Contaminants in cetaceans from UK waters: Status as assessed within the cetacean strandings investigation programme from 1990 to 2008. Mar. Pollut. Bull. 64: 1485–1494.

Lawson, N.M. and R.P. Mason. 1998. Accumulation of mercury in estuarine food chains. Biogeochemistry. 40: 235–247.

Lemes, M., F. Wang, G.A. Stern, S.K. Ostertag and H.M. Chan. 2011. Methylmercury and selenium speciation in different tissues of beluga whales (*Delphinapterus leucas*) from the western Canadian Arctic. Environ. Toxicol. Chem. 30: 2732–2738.

Leonzio, C., S. Focardi and C. Fossi. 1992. Heavy metals and selenium in stranded dolphins of the Northern Tyrrhenian (NW Mediterranean). Sci. Total Environ. 119: 77–84.

Mason, R.P., W.F. Fitzgerald and F.M.M. Morel. 1994. The biogeochemical cycling of elemental mercury: anthropogenic influences. Geochem. Cosmochim. Acta. 58(15): 3191–3198.

Mason, R.P., J.R. Reinfelder and F.M. Morel. 1996. Uptake, toxicity, and trophic transfer of mercury in a coastal diatom. Environ. Sci. Technol. 30: 1835–1845.

Mason, R.P., J.M. Laporte and S. Andres. 2000. Factors controlling the bioaccumulation of mercury, methylmercury, arsenic, selenium, and cadmium by freshwater invertebrates and fish. Arch. Environ. Contam. Toxicol. 38: 283–297.

Mason, R.P. and G.-R. Sheu. 2002. Role of the ocean in the global mercury cycle. Global Biogeochem. Cycles. 16(4): 40-1–40-14.

Miles, C.J., H.A. Moye, E.J. Phlips and B. Sargent. 2001. Partitioning of monomethylmercury between freshwater algae and water. Environ. Sci. Technol. 35: 4277–4282.

Moore, S.E. 2008. Marine mammals as ecosystem sentinels. J. Mammal. 89: 534–540.

National Research Council. 1996. The Bering Sea Ecosystem. The National Academies Press, Washington, DC, USA.

Neathery, M.W. and W.J. Miller. 1975. Metabolism and toxicity of cadmium, mercury, and lead in animals: A review. J. Dairy Sci. 58: 1767–1781.

Newell, R.C. 2013 Adaptation to environment: essays on the physiology of marine animals. Elsevier. 554 p.

Ng, T.T., C. Amiard-Triquet, P.S. Rainbow, J.C. Amiard and W.X. Wang. 2005. Physico-chemical form of trace metals accumulated by phytoplankton and their assimilation by filter-feeding invertebrates. Mar. Ecol. Prog. Ser. 299: 179–191.

Nigro, M., A. Campana, E. Lanzillotta and R. Ferrara. 2002. Mercury exposure and elimination rates in captive bottlenose dolphins. Mar. Pollut. Bull. 44: 1071–1075.

Noël, M., S. Jeffries, D.M. Lambourn, K. Telmer, R. Macdonald and P.S. Ross. 2016. Mercury accumulation in harbour seals from the Northeastern Pacific Ocean: The role of transplacental transfer, lactation, age and location. Arch. Environ. Contam. Toxicol. 70: 56–66.

Nomiyama, K., S. Murata, T. Kunisue, T.K. Yamada, H. Mizukawa, S. Takahashi et al. 2010. Polychlorinated biphenyls and their hydroxylated metabolites (OH-PCBs) in the blood of toothed and baleen whales stranded along Japanese Coastal Waters. Environ. Sci. Technol. 44: 3732–3738.

Okay, O.S., P. Donkin, L.D. Peters and D.R. Livingstone. 2000. The role of algae (*Isochrysis galbana*) enrichment on the bioaccumulation of benzo [a] pyrene and its effects on the blue mussel *Mytilus edulis*. Environ. Pollut. 110: 103–113.

Pedrero, Z., L. Ouerdane, S. Mounicou, R. Lobinski, M. Monperrus and D. Amouroux. 2012. Identification of mercury and other metals complexes with metallothioneins in dolphin liver by hydrophilic interaction liquid chromatography with the parallel detection by ICP MS and electrospray hybrid linear/orbital trap MS/MS. Metallomics. 4: 473–479.

Polizzi, P., M. Romero, L.C. Boudet, K. Das, P. Denuncio, D. Rodríguez et al. 2014. Metallothioneins pattern during ontogeny of coastal dolphin, *Pontoporia blainvillei*, from Argentina. Mar. Pollut. Bull. 80: 275–281.

Pompa, S., P.R. Ehrlich and G. Ceballos. 2011. Global distribution and conservation of marine mammals. Proceedings of the National Academy of Sciences of the United States of America. 108: 13600–13605.

Ralston, N.V.C., J.L. Blackwell and L.J. Raymond. 2007. Importance of molar ratios in selenium-dependent protection against methylmercury toxicity. Biol. Trace Elem. Res. 119: 255–268.

Ralston, N.V.C. 2008. Selenium health benefit values as seafood safety criteria. EcoHealth. 5: 442–455.

Reif, J.S., A.M. Schaefer and G.D. Bossart. 2015. Atlantic bottlenose dolphins (*Tursiops truncatus*) as a sentinel for exposure to mercury in humans: Closing the loop. Vet. Sci. 2: 407–422.

Reinfelder, J.R., N.S. Fisher, S.N. Luoma, J.W. Nichols and W.X. Wang. 1998. Trace element trophic transfer in aquatic organisms: a critique of the kinetic model approach. Sci. Total Environ. 219: 117–135.

Riedman, M. 1990. Pinnipeds: Seals, Sea Lions, and Walruses. University of California Press: Berkeley. 149 p.

Romero, M.B., P. Polizzi, L. Chiodi, K. Das and M. Gerpe. 2016. The role of metallothioneins, selenium and transfer to offspring in mercury detoxification in Franciscana dolphins (*Pontoporia blainvillei*). Mar. Pollut. Bull. 1: 650–654.

Ross, P.S. 2000. Marine mammals as sentinels in ecological risk assessment. Hum. Ecol. Risk Assess. 6: 29–46.

Schaefer, A.M., H.C.W. Stavros, G.D. Bossart, P.A. Fair, J.D. Goldstein and J.S. Reif. 2011. Associations between mercury and hepatic, renal, endocrine, and hematological parameters in Atlantic bottlenose dolphins (*Tursiops truncatus*) along the eastern coast of Florida and South Carolina. Arch. Environ. Contam. Toxicol. 61: 688–695.

Seixas, T.G., H.A. Kehrig, G. Fillmann, A.P. Di Beneditto, C.M. Souza, E.R. Secchi et al. 2007. Ecological and biological determinants of trace elements accumulation in liver and kidney of *Pontoporia blainvillei*. Sci. Total Environ. 385: 208–220.

Siscar, R., S. Koenig, A. Torreblanca and M. Solé. 2014. The role of metallothionein and selenium in metal detoxification in the liver of deep-sea fish from the NW Mediterranean Sea. Sci. Total Environ. 466: 898–905.

Smith, K.F., K. Acevedo-Whitehouse and A.B. Pedersen. 2009. The role of infectious diseases in biological conservation. Anim. Conserv. 12: 1–12.

Sonne, C. 2010. Health effects from long-range transported contaminants in Arctic top predators: An integrated review based on studies of polar bears and relevant model species. Envir. Int. 36: 461–491.

State of Alaska Epidemiology Bulletin. 2010. Alaska hair biomonitoring program update, July 2002–May 2010. Division of Health, Department of Health and Social Services. 3601 C Street, Ste 540, Anchorage, AK, 99503. Bulletin 18, June 24, 2010. http://www.epi.hss.state.ak.us/bulletins/docs/b2010__18.pdf.

Tillander, M., J.K. Mioettinen and W. Koisisto. 1972. Excretion rate of methylmercury in the sea: (*Pusa hispida*). pp. 303–305. *In*: Ruivo, I. (ed.). Marine Pollution and Sea Life, Fishing News Ltd., London, UK.

Viarengo, A., B. Burlando, F. Dondero, A. Marro and R. Fabbri. 1999. Metallothionein as a tool in biomonitoring programmes. Biomarkers. 4: 455–466.

Wagemann, R. and D. Muir. 1984. Concentrations of Heavy Metals and Organochlorines in Marine Mammals of Northern Waters: Overview and Evaluation. Western Region, Department of Fisheries and Oceans, Canada.

Wagemann, R., R.E.A. Stewart, W.L. Lockhart, B.E. Stewart and M. Povoledo. 1988. Trace metals and methylmercury: associations and transfer in harp seal (*Phoca groenlandica*) mothers and their pups. Mar. Mammal Sci. 4: 339–355.

Wagemann, R., W.L. Lockhart, H. Welch and S. Innes. 1995. Arctic marine mammals as integrators and indicators of mercury in the Arctic. Water Air Soil Pollut. 80: 683–693.

Wagemann, R., S. Innes and P.R. Richard. 1996. Overview and regional and temporal differences of heavy metals in arctic whales and ringed seals in the Canadian Arctic. Sci. Total Environ. 186: 41–66.

Wagemann, R., E. Trebacz, G. Boila and W.L. Lockhart. 2000. Mercury species in the liver of ringed seals. Sci. Total Environ. 261: 21–32.

Wang, W.X. and N.S. Fisher. 1998. Accumulation of trace elements in a marine copepod. Limnol. Oceanogr. 43: 273–283.

Wang, W.X. and P.S. Rainbow. 2005. Influence of metal exposure history on trace metal uptake and accumulation by marine invertebrates. Ecotoxicol. Environ. Saf. 61: 145–159.

Watras, C.J., R.C. Back, S. Halvorsen, R.J.M. Hudson, K.A. Morrison and S.P. Wente. 1998. Bioaccumulation of mercury in pelagic freshwater food webs. Sci. Total Environ. 219: 183–208.

Weihe, P. and H.D. Joensen. 2012. Dietary recommendations regarding pilot whale meat and blubber in the Faroe Islands. Int. J. Circumpolar. Health. 71: 18594.

WHO. 1990. Methylmercury. Environmental Health Criteria 101. World Health Organization, Geneva.

Winship, K.A. 1985. Organic mercury compounds and their toxicity. Adverse Drug React Acute Poisoning Rev. 5: 141–180.

Wintle, N., D. Duffield, R. Jones and J. Rice. 2011. Total mercury in stranded marine mammals from the Oregon and southern Washington coasts. Mar. Mamm. Sci. 27: 268–278.

Yang, J., T. Kunito, Y. Anan, S. Tanabe and N. Miyazaki. 2004. Total and subcellular distribution of trace elements in the liver of a mother–fetus pair of Dall's porpoises (*Phocoenoides dalli*). Mar. Pollut. Bull. 48: 1122–1129.

Zhou, Q., J. Zhang, J. Fu, J. Shi and G. Jiang. 2008. Biomonitoring: an appealing tool for assessment of metal pollution in the aquatic ecosystem. Anal. Chim. Acta. 606: 135–150.

5

Ecotoxicology of Pharmaceutical and Personal Care Products (PPCPs)

Enrico Mendes Saggioro,[1,]* Danielle Maia Bila[2]
and *Suéllen Satyro[3]*

Introduction

Micropollutants have been of concern in recent years due to their occurrence in the aquatic environment. Also described as contaminants of emerging concern (CEC), micropollutants consist of a broad and expanding range of anthropogenic, as well as natural substances. Micropollutants, such as pharmaceuticals and personal care products (PPCPs), industrial chemicals and pesticides, are not yet included in lists of regulated substances (Luo et al. 2014).

PPCPs comprise several groups of organic compounds such as antibiotics, hormones, anti-inflammatory, antiepileptic, blood lipid regulators, β-blockers, contrast media, cytostatic, antimicrobial agents, synthetic musks, insect repellents, preservatives and sunscreen UV filters (Liu and Wong 2013). The occurrence of micropollutants in the aquatic environment has been frequently associated to many adverse effects, including short- and long-term toxicity, endocrine disrupting effects and microorganism antibiotic resistance (Fent et al. 2006, Pruden et al. 2006).

[1] Sanitation and Environment Health Department, Sergio Arouca National School of Public Health, Oswaldo Cruz Foundation, Rua Leopoldo Bulhões, 1480, Manguinhos, CEP: 21041210, Rio de Janeiro, RJ, Brazil.
[2] Department of Environmental and Sanitary Engineering, State University of Rio de Janeiro, Rio de Janeiro, RJ, Brazil.
E-mail: danielebilauerj@gmail.com
[3] Department of Chemical and Biological Engineering, University of British Columbia, 2360 East Mall, Vancouver, BC, Canada.
E-mail: satyro@mail.ubc.ca
* Corresponding author: enrico.saggioro@ensp.fiocruz.br

Most micropollutants are ubiquitous, found in waters from all over the world at low concentrations (from ng·L⁻¹ to µg·L⁻¹) (Saggioro et al. 2014), probably as a consequence of imperfect manufacturing processes and/or leaching from final products, or yet, because of incomplete PPCPs removal in wastewater treatment plants (WWTP) (Daughton and Ternes 1999, Li 2014). Incomplete human metabolism and excretion into waste are also an important source of PPCPs release to aquatic environments (Kümmerer 2009). Domestic sewage treatment plants have been recognized as the main route of introduction of PPCPs substances, resulting from human use, into the aquatic environment (Ternes 1998) (Fig. 1).

Among PPCPs, several compounds are released into the environment. Animals and humans are exposed, not to individual contaminants, but to complex mixtures of different action mode. Consequently, the action of these PPCPs may cause additive or synergistic effects (Birkett and Lester 2003). To describe PPCPs ecotoxicology, 4 classes of pharmaceutical compounds and 2 classes of personal care products (PCPs) were selected for discussion in this chapter, based on ecotoxicological effects already studied in the literature, data on population consumption, release percentages and their occurrence in the environment. The chosen pharmaceutical compounds were Carbamazepine (CBZ), Ibuprofen (IBP), Erythromycin (ERY) and 17α-ethinylestradiol (EE2), and the selected personal care products were Triclosan (TCS) and Parabens.

The great concern regarding CBZ is that its high environmental occurrences can be assigned to its extensive use in day-to-day life and the low efficiencies of the biological methods employed in WWTPs (> 10%) (Calisto et al. 2011).

Similarly, IBP is the third-most popular drug in the world, an essential nonprescription drug often used at high therapeutic doses (600–1200 mg·d⁻¹) and displays a significant excretion level, of 70–80% of the therapeutic dose (Buser et al. 1999). Due to its wide usage, its occurrence in the aquatic environment has been

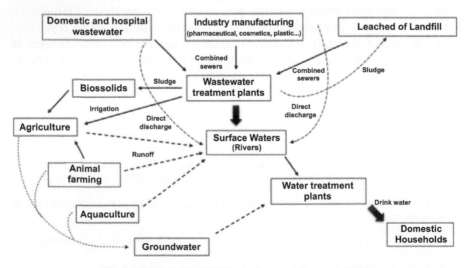

Fig. 1. PPCPs pathway into the environment (Luo et al. 2014).

frequently detected worldwide, such as in rivers and streams across North America (Kolpin et al. 2002), Europe (Buser et al. 1999), North Korea (Kim et al. 2007), Japan (Nakada et al. 2006) and Taiwan (Lin and Tsai 2009).

EE2 is the most common component used in oral contraceptives and hormone replacement therapy, and contraceptives contain 30–50 µg of EE2 per pill (Beausse 2004, Johnson et al. 2000). This compound is one of the most potent endocrine disrupting compounds (EDC) found in the aquatic environment.

Finally, ERY is an antibiotic heavily used in fish farms (Esposito et al. 2007, Chanda et al. 2011, Woo and Bruno 2011, Patil et al. 2016) and greatly affects the water treatment system, since it inhibits ammonification, nitrification and nitration, and also affects heterotrophs, like filamentous bacteria, causing floc disintegration and breakage of filaments (Alighardashi et al. 2009, Louvet et al. 2010).

TCS and Parabens are of high relevance, since they can disrupt human and animal endocrine systems. The former is employed as an antiseptic agent in a vast array of personal care and consumer products. This extensive use results in its direct discharge into sewage systems and receiving surface waters (Barceló et al. 2003). As a bactericidal substance, its continuous release to the environment can promote resistance and changes in the microbial community structure (Daughton and Ternes 1999). Contaminants displaying lipophilic characteristics, such as TCS (log K_{OW} ~ 4.76; USFDA 2008) are not easily eliminated by fish through transformation and diffusion, thus offering a high potential risk for both aquatic organisms and humans (Adolfsson-Erici et al. 2002). Regarding Parabens, these are used daily in various human activities and are continuously released into the aquatic environment. Several compounds belonging to this group mimic endogenous hormones, thus presenting estrogenic activity. The literature reports that these compounds exhibit estrogenic activity in both *in vitro* and *in vivo* assays (Darbre et al. 2002, Routledge et al. 1998b).

Carbamazepine Ecotoxicology

Carbamazepine (CBZ; 5H-dibenzo[b,f]azepine-5-carboxamide) belongs to a class of anticonvulsant medications used to reduce abnormal electrical activity in the brain and, thus, control certain types of seizures (Mohapatra et al. 2014). CBZ is also used to restore episodes of mania or mixed episodes in patients with bipolar disorder. Its mechanism blocks the sodium channels, reducing the action potential of neurons, and can also antagonize adenosine receptors and inhibit the accumulation of cyclic adenosine 3',5'-monophosphate (cAMP) (Jarvis et al. 2014). CBZ metabolization *via* the Cytochrome P450 (CYP) mechanism can generate an active compound (CBZ-10,11-epoxide), as well as other inactive glucuronide compounds. It is estimated that about 1,014 tons of CBZ are annually consumed worldwide (Zhang et al. 2008). CBZ has been detected in a variety of environmental matrices, such as WWTP (Bahlmann et al. 2009), ground (Focazio et al. 2008), surface (Tixier et al. 2003) and even in treated drinking water (Heberer et al. 2002).

PCPPs, including CBZ, have also been found in the aquatic environment as mixtures, not as a single compound (Cleuvers 2003). In this context, two models for risks assessment can be applied in ecotoxicological studies for the prediction of mixture toxicity. The first, the concentration addition model (similar action) is used when the compounds produce the same toxicological response (e.g., death) in the mixture but do not act in target sites, as specific receptors. Concentration addition could show substances that contribute to cumulative toxicological effects even being below their individual No Effect Concentration (NOEC) (Cleuvers 2003), as demonstrated in Eq. 1:

$$\sum_{i=1}^{n} \frac{c_i}{EC_{Xi}} = 1 \tag{1}$$

where, Ci is the concentration of the individual compound in the mixture that produces total effect of X%, and EC_{Xi} is the concentration of single compound that produces the same effect X when present alone in the aqueous solution.

The second model is known as an independent action, in which the compounds act in the target sites, but in different receptors of the organism. Each substance used in concentration below its own NOEC does not contribute to the cumulative toxicological effect of the mixture. In this case, the substances can act as antagonist or agonist producing different effects. The action occurs independently as Eq. 2:

$$E_{(Cmix)} = 1 - [(1 - E_{(C1)})((1 - E_{(C2)})] \tag{2}$$

where, $E_{(Cmix)}$ is the mixed total effect, while the $E_{(C1)}$ and $E_{(C2)}$ are the individual effects of the substances.

In this regard, carbamazepine and clofibrinic acid were evaluated by these models in mixtures concerning their ecotoxicological effects on *Daphnia magna* and algae (*Desmodesmus* and *Lemna*) (Cleuvers 2003). In the *Daphnia* tests, the compounds showed the concept of concentration addition because their effect, when together (95% immobilization), were highest than when tested alone (1% and 16% immobilization for clofibrinic acid and CBZ, respectively). However, algae testing revealed better adjustment to the concept of independent action in the mixture effect (Cleuvers 2003).

Apart from EC_{50} determinations for risk assessments and the prediction of combination effects of the evaluated compounds, several other endpoints can also be evaluated in the ecotoxicological studies. According to EC_{50} results, CBZ is toxic to cnidarians (EC_{50} 1–10 mg L^{-1}) and nontoxic to crustaceans and fish (EC_{50} > 100 mg L^{-1}) (Cleuvers 2003).

As pharmaceutical compounds continuously enter the environment, it is essential to carry out chronic tests to predict possible long-term effects. Life-history consequences on multigenerational studies can provide detailed information about drugs' effects on non-target organisms (Dietrich et al. 2010). For example, CBZ at low concentrations can act as a reproduction stimulant in *Daphnia pulex*, with high juvenile somatic growth, increase of the number of offspring per female and earlier maturation (Lürling et al. 2006). On the other hand, high CBZ concentrations have been shown to promote decreasing rates of population growth owing to mortality and delayed periods to bear the first offspring (Lürling et al. 2006, Lamichhane et al. 2013). The evaluation of sex ratios after CNZ exposure is considered one of the most important sub-lethal endpoints in this regard, even more so than fecundation rates, since almost all *Daphnia* broods exposed to CBZ were females, while males were only observed after the third generation (Lürling et al. 2006). In contrast, multigenerational studies have also reported tolerance of second generation Daphnids. The successive generation could develop drug resistance. Long-term exposure to sublethal concentrations can provide genetic resistance by transgenerational effects mechanism (Dietrich et al. 2010, Lamichhane et al. 2013).

Behavioral changes are another sub-lethal endpoint that can aid in understanding toxicological drug effects and provide data for toxicological impact analyses. For example, CBZ exposure was shown to alter the feeding behavior and swimming speed in Japanese medaka fish (*Oryzias latipes*) (Nassef et al. 2010b). The hypothesis is that CBZ alters the release of acetylcholine (ACh), which is modulated in the synaptic cleft by acetylcholinesterase (AChE) that promotes ACh hydrolysis into choline and acetate (Kwong 2002) *via* inhibition of Na^+ channel activity. Alterations in AChE and hormone levels can in fact lead to behavior changes, food consumption, reproduction activity, energy metabolism and, finally, declines in the numbers of several species (Xuereb et al. 2009). In another study, CBZ at 100 or 1000 µg L^{-1} inhibited AChE activity in the monogonont rotifer (*Brachionus koreanus*), as well as decreased AChE mRNA expression under concentration and time-dependent CBZ exposure (Rhee et al. 2013).

CBZ has also been implicated in altering the brain physiology of juvenile Atlantic salmon, through high up-regulation of somatolaction, prolactin and growth hormones (Hampel et al. 2014). The transcription up-regulation can be explained by the CBZ capacity to inhibit histone deacetylases (HDACs) by gene expression acetylation, responsible for suppressing transcription genes and maintaining pituitary hormones genes (Kouzarides 2007, Hobara et al. 2010).

The liver is the main detoxification mechanism for drug elimination. Enzymes belonging to the Cytochrome P450 family (CYP) play an important role in the biotransformation of xenobiotics/toxins in the organism, although CYP metabolism can release reactive oxygen species (ROS), which can be harmful to cells. CBZ can interact with CYP1A metabolism as verified by the inhibition of the EROD activity (EC_{50} 24 h = 318 µM), affecting xenobiotic metabolism (detoxification mechanisms) and improving CBZ toxicity action (Laville et al. 2004). Interaction and inhibition of CYP1A is established by covalent binding of reactive metabolic epoxide-CBZ, demonstrating that fish can metabolize CBZ (Laville et al. 2004). However, Li et al. (2011) did not find significant CYP1A activity after exposing rainbow trout to mg.L^{-1} of CBZ for 4 days, concluding that CBZ is not metabolized by this isoenzyme. However, CYP2C9 and CYP3A4 isoenzymes are the in-charge cytochromes for pharmaceuticals metabolism in humans. Thus, it has been reported that CBZ was able to increase CYP3A-related monooxygenase activity and promote lipid peroxidation (LPO) in trout hepatocytes cells (Gagné et al. 2006), in the annelid *Hediste diversicolor* (Pires et al. 2016) and in clams (Almeida et al. 2015).

In addition to effects on the hepatocyte metabolic system disorders, CBZ effects have also been studied regarding fish reproduction, since male fish gametes are directly exposed to pharmaceutical pollutants prior to fecundation, due to gametes release in the water. In one study, carp spermatozoa showed a dose-dependent decrease of spermatozoa motility and velocity after exposure to CBZ (Li et al. 2010). Carp spermatozoa LPO and antioxidant enzymes (Glutathione peroxidase (GPx), superoxide dismutase (SOD), and glutathione reductase (GR)) were also significantly affected by an increase of oxidative stress and inhibition of antioxidant system (Li et al. 2010). Particularly, male gametes are susceptible to stress, due to low polyunsaturated fatty acid and scavenging enzyme content. This promotes a loss of capacity to regulate intracellular Ca^{+2} and cyclic AMP that are responsible for spermatozoa motility in the water and fertilization ability (Li et al. 2010).

Aerobic respiration produces reactive oxygen species (ROS), which may potentially generate oxidative stress. Under homeostasis conditions, antioxidant defense systems can protect the organism from cellular damage (Matés et al. 1999). However, upon xenobiotic exposure, ROS production is increased, which can cause lipid peroxidation, DNA damage and protein carbonylation, leading to oxidative stress (Chen et al. 2017).

A positive LPO has been attributed to the presence of nucleophilic groups in the CBZ molecule. However, Vernouillet et al. (2010) observed opposite results in *Hydra attenuata*, exposed during 6 h with *T. platyurus* previously exposed to contaminated algae (*P. subcapitata*) to 150 mg.L^{-1} CBZ, with the induction of CYP3A and decreased LPO. In this case, low LPO levels due to CBZ exposure was attributed to the fact that CBZ may act as a radical scavenger, preventing fatty acid oxidation or inhibiting the production of cytosolic phospholipase A_2, which decreases the amount of available arachidonic acid to the metabolism.

The investigation of variations in the antioxidant enzymatic systems of aquatic organisms has been proven to be an interesting tool to predict tissue damage by pharmaceutical pollutants, especially in fish, that appears to possess receptors and enzymatic systems similar to mammals (Malarvizhi et al. 2012). In this context, fish exposed to CBZ have displayed increased antioxidant enzymes activities, such as SOD, CAT (catalase), GR (glutathione reductase) and GPx in the liver, muscle and intestine of rainbow trout specimens (*Oncorhynchus mykiss*) (Li et al. 2011), as well as GR and GST in pumpkinseed sunfish intestines (Brandão et al. 2013). SOD and CAT are the first line of antioxidant defense to prevent lipid peroxidation events (Matés et al. 1999). SOD aids in the production of O_2 and H_2O_2 from the superoxide radical (O_2^-), whereas CAT is responsible for catalyzing H_2O from H_2O_2 produced by SOD (Matés et al. 1999).

High antioxidant enzyme activity is attributed to adaptive responses to oxidative stress, with possible protective effects against LPO. However, some studies have observed down-regulated antioxidant enzymes in fish brain and gills after CBZ exposure (Li et al. 2011). LPO protection effects due to antioxidant defense enzymes seem to be decreased in gills and brain after CBZ exposure, since these organs display high LPO levels demonstrating particular susceptibility to CBZ (Li et al. 2011). The antioxidant defense system in the liver is well developed to metabolize and eliminate xenobiotics, whereas gills are directly exposed to CBZ without absorption or distribution throughout fish tissues, and low levels of antioxidant enzymes are found in the brain (Li et al. 2011). In the same way, gills have been shown to be significantly affected by CBZ in the freshwater bivalve *Corbicula fluminea*, where low levels of SOD and GR were observed, while malondialdehyde (MDA) was significantly up-regulated (Chen et al. 2014).

Antioxidant enzyme levels can also be influenced by CYP activity, LPO and CBZ bioaccumulation. On the one hand, CBZ exposure can promote high SOD activity with no LPO signs, indicating that CBZ is well-metabolized. On the other hand, high CBZ levels can promote both bioaccumulation and LPO, because this compound is able to inhibit SOD and CYP3A4 (Almeida et al. 2015, Freitas et al. 2016, Pires et al. 2016).

In addition to fish, several algae have displayed altered antioxidant enzyme activity after CBZ exposure. Green algae *Scenedesmus obliquus* and *Chlorella pyrenoidosa*, for example, showed increases in both SOD and CAT activity when exposed to CBZ (Zhang et al. 2012). A pro-oxidant CBZ effect was also found in the green algae *Dunaliella tertiolecta*, where high MDA levels and low chlorophyll alpha (Chl-α) content were observed (Tsiaka et al. 2013).

In vitro toxicity tests using isolated cell cultures are an excellent tool to reduce test organisms usage. They are also a low cost, reliable and quick way to obtain verifiable results to aid in the understanding of the mechanisms involved in molecular responses to toxicants (Gagnaire et al. 2004). For example, sub-lethal endpoints evaluated using Vero monkey cells demonstrated high sensitivity to CBZ (EC_{50} = 19 μM) and adequate predictions on the effects on a mammalian target, probably because CBZ was designed to act in humans (Jos et al. 2003). Neutral red assays, cell metabolic activity (MTT assay), intracellular lactate dehydrogenase (LDH) leakage and cell proliferation evaluated in the monkey cell model were inhibited by CBZ exposure, with the first two endpoints being most sensitive (EC_{50} ranging from 19 to 100 μM) (Jos et al. 2003). Alterations in mitochondrial function (MTT assay) and cell membrane integrity (Trypan blue exclusion test) in zebra mussel cells (haemocytes, gill and digestive gland) have also been reported (Parolini et al. 2011b). Gill cells are a main target for CBZ, expressively reducing mitochondrial activity and cell viability (Parolini et al. 2011b).

Another proposed assay to replace *in vivo* tests is the fish embryo toxicity (FET) test, also an alternative to acute fish tests, which has also been applied to evaluate CBZ exposure effects. The No Observed Effect Concentration (NOEC) FET test for CBZ (30.6 mg·L^{-1}–72 h) was similar to that observed for Zebrafish (*Danio rerio*) (25 mg·L^{-1}–10 d). Furthermore, rat embryos exposed to CBZ suffered pericardial edema and delayed heartbeat as the main sensitive endpoints in the FET test (van den Brandhof and Montforts 2010). In the same way, Japanese medaka fish embryos can also be an excellent model to predict toxic effects by the *ovo* nanoinjection technique, allowing for toxicity evaluation of chemicals during early development stages (Hano et al. 2005). In this regard, CBZ altered the survival of medaka embryos with an EC_{50} at 13.1 ng/egg. Hatching time and hemorrhaged embryos significantly increased under CBZ exposure. Hatching process delays can be explained by CBZ inhibition of the hatching enzyme chorionase, which is responsible for breaking the eggshell for larva emergence. The hemorrhage effect is probably due to the alterations of sodium-potassium and calcium pumps, which cause perturbations in the plasma membrane (Nassef et al. 2010a).

Mesocosm experiments also allow for the understanding of pollutant influences on the invertebrate community and ecosystem dynamics, and has been applied in CBZ investigations, specifically a mesocosm model with gastropods, zooplanktons, filamentous algae and phytoplankton, evaluated at environmentally CBZ relevant concentrations (Jarvis et al. 2014). Unexpectedly, invertebrate richness and overall diversity increased after 31 days but sediment organic matter decreased (the main source energy in aquatic systems). The perturbations of freshwater communities can lead to competition and alterations of ecosystems dynamics, including dissolved nutrient concentrations, primary production and decomposition (Jarvis et al. 2014), and further indicate deleterious CBZ effects.

Ibuprofen Ecotoxicology

Ibuprofen (IBP; (rac)-2-(4-isobutylphenyl)propionic acid) is a non-steroidal anti-inflammatory drug (NSAID) widely used as an analgesic and in the treatment of fever and rheumatic disorders (Hutt and Caldwell 1983). IBP has been designed to inhibit a metabolic pathway in the synthesis of bioactive fatty acids commonly known as eicosanoids (e.g., prostaglandins and leukotrienes), which, in mammals and invertebrates, function as auto/paracrine signalers involved in reproduction and ion transport (Hayashi et al. 2008). Therefore, it is expected that chronic exposure to IBP in the aquatic environment could affect the reproduction of aquatic animals (Paíga et al. 2013). In addition, prolonged exposure to pharmaceutical compounds at low concentrations may also promote behavior changes, such as alterations in feeding or predator avoidance behaviors.

An amphipod, *Gammarus pulex*, exposed to IBP at low concentrations (10 ng·L^{-1}) displayed 50% decreased activity compared to controls (De Lange et al. 2006). This can be explained by the IBP mode of action, which causes prostaglandin (PG) biosynthesis inhibition. PG promotes muscle contractions or atony in different tissues. Therefore, abnormal patterns of muscle contractions cause decreased feeding (Quinn et al. 2008), leading to less energy intake and causing adverse effects on growth and reproduction (De Lange et al. 2006). IBP also altered these endpoints in *D. magna*, with significantly affected reproduction in the form of reduced fecundity (Heckmann et al. 2007).

IBP also inhibits the cyclooxygenases (COX) responsible for converting the precursor arachidonic acid to eicosanoids, which act as autocrine or paracrine signalers (local action) in the regulation of invertebrate reproduction (interfering in vitellogenesis and ovulation) (Heckmann et al. 2007, Hayashi et al. 2008). However, after IBP exposure is terminated, reproductive functions might recover (Hayashi et al. 2008). Interestingly, the somatic growth of chronically IBP-exposed *D. magna* populations was shown to increase during IBP exposure. This can be explained by the "Principle of Allocation" since the blocked reproduction explained above would allow for energy to be invested in somatic growth (Heckmann et al. 2007).

Reproductive alterations have also been reported in several food chain levels, including in teleosts. For example, chronic IBP exposure in Japanese medaka fish significantly increased egg numbers per reproductive event while decreasing spawning rates. This is explained by the fact that the liver is responsible for vitellogenin (VTG) production; increased liver size (determined by the hepatosomatic index—HIS) increases VTG production, which, in turn, influences egg numbers, development and spawning per reproductive event (Flippin et al. 2007, Han et al. 2010).

Reproductive disorders can also be attributed to high levels of estradiol caused by IBP exposure. For example, IBP was shown to promote the increase of 17β-estradiol (E2) and CYP19A (aromatase) activity in H295R cells while testosterone (T) levels decreased (Han et al. 2010). High aromatase activity stimulates the conversion of T to E2, leading to alterations in T and E2 concentrations in the organisms (Han et al. 2010). Another endocrine disrupt endpoint is alkali-labile phosphate (ALP), which indirectly assesses vitellogenin-like proteins. This endpoint was found to be altered in both female and male mussels exposed to IBP, which displayed significantly enhanced of ALP levels, particularly males (Gonzalez-Rey and Bebianno 2012). Using the same approach, IBP was shown to negatively interfere in several endpoints in zebrafish, such as embryonic development, hatching delays (inhibition of the chorionase enzyme), organogenesis (pericardial edema, lower heart rate, and malformations), larval growth and survival (David and Pancharatna 2009).

Cytogenotoxicity has also been related to IBP exposure, inducing apoptosis in bivalve zebra mussel hemocytes (Parolini et al. 2009) and zebrafish erythrocytes (Rocco et al. 2010). Destabilization of the lysosomal membrane stimulates oxidative stress, with consequent DNA fragmentation and cell death (Parolini et al. 2009). Although it has been postulated that IBP concentrations may cause DNA damage, leading to apoptosis, negative correlations between lysosomal membrane stability and genotoxicity endpoints have been observed after exposure to low IBP concentrations This contributes to the hypothesis that low IBP concentrations can promote DNA damage by the creation of adducts without significant ROS formation, while high IBP concentrations cause oxidative stress, DNA alterations and cell death (Parolini et al. 2009).

IBP metabolites derived from acyl glucuronides display electrophilic properties and can form covalent bonds with nucleophilic amino acid groups, present in intra- and extracellular proteins (Gómez-Oliván et al. 2014). In addition, IBP exposure can also modify the enzymes responsible for the antioxidant system, an important barrier in protecting organisms against damage caused by LPO. CAT, SOD, GR and GPx have been shown to increase in a time-dose dependent manner, returning to base levels at the end of IBP exposure at several aquatic species (Parolini et al. 2009, Gonzalez-Rey and Bebianno 2012, Aguirre-Martínez et al. 2015). The same was observed for LPO in the digestive gland in an aquatic bivalve mollusk species *Corbicula fluminea* and *Mytilus galloprovincialis* (Gonzalez-Rey and Bebianno 2012, Aguirre-Martínez et al. 2015). However, gill tissue showed more pronounced alterations than the digestive gland, presenting delayed antioxidant system responses, with the down-regulation of CAT gene expression (Gonzalez-Rey et al. 2014) after IBP exposure.

IBP exposure also acts on enzymes responsible for xenobiotic detoxification (phase I and II enzymes). Phase I enzyme activities are enhanced after IBP contact. More specifically, the biosynthesis of isoforms CYP1A and CYP3A is induced (Thibaut and Porte 2008, Aguirre-Martínez et al. 2015). GST activity also displayed a marked enhancement after IBP exposure, indicating a probable detoxification mechanism *via* conjugation phase II reactions (Parolini et al. 2011a, Aguirre-Martínez et al. 2015). Increased levels of GR activity can indicate the need for reduced glutathione (GSH) from oxidized glutathione (GSSG) to act as a substrate. GSH is one of the major lines of antioxidant defense capable of acting at the same time as a direct ROS scavenger (nonenzymatically) or as an antioxidant enzyme cofactor (for GPx and GST) (Gómez-Oliván et al. 2014). High LPO levels and GR activity are a strong indicator that the antioxidant system is not able to neutralize the presence of pro-oxidant agents (Gonzalez-Rey and Bebianno 2012). Chronic IBP exposure can also lead to adaptation conditions of the organisms or homeostasis imbalance, which promotes oxidative stress leading to lipid membrane, protein and nucleic acids (DNA and RNA) injuries.

Toxicogenomic studies are an excellent tool to understand how pollutants can affect the genomic level, while transcriptomic techniques aid in the investigation of xenobiotic interactions and mechanisms under gene expression view. In this context, alterations in gene expression due to IBP exposure have been extensively studied in Daphnids. IBP-exposed *Daphnia magna*, for example, revealed up-regulation of the leukotriene B4 12-hydroxydehydrogenase (*Ltb4dh*) gene, which promotes the metabolism of leukotriene B4, responsible for arachidonic acid biosynthesis (Heckmann et al. 2006).

The expression of genes traditionally involved with pollutant metabolism is also affected by IBP. For example, *CYP4* gene expression in *Daphnia magna* decreased after IBP exposure, demonstrating changes in the biotransformation and excretion rate of toxicants (Heckmann et al. 2006, Bang et al. 2015). *CYP360A* (homologue to the mammalian *CYP3A*) and *GST* gene expressions were also inhibited after exposure to low IPB concentrations, whereas at high concentrations and prolonged exposure, they demonstrated significant stimulation (Wang et al. 2016).

Metabolomic approaches can also aid in understanding other factors able to impair *D. magna* development caused by IBP. For example, IBP exposure at low concentrations induced a significant decrease in certain essential amino acids, such as leucine, arginine and lysine in crustaceans, which may also affect growth and osmoregulation (Kovacevic et al. 2016).

Triclosan Ecotoxicity

Triclosan (CAS 3380-34-5; 5-chloro-2-(2,4-dichlorophenoxy)phenol; Irgasan®; TCS) is a chlorinated phenoxyphenol used as an antiseptic agent in a vast array of personal care (e.g., toothpaste, acne cream, deodorant, shampoo, toilet soap) and consumer products (children's toys, footwear, kitchen cutting boards). TCS was first detected in the environment in the early 2000s, in Spain (Agüera et al. 2003), Canada (Metcalfe et al. 2003), EUA (McAvoy et al. 2002) and Japan (Harada et al. 2008). TCS is absorbed from the gastrointestinal tract and across the skin (Black et al. 1975, Black and Howes 1975, Siddiqui and Buttar 1979, Moss et al. 2000, Dayan 2007).

Adolfsson-Erici et al. (2002) published the first results pointing to the presence of TCS in human breast milk. Subsequently, Dayan (2007) detected TCS in more than 80% of analyzed human breast milk, with a daily baby intake of 74 $\mu g \cdot kg^{-1} \cdot d^{-1}$, according to the author's calculations. Although some studies indicate non-toxic effects of TCS (Russell and Montgomery 1980, Rodrigues et al. 2007), in the last 10 years, a massive amount of studies have been undertaken to prove the existence of toxicity effects, as detailed below.

Harada et al. (2008) observed that TCS can affect different aquatic web levels including algae (*Pseudokirchneriella subcapitata*, $EC50_{96h}$ = 0.012 mg·L^{-1}), protozoa (*Tetrahymena pyriformis*, $EC50_{96h}$ = 0.21 mg·L^{-1}), crustaceans (*D. magna*, $EC50_{48h}$ = 0.26 mg·L^{-1}), bacteria (*Vibro fischeri*, $EC50_{15min}$ = 0.52 mg·L^{-1}) and amphibians (*Xenopus laevis*, $LC50_{96h}$ = 0.82 mg·L^{-1}).

Yang et al. (2008) observed the inhibition of the microalgae *P. subcapitata* growth in the presence of TCS ($IC50_{72h}$ = 0.53 µg·L^{-1}), and Delorenzo and Fleming (2007), while evaluating several PPCPs regarding toxicity to the marine algae *Dunaliella tertiolecta*, observed that TCS was the only compound that yielded toxicity at usual environmental concentrations ($EC50_{96h}$ = 3.55 µg·L^{-1}). According to Yang et al. (2008), TCS also affected the photosynthesis ($EC50_{24h}$ = 3.7 µg L^{-1}) and the reproduction system ($EC50_{24h}$ = 1.9 µg L^{-1}) of the chlorophyte *Scenedesmus vacuolatus*, while the diatom *Nitzschia palea* was affected by TCS both in suspension ($EC50_{24h}$ = 390 µg·L^{-1}) and in biofilm form ($EC50_{24h}$ = 430 µg·L^{-1}). Periphyton communities, on the other hand, were more resistant to TCS ($EC50_{24h}$ = 900 µg·L^{-1}).

Regarding benthic invertebrates, which are essential to the aquatic chain and can transfer anthropogenic contaminants from sediments and are, thus, important ecotoxicological indicators, Dussault et al. (2008) evaluated the LC and EC during 10 days concerning several PPCPs, and observed that TCS was the most toxic for *Chironomus tentans* ($LC50_{10d}$ = 0.4 mg·L^{-1}; $LC50_{10d}$ = 0.28 mg·L^{-1}) and *Hyalella azteca* ($LC50_{10d}$ = 0.2 mg·L^{-1}; $LC50_{10d}$ = 0.25 mg·L^{-1}).

TCS levels higher than 500 nM were also shown to be acutely toxic during embryo development of sea urchin *Psammechinus miliaris*. Observed abnormalities were related to the development of the arms and a slight edema around the larval body, which appears to result from abnormal skeletogenesis of skeletal rods (Anselmo et al. 2011).

Morisseau et al. (2009) observed that TCS also inhibits carboxylesterases (CES1 and CES2), widely distributed enzymes throughout the body that catalyze the hydrolysis of esters, amides, thioesters, and carbamates (Laizure et al. 2013). Lin et al. (2010) suggested that the earthworm *Eisenia andrei* has the capacity to tolerate the oxidative stress and activate the antioxidant system at the first stage of stress at all doses of TCS (0–300 mg·kg^{-1}). CAT activity increased after 2-d (days) TCS exposure and subsequently returned to controlled levels in the control. A significant interaction between TCS dose and duration of exposure was observed regarding CAT and GST activity.

Acute tests demonstrated that the crustacean *Thamnocephalus platyurus* ($LC50_{24h}$ = 0.47 mg·L^{-1}) is more sensitive than Japanese medaka fish ($LC50_{96h}$ = 0.60 mg·L^{-1}) (Kim et al. 2009). However, Nassef et al. (2010b) observed that low TCS concentrations have significant effects on the swimming and feeding behaviors of Japanese medaka fish, suggesting that behavior is a more sensitive indicator of toxicity than mortality. In another study on Japanese medaka fish, embryonic development delays were observed in the presence of TCS, and evolved a spinal curvature in the newly-hatched larvae, with significantly increased hemorrhage, yolksac and heart beat rate (Nassef et al. 2010b).

TCS also showed deleterious effects, such as embryotoxicity, hatching delay and biomarker levels alterations, in both adults and early stage zebrafish. Acute toxicity was detected both in adults (LC50$_{96h}$ = 0.34 mg·L^{-1}) and embryos (LC50$_{96h}$ = 0.42 mg·L^{-1}). Embryotoxicity was revealed by delays in otolith formation, eye and body pigmentation, spine malformations, pericardial oedema and undersize. Cholinesterase (ChE), lactate dehydrogenase (LDH) and glutathione S-transferase (GSH) levels increased in the early stages (Oliveira et al. 2009). TCS exposure was also related to cardiac problems in zebrafish at environmentally relevant concentrations, where individuals presented pericardial edema and alterations in heart structure (Saley et al. 2016).

TCS exposure induced morphological malformations in *Bufo gargarizans* (an endemic frog species in China) embryos, including hyperplasia, abdominal edema, and axial flexures. This resulted not only in delayed growth and development but also caused teratogenic effects (Chai et al. 2016).

Wheat seedlings (*Triticum aestivum* L.) exposed for 21 days to TCS were damaged by the accumulation of chlorophyll (CHL), the synthesis of soluble protein (SP), and the activity of peroxidase (POD) and SOD (An et al. 2009).

In mammals, Welk et al. (2007) observed that mouthwash containing TCS can cause tissue damage on explants of neonatal rat peritoneum. In addition, TCS doses significantly decreased the live birth index and 6-d survival index of Wistar Rat (Rodríguez and Sanchez 2010). Intrauterine exposure of the Wistar Rat fetus produced a marked decrease in the sex ratio (male:female), with the number of male offspring significantly lower than number of females. Developmental effects of TCS at high concentrations may be associated with disruption of thyroid hormones homeostasis (Chai et al. 2016). However, Zorrilla et al. (2009) did not observe TCS effects on puberty or the development of the male reproductive tract of Wistar rats. TCS also induced hypothyroxinemia and hepatic enzyme induction in rat models (Crofton et al. 2007, Zorrilla et al. 2009, Paul et al. 2010) (Long-Evans and Wistar). According to Paul et al. (2010), TCS upregulates mRNA expression and activity of some phase I and phase II hepatic enzymes in rats who received TCS by gavage. T4 and T3 decreased, while TSH showed no alterations. TCS might initiate hypothyroxinemia with the activation of hepatic constitutive active/androstane receptor (CAR) and pregnane X (PXR) receptor.

Cytochrome P450 enzymes (CYP1A and CYP3A) and GST responses to TCS exposure in yellow catfish (*Pelteobagrus fulvidraco*) were evaluated (Ku et al. 2014). Results indicated that TCS significantly elevated CYP1A and GST but decreased CYP3A expression, EROD (ethoxyresorufin-*O*-deethylase) activity and MDA (malondialdehyde) content. TCS may be used as a substrate for phase II enzymes in different organisms, like earthworm *Eisenia andrei* (Lin et al. 2010), male Wistar rats (Moss et al. 2000) and marine bivalve *Mytilus galloprovincialis* (Canesi et al. 2007).

Another concern regarding TCS is its degradation products. Since TCS is structurally similar to other polychlorinated phenoxyphenols, it can cyclize into toxic polychlorodiben-zo-p-dioxins, and 2,4-dichlorophenol, 2,8-dichlorodibenzop-dioxin (Singer et al. 2002), and methyl triclosan (Farré et al. 2008) can be formed during TCS degradation. Farré et al. (2008) assessed TCS ($EC50_{30min}$ = 0.28 µg·mL^{-1}) and methyl triclosan ($EC50_{30min}$ = 0.21 µg·mL^{-1}) toxicity in domestic wastewater using *V. fischeri*.

Regarding TCS genotoxicity, studies have evaluated several organisms, such as *E. andrei*, through a comet assay (Lin et al. 2010), with significant changes in the length and diameter of the comet head (LDR) detected with increasing TCS doses. This was associated with necrotic or apoptotic DNA fragmentation. Increased genotoxicity with increasing doses of TCS on *E. andrei* was also observed by Lin et al. (2014), in which TCS was also related with heat shock protein (HSP70) up-regulation. The same was observed in hemocytes of the freshwater bivalve zebra mussel (*Dreissena polymorpha*) during *in vivo* tests (Binelli et al. 2010). Lin et al. (2012) attributed the DNA damage on *E. andrei* to ROS production, specifically O_2^-, which can act as a univalent oxidant or a reductant and can cause deleterious effects on macromolecules such as DNA, RNA, and proteins.

Genomic analyses have demonstrated that zebrafish embryos (24-h post-fertilization) exposed to TCS were at the early stage of somitogenesis, and three genes (*Oct4*, *Sox2* and *Nanog*) were shown to be up-regulated in treated groups when compared with the controls (Chen et al. 2015).

Proteomic analyses can also be useful to evaluate PCPPs toxicity. In one study, Riva et al. (2012) used proteomic analyses to track TCS toxicity in zebra mussel, and observed that TCS exposure increased the expression of both tubulin subunits, α and β which are involved in the cytoskeletal structure and the mechanism of Ca^{2+}-binding. It seems that TCS interferes with intracellular Ca^{2+} homeostasis (Ahn et al. 2008, Tamura et al. 2011). Riva et al. (2012) also found an overexpression of myosin light chain, a protein related to cytoskeletal motility. Alterations in the expression of any of the cytoskeletal proteins can cause several adverse effects to the cells (Nawaz et al. 2005).

Significant cytotoxicity is also linked to TCS. For example, TCS exposure to non-induced human mesenchymal stem cells (hMSCs) inhibited adipocyte differentiation of hMSCs in a concentration-dependent manner (Guo et al. 2012). Inhibitory effects were confirmed by a decrease in gene expression of specific adipocyte differentiation biomarkers, including adipocyte protein 2, lipoprotein lipase, and adiponectin. An important observation made by the authors of that study is that TCS inhibits adipocyte differentiation of hMSCs under concentrations that are not cytotoxic and in the range usually observed in human blood.

TCS has been shown to cause effects on the mitochondria of zebrafish embryos, including oxygen consumption rate increase, inhibition of ATP-linked respiration and spare respiratory capacity, inhibiting mitochondrial ATP production (Shim et al. 2016, Raftery et al. 2017).

Long-term TCS exposure is also postulated to increase the multiplicity, size, and incidence of liver tumors (hepatocellular carcinoma, HCC) in mice (Male C57BL/6) (Yueh et al. 2014). TCS-mediated liver regeneration and fibrosis preceded HCC development and may constitute the primary tumor-promoting mechanism through which TCS acts. TCS exposure was also related to lipid accumulation in liver of zebrafish larvae (Ho et al. 2016).

Erythromycin Ecotoxicology

Erythromycin (CAS 114-07-8; Erythromycinum; ERY) is a macrolide antibiotic which acts against gram-positive cocci by binding irreversibly to the 50S subunit of bacterial ribosomes interfering with bacterial protein synthesis (González-Pleiter et al. 2013). It is used to treat certain bacterial infections such as respiratory tract, including bronchitis, pneumonia, Legionnaires' disease, and pertussis, diphtheria, sexually transmitted diseases (STD), including syphilis, ear, intestine, gynecological, urinary tract, and skin infections, and is also used in recurrent rheumatic fever prevention (ASHP 2017).

ERY was recently detected in surface waters in Germany (Burke et al. 2016), USA (Fairbairn et al. 2016), Greece (Nannou et al. 2015), China (Dong et al. 2016a, Yao et al. 2017), Italy (Calamari et al. 2003), and in coastal marine waters in the southern sea of Korea (Kim et al. 2017), in WWTP in China (Dong et al. 2016b) and Canada (Xiu-Sheng Miao et al. 2004), as well as in surface sediments in Brazil (Beretta et al. 2014).

ERY has toxic effects at environmentally relevant levels for the luminescent terrestrial bacterium *Photorhabdus luminescens* (EC_{50} = 0.022 mg·L^{-1}) and for the algae *P. subcapitata* (EC_{50} = 0.35 mg·L^{-1}) (González et al. 2016). No effects were observed in zebrafish (*Danio rerio*) or in the bacteria *Vibrio fischeri*, but positive effects were found for the crustaceans *Thamnocephalus platyurus* ($LC50_{24h}$ = 17.68 mg·L^{-1}), *Ceriodaphnia dubia* ($EC50_{48h}$ = 10.23 mg·L^{-1}) and *D. magna* ($EC50_{24h}$ = 22.45 mg·L^{-1}), as well as for the rotifer *Brachionus calyciflorus* ($LC50_{24h}$ = 27.53 mg·L^{-1}). Chronic tests showed a higher toxicity for *P. subcapitata* ($EC50_{24h}$ = 0.020 mg·L^{-1}), *C. dubia* ($EC50_{48h}$ = 0.94 mg·L^{-1}) and *B. calyciflorus* ($LC50_{24h}$ = 0.22 mg·L^{-1}). The AMES test that asses the mutagenic potential, was negative for ERY (Isidori et al. 2005).

According to Nie et al. (2013), ERY caused reductions in ascorbate (AsA) and GSH biosynthesis, ascorbate–glutathione cycle, xanthophylls cycle and antioxidant enzyme activities on algae *P. subcapitata*.

In plants, many photosynthesis-related processes, primary photochemistry, electron transport, photophosphorylation and carbon assimilation in *Selenastrum capricornutum* have been shown to be inhibited by low ERY concentrations (0.06 mg·L^{-1}) (Liu et al. 2011). ERY has also been demonstrated to cause phytotoxicity (root elongation deviation) in lettuce and carrots crops (Pan and Chu 2016).

Growth of *Microcystis flos-aquae* was significantly inhibited at high levels of ERY, which in high concentration also increase the SOD and CAT activities. However, the increased levels of these antioxidant enzymes were not enough to degrade the excess of ROS, causing an increase on de MDA levels and lipid peroxidation (Wan et al. 2015).

Concentration-dependent bradycardia in *in vitro* (Sprague-Dawley) embryonic rat heart function was observed in individuals exposed to ERY (Nilsson and Webster 2014). It was suggested that cardiotic effects caused by ERY started on the heart mitochondria, since it induced ROS formation, mitochondrial membrane permeabilization and mitochondrial swelling, and finally cytochrome *c* release in cardiomyocyte mitochondria (Salimi et al. 2016).

Genotoxicity tests indicated DNA damage (chicken DT40 cells) after ERY exposure, which could be eliminated by nucleotide excision repair (Liu et al. 2012). Blue mussels (*Mytilus edulis*) hemocytes exposed to ERY had a severe decrease in phagocytosis, and a substantial DNA damage when in high concentration (Lacaze et al. 2015).

17α-Ethinylestradiol Ecotoxicology

Natural and synthetic hormones are considered the most potent estrogenic compounds available, and may adversely affect several animal species even at low concentrations (ng L^{-1} range). The occurrence of natural hormones, 17β-estradiol (E2), estrone (E1) e estriol (E3) and the synthetic hormone, 17α-ethinylestradiol (EE2), in the aquatic environment, including raw and treated sewage, surface water, groundwater and drinking water, has been extensively reported in the literature (Routledge et al. 1998a, Janex-Habibi et al. 2009, Luo et al. 2014).

EE2, like other steroidal hormones, has a chemical structure comprising 17 carbon atoms, consisting of a phenolic, two cyclohexane and one cyclopentane ring. Estrogens differ by the group in the C17 position of the cyclopentane ring. EE2 presents an ethynyl group on C17. Steroidal hormones are characterized by their phenolic A ring, which has the hydroxyl group at C3, conferring estrogenic activity (Birkett and Lester 2003).

Estrogenic substances can be identified by their ability to bind to the estrogen receptor (ER) and to induce or attenuate a response. Several assays have been used to assess the estrogenic activity of suspected estrogenic substances or complex mixtures in environmental samples (surface water, sediments raw and treated sewage) (Beck et al. 2006, Bergamasco et al. 2011, Dias et al. 2015, Li et al. 2015, Conley et al. 2017). *In vitro* assays use a variety of endpoints, such as estrogen receptor transcription and cell proliferation assays, and include determination of effects on organ weights, cell differentiation, protein expression, and enzyme activities (Zacharewski 1997). Experimental studies confirm that EE2 is capable of elucidating the deleterious effects observed in wild animals at concentration that have been measured in surface water. The irreversible effects observed in animals by the environmentally relevant EE2 concentrations demonstrate the ecological impact of aquatic contamination by estrogens.

Based on a review of human excretion carried out in the literature (Johnson and Williams 2004), developed a model to estimate the excretion of EE2 in domestic sewage. In this model, about 43% of the total ingested EE2 is metabolized within the body and 57% is excreted in feces and urine. The authors considered an average intake of 26 µg d^{-1} EE2 in the contraceptive pills by the female population for the study region. The total of EE2 excreted by the considered ingesting was estimated to be 10.5 µg d^{-1} (range 9.6–11.3 µg d^{-1}) in raw sewage.

Most of the estrogens excreted by the human population are in the form of biologically inactive conjugates (sulfates and glucuronides). However, free estrogen is also present in the daily excretion due to transformations by the natural intestinal flora prior to excretion. Furthermore, these conjugated compounds must be deconjugated during the sewage treatment process, yielding the free steroids into the effluent. Studies show that deconjugation occurs during the biological process in WWTP (Routledge et al. 1998a, Ternes et al. 1999, Johnson and Sumpter 2001, Johnson and Williams 2004).

Raw and treated sewage are one of the main sources of xenoestrogens in the aquatic environment. Due to incomplete removal on WWTP, estrogens are continuously released into the aquatic environment (Desbrow et al. 1998, Ternes et al. 1999). Both natural and synthetic estrogens are mainly responsible for the estrogenic activity observed in WWTP effluents (Jobling et al. 1998, Routledge et al. 1998b, Solé et al. 2003).

Several studies have reported the occurrence of EE2 in domestic sewage, WWTP effluent and surface water worldwide. EE2 concentrations in raw sewage ranged from 0.5 to 150 ng L^{-1} in Canada, China, Spain, France, and the USA (Drewes et al. 2003, Janex-Habibi et al. 2009, Atkinson et al. 2012, Martín et al. 2012, Ye et al. 2012), in WWTP effluents ranged from 0.1 to 120 ng L^{-1} in Canada, China, Spain, France, and the USA (Drewes et al. 2003, Janex-Habibi et al. 2009, Atkinson et al. 2012, Martín et al. 2012, Ye et al. 2012) and in surface water ranged from < 0.5 to 30 ng L^{-1} in China, South Korea, Indonesia, Malaysia and Thailand (Kim et al. 2009, Duong et al. 2010, Liu et al. 2015). However, in other countries, such as Brazil, significantly higher concentrations were detected, reaching values of 3,000 ng L^{-1} in raw sewage (Pessoa et al. 2014) and 1,000 ng L^{-1} in WWTP effluents (Pessoa et al. 2014).

The hypothesis that chemicals present in the environment can cause endocrine disruption in animals was first evidenced in the early 1900s. Allen and Doisy (1923) and (Doodds et al. 1938) investigated the effects on the endocrine system of laboratory animals by estrogenic substances. Allen and Doisy (1923) developed a mouse and rat assay to determine the estrogenic activity of chemicals by assessing uterine weight change, vaginal cornification and female sexual receptivity after exposure to the substances tested (industrial by-products). This is one of the first assays developed to detect estrogenic activity. Important events have been related to the effects of human exposure to EDC. Between the 1940s and 1970s, the potent synthetic estrogen diethylstilbestrol (DES) was prescribed by medical experts to block spontaneous abortions. However, children born to mothers who used DES went through puberty developed dysfunction in the reproductive system, reduced fertility and cancer in the reproductive system (Colborn et al. 1993, Birkett and Lester 2003).

The estrogenic response of steroid estrogens was determined by several *in vitro* and *in vivo* assays and their potency demonstrated to be over a thousand times greater than any xenoestrogen (organochlorine pesticides, phthalates, alkyphenols) (Routledge et al. 1998b, Legler et al. 2002). Studies indicate that EE2 and E2 are more potent than E1 and E3. However, EE2 was 2 to 30 times more potent than E2 (Folmar et al. 2002, Thorpe et al. 2003, 2006, Van Den Belt et al. 2004, Brian et al. 2005). Studies comparing the results of *in vitro* (Yeast Estrogen Screen—YES and Michigan Cancer Foundation-7—MCF-7) and *in vivo* (vitellogenin induction) assays and estrogenic response of EE2 have been normalized to E2. The estrogenic potencies vary depending on the type of bioassay used and the endpoint measurements.

Van Den Belt et al. (2004) observed a difference between relative estrogenic potency (EC_{50}-E2/EC_{50}-EE2) in *in vitro* and *in vivo* assays. EE2 is more potent in *in vivo* than *in vitro* assays. EC_{50} values for VTG induction and YES assay of 0.021 ± 0.0007 nmol L^{-1} and 0.174 ± 0.040 nmol L^{-1}, respectively, were found for EE2. *In vitro* assays may not perfectly reflect the *in vivo* response of aquatic species to the same substance (Zacharewski 1997, Van Den Belt et al. 2004).

Studies have reported that the incidence of widespread intersex and induction of vitellogenin synthesis in male fish are correlated to the discharge of WWTP effluent into surface waters (Desbrow et al. 1998, Routledge et al. 1998a). For example, Rodgers-Gray et al. (2001) observed an increase in plasma VTG levels in fish (*Rutilus rutilus*) when exposed to effluents in the UK, in which estrogens E2, E1 and EE2 were present at concentrations of 4, 50 and 1.7–3.4 ng L^{-1}, respectively. Studies show that the deleterious effects of estrogens were observed at very low concentrations (the order of ng L^{-1}).

The exposure to estrogenic substances associated with WWTP effluent discharges has been shown to cause intersex in wild populations of the fish of river when exposure occurs during the critical period of sexual differentiation. Studies on different fish species, such as *Cyprinus carpio* (Gimeno et al. 1998) and *Rutilus rutilus* (Jobling et al. 1998), observed the appearance of the female characteristics and the disappearance of male characteristics in the gonadal tissue, as well as induction in VTG production.

Steroid estrogens have been appointed as the main responsible for the endocrine disruption observed in wild animals. Several studies have reported the ability of EE2 to affect the endocrine system of exposed wild animals by incidence of intersexuality (fish with gonads containing male and female tissue, and/or feminized reproductive ducts), change in mating behavior, delay in sexual maturity, delay in sexual development, decreased egg fertilization and change in sexual reproductive behavior even at low concentrations. Exposure during development affects fertility and both reproductive and non-reproductive behavior in mammals and fish. Table 1 presents a compilation of literature studies that describe the effects caused by EE2 on different animal species.

Steroid estrogens have been pointed out as the main responsible for the induction of vitellogenin production observed in several fish species (Schmid et al. 2002, Soares et al. 2009, Söffker et al. 2012). EE2 has been shown to induce VTG production in male fish at 0.1 to 0.5 ng L^{-1} (Purdom et al. 1994). Studies suggest that environmentally relevant concentrations of EE2 in surface water have been shown to induce a large set of deleterious effects in fish species.

According to Schmid et al. (2002), high levels of VTG in plasma can cause fish mortality. In their study, *Pimephales promelas* fish were exposed to 50 ng L^{-1} of 17α-ethinylestradiol for 35 days, followed by the same depuration period. The authors observed 100% mortality between days 20 and 36 of the exposure phase when increased VTG levels in the plasma were observed.

Zebrafish embryos were exposed to 1.2 and 1.6 ng L^{-1} EE2 from day 1 to day 80 post-fertilization (Volkova et al. 2015). Low doses of EE2 resulted in persistent changes in the behavior and fertility of zebrafish. Furthermore, even after remediation in clean water for 82 days until adulthood, the effects on non-reproductive behavior and fertility persisted.

Table 1. Adverse effects of EE2 in different organisms.

Species	Life stage	Observed effects	EE2 concentration/ Exposure period	Reference
Pimephales promelas	Adult males	Vitellogenin gene (vtg) induction and fish mortality	50 ng L^{-1} for 35 days	Schmid et al. 2002
Danio rerio	Embryonic development	Changes in non-reproductive behavior and fertility	1.2 and 1.6 ng.L^{-1} for 82 days	Volkova et al. 2015
Danio rerio	Embryonic development and adult males	Developmental abnormalities of eggs and embryos, increased embryo mortality, Induction of the vtg gene in male fish	0.5, 1 and 2 ng L^{-1} (measured concentrations of 0.19, 0.24 and 1 ng L^{-1}, respectively)	Soares et al. 2009
Danio rerio	Adult males	vitellogenin gene (vtg) induction	0.4 and 2.2 ng L^{-1} 14 days	Söffker et al. 2012
Danio rerio	Adult males	Impact on reproduction and sexual behavior in male fish	0,5 and 25 ng L^{-1} for 14 days	Reyhanian et al. 2011
Mangrove rivulus, Kryptolebias marmoratus	Embryonic Development and adult	Impacts growth, reproduction and steroid hormone levels	0.4 and 120 ng L^{-1} for 28 days post-hatching	Voisin et al. 2016
Protosalanx hyalocranius	Embryonic Development	Increased embryo mortality, teratogenesis, and hatching retardation	Range 0.05 and 1 mg L^{-1} for up to 27 days	Hu et al. 2017
Xenopus tropicalis	Adult amphibians after larval exposure	Reproductive organ development, fertility, and sexual behavior	1.8, 18, 181 ng L^{-1}	Gyllenhammar et al. 2009

Figure 2 displays the potential adverse effects in fish associated with environmentally relevant concentrations of EE2 in surface waters.

Studies have shown that environmentally relevant concentrations of EE2 are not lethal to *Protosalanx hyalocranius* embryos, although they cause impacts on embryo development (increased embryo mortality, teratogenesis, and hatching retardation) (Hu et al. 2017). In amphibians, larval exposure to environmentally relevant concentrations of EE2 (1.8 ng L^{-1}) induced male to female sex-reversal of male *Xenopus tropicalis* frogs, leading to reduced fertility in the adult frogs (Gyllenhammar et al. 2009).

In January 2012, the European Commission proposed limits on the annual average concentrations of EE2 in surface water to 0.035 ng L^{-1} (Gilbert 2012, Owen and Jobling 2012). However, Members of the European Parliament's environment committee, or MEPs, reject restricting pharmaceuticals in water ("MEPs reject

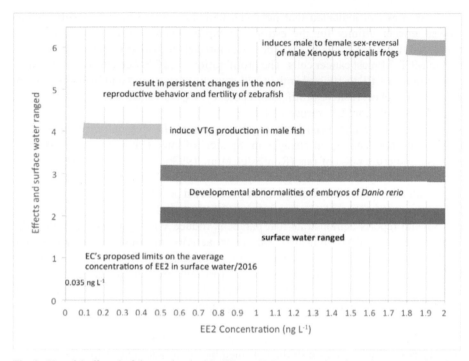

Fig. 2. Harmful effects in fish associated with different EE2 concentrations in surface waters. (Purdom et al. 1994, Gyllenhammar et al. 2009, Kim et al. 2009, Soares et al. 2009, Duong et al. 2010, Owen and Jobling 2012, Gilbert 2012, Liu et al. 2015, Volkova et al. 2015).

restricting pharmaceuticals in water—POLITICO," n.d.). Due to pressure from the pharmaceutical industry, EE2 was added to the water priority substances list, as well as diclofenac and estradiol (Directive 2011), but were not given concentration limits in surface waters. In addition, the high costs required for the modernization of WTP aiming an increase in removal efficiency of these pharmaceuticals were also considered. These three pharmaceuticals were the first to be included in the water priority substances list (Directive 2011).

Paraben Ecotoxicology

Parabens are alkyl esters of para-hydrobenzoic acid, differing only in the ester group, which may be a methyl, an ethyl, a propyl, a butyl, an isobutyl, an isopropyl or a benzyl group. Parabens are compounds used as antimicrobial preservatives in cosmetics, food, drinks pharmaceuticals and PPCPs (Soni et al. 2005).

According to Routledge et al. (1998b), methyl and propyl parabens are 10^{-4} and 10^{-7} less potent than 17β-estradiol *in vitro* YES assay, respectively. In addition, their estrogenicity increases with the increase of the ester group chain. *In vitro* studies show that parabens are weakly estrogenic. However, they result in additive effects when in mixtures with other estrogenic substances (Routledge et al. 1998b, Miller et al. 2001, Rajapakse et al. 2002, Canosa et al. 2006, Kjærstad et al. 2010).

In vivo assays indicated that parabens with longer and branched side chains showed greater affinity for the estrogen receptor. Okubo et al. (2001) reported estrogenic activity of ethyl-, propyl-, butyl-, isopropyl- and isobutyl-benzyl paraben in human MCF-7 breast cancer cells. The proliferation of MCF-7 cells was induced at a concentration of 10^5 to 10^7 higher than 17β-estradiol. Isopropyl- and isobutylparaben showed the highest relative proliferation potency, EC 50 values were 5.7×10^{-7} mol L^{-1} and 6.8×10^{-7} mol L^{-1}, respectively.

Parabens have also been shown to be estrogenic *in vivo* uterotrophic assays. Studies indicate histological changes in the uteri of mice (Lemini et al. 2004) and increase in uterine mass of rats (Routledge et al. 1998b, Darbre et al. 2002). In the study of Routledge et al. (1998b), methyl- and butylparaben were analyzed in a rat uterotrophic assay, but only butylparaben produced a positive uterotrophic response. Contudo was 100,000 times less potent than 17β-estradiol.

Several reports demonstrate that parabens induce VTG synthesis in male fish. Pedersen et al. (2000) indicated estrogenic activity of *p*-hydroxybenzoate and ethyl-, n-propyl- and n-butylparaben (the range of concentration at 100 and 300mg. kg^{-1}), which promoted vitellogenin induction in rainbow trout assay. According to Bjerregaard et al. (2003), propylparaben induced an increase in VTG synthesis in a rainbow trout *Oncorhynchus mykiss* after oral exposure of 22 mg kg^{-1} 2 d^{-1} *via* food and water.

Parabens also act as antimicrobials for mechanisms of action by inhibiting the transport of substances into the cell membrane, in addition to interfering with mitochondrial functions (Soni et al. 2005).

Regarding paraben toxicity, benzyl-paraben is known to be the most toxic, while methyl-paraben and ethyl-paraben are the least toxic (Soni et al. 2001). Methyl- and ethyl-paraben are also toxic and show 48 h median effective concentration (EC50–48 h) values ranging from 62 to 19 mg L^{-1} in the *Daphnia magna* acute test. For benzyl paraben, the range of EC50 (48 h) values was 6.6 to 2 mg L^{-1} for this organism (Yamamoto et al. 2007, Dobbins et al. 2009, Terasaki et al. 2009).

Yamamoto et al. (2011) observed that propyl-paraben was more toxic than ethyl- and methyl-paraben for organisms at two trophic levels. In the following order of parabens, methyl, ethyl- and n-propyl-paraben, the EC50 (72 h) values for green algae (*Psuedokirchneriella subcapitata*) were 80, 52 and 36 mg L^{-1}. In the case of medaka fish (*Oryzias latipes*), the LC50 (96 h) values were 63, 14 and 4.9 mg L^{-1}. Thus, this contaminant has shown to be deleterious to different organisms, and is an issue in the environment.

Conclusions

Studies indicate that humans and wildlife are exposed to different PPCPs chemicals, in different concentrations, through various routes. The four classes of pharmaceutical compounds and two classes of personal care products (PCPs) selected for discussion herein show environmental relevance and have already been studied in the literature. In addition, data is available on population consumption, release percentages and their occurrence in the environment. Sub-lethal effects for all compounds have been confirmed in several studies, at even very low concentrations. Among these, behavior alterations, reproduction changes, interference of enzymes phase I metabolization (CYP), alterations of enzymes responsible for antioxidant systems (GST, CAT, GPx, GSH, SOD, GR), lipid peroxidation and genotoxicity were the main endpoints caused by PPCPs in different levels of the food chain. Given this, there is a strong need to understand the additive and synergistic effects of such mixtures and to continue their evaluation in both *in vitro* and *in vivo* assays in order to further elucidate their mechanism of action and toxic effects.

References

Adolfsson-Erici, M., M. Pettersson, J. Parkkonen and J. Sturve. 2002. Triclosan, a commonly used bactericide found in human milk and in the aquatic environment in Sweden. Chemosphere. 46: 1485–1489. Doi:10.1016/S0045-6535(01)00255-7.

Agüera, A., A.R. Fernández-Alba, L. Piedra, M. Mézcua and M.J. Gómez. 2003. Evaluation of triclosan and biphenylol in marine sediments and urban wastewaters by pressurized liquid extraction and solid phase extraction followed by gas chromatography mass spectrometry and liquid chromatography mass spectrometry. Anal. Chim. Acta. 480: 193–205. Doi:10.1016/S0003-2670(03)00040-0.

Aguirre-Martínez, G.V., A.T. DelValls and M. Laura Martín-Díaz. 2015. Yes, caffeine, ibuprofen, carbamazepine, novobiocin and tamoxifen have an effect on *Corbicula fluminea* (Muller, 1774). Ecotoxicol. Environ. Saf. 120: 142–154. Doi:10.1016/j.ecoenv.2015.05.036.

Ahn, K.C., B. Zhao, J. Chen, G. Cherednichenko, E. Sanmarti, M.S. Denison et al. 2008. *In vitro* biologic activities of the antimicrobials triclocarban, its analogs, and triclosan in bioassay screens: receptor-based bioassay screens. Environ. Health Perspect. 116: 1203–10. Doi:10.1289/ehp.11200.

Alighardashi, A., D. Pandolfi, O. Potier and M.N. Pons. 2009. Acute sensitivity of activated sludge bacteria to erythromycin. J. Hazard. Mater. 172: 685–692. Doi:10.1016/j.jhazmat.2009.07.051.

Allen, E. 1983. Landmark article Sept 8, 1923. An ovarian hormone. Preliminary report on its localization, extraction and partial purification, and action in test animals. By Edgar Allen and Edward A. Doisy. JAMA J. Am. Med. Assoc. 250: 2681–2683. Doi:10.1001/jama.250.19.2681.

Almeida, A.F.R., V. Calisto, V.I. Esteves, R.J. Schneider, A.M.V.M. Soares and E. Figueira. 2015. Chronic toxicity of the antiepileptic carbamazepine on the clam *Ruditapes philippinarum*. Comp. Biochem. Physiol. Part—C Toxicol. Pharmacol. 172-173: 26–35. Doi:10.1016/j.cbpc.2015.04.004.

An, J., Q. Zhou, Y. Sun and Z. Xu. 2009. Ecotoxicological effects of typical personal care products on seed germination and seedling development of wheat (*Triticum aestivum* L.). Chemosphere. 76: 1428–1434. Doi:10.1016/j.chemosphere.2009.06.004.

Anselmo, H.M.R., L. Koerting, S. Devito, J.H.J. van den Berg, M. Dubbeldam, C. Kwadijk et al. 2011. Early life developmental effects of marine persistent organic pollutants on the sea urchin *Psammechinus miliaris*. Ecotoxicol. Environ. Saf. 74: 2182–2192. Doi:10.1016/j.ecoenv.2011.07.037 .

ASHP. 2017. Erythromycin: MedlinePlus Drug Information [WWW Document]. Am. Soc. Heal. Pharm. | U.S. Natl. Libr. Med. URL https://medlineplus.gov/druginfo/meds/a682381.html (accessed 5.2.17).

Atkinson, S.K., V.L. Marlatt, L.E. Kimpe, D.R.S. Lean, V.L. Trudeau and J.M. Blais. 2012. The occurrence of steroidal estrogens in south-eastern Ontario wastewater treatment plants. Sci. Total Environ. 430: 119–125. Doi:10.1016/j.scitotenv.2012.04.069.

Bahlmann, A., M.G. Weller, U. Panne and R.J. Schneider. 2009. Monitoring carbamazepine in surface and wastewaters by an immunoassay based on a monoclonal antibody. Anal. Bioanal. Chem. 395: 1809–1820. Doi:10.1007/s00216-009-2958-7.

Bang, S.H., J.-Y. Ahn, N.-H. Hong, S.S. Sekhon, Y.-H. Kim and J. Min. 2015. Acute and chronic toxicity assessment and the gene expression of Dhb, Vtg, Arnt, CYP4, and CYP314 in *Daphnia magna* exposed to pharmaceuticals. Mol. Cell. Toxicol. 11: 153–160. Doi:10.1007/s13273-015-0013-7.

Barceló, D., M. Petrović, E. Eljarrat, M.J.L. De Alda and A. Kampioti. 2003. Analysis and removal of emerging contaminants in wastewater and drinking water. TrAC Trends Anal. Chem. 22: 685–696. Doi:10.1016/S0165-9936(03)01105-1.

Beausse, J. 2004. Selected drugs in solid matrices: A review of environmental determination, occurrence and properties of principal substances. TrAC—Trends Anal. Chem. 23: 753–761. Doi:10.1016/j. trac.2004.08.005.

Beretta, M., V. Britto, T.M. Tavares, S.M.T. da Silva and A.L. Pletsch. 2014. Occurrence of pharmaceutical and personal care products (PPCPs) in marine sediments in the Todos os Santos Bay and the north coast of Salvador, Bahia, Brazil. J. Soils Sediments. 14: 1278–1286. Doi:10.1007/s11368-014-0884-6.

Binelli, A., M. Parolini, A. Pedriali and A. Provini. 2010. Antioxidant activity in the zebra mussel (*Dreissena polymorpha*) in response to triclosan exposure. Water, Air, Soil Pollut. 217: 421–430. Doi:10.1007/s11270-010-0597-4.

Birkett, J.W. and J.N. Lester. 2003. Endocrine Disrupters in Wastewater and Sludge Treatment Processes, America.

Bjerregaard, P., D.N. Andersen, K.L. Pedersen, S.N. Pedersen and B. Korsgaard. 2003. Estrogenic effect of propylparaben (propylhydroxybenzoate) in rainbow trout *Oncorhynchus mykiss* after exposure via food and water. Comp. Biochem. Physiol. -C Toxicol. Pharmacol. 136: 309–317. Doi:10.1016/j. cca.2003.10.004.

Black, J.G. and D. Howes. 1975. Percutaneous absorption of Triclosan from toilet preparations. J. Soc. Cosmet. Chem. 26: 205–215.

Black, J.G., D. Howes and T. Rutherford. 1975. Percutaneous absorption and metabolism of Irgasan® DP300. Toxicology. 3: 33–47. Doi:10.1016/0300-483X(75)90006-2.

Brandão, F.P., S. Rodrigues, B.B. Castro, F. Gonçalves, S.C. Antunes and B. Nunes. 2013. Short-term effects of neuroactive pharmaceutical drugs on a fish species: Biochemical and behavioural effects. Aquat. Toxicol. 144-145: 218–229. Doi:10.1016/j.aquatox.2013.10.005.

Brian, J.V., C.A. Harris, M. Scholze, T. Backhaus, P. Booy, M. Lamoree et al. 2005. Accurate prediction of the response of freshwater fish to a mixture of estrogenic chemicals. Environ. Health Perspect. 113: 721–728. Doi:10.1289/ehp.7598.

Burke, V., D. Richter, J. Greskowiak, A. Mehrtens, L. Schulz and G. Massmann. 2016. Occurrence of antibiotics in surface and groundwater of a drinking water catchment area in Germany. Water Environ. Res. 88: 652–659. Doi:10.2175/106143016X14609975746604.

Buser, H.-R., T. Poiger and M.D. Müller. 1999. Occurrence and environmental behavior of the chiral pharmaceutical drug ibuprofen in surface waters and in wastewater. Environ. Sci. Technol. 33: 2529–2535. Doi:10.1021/es981014w.

Calamari, D., E. Zuccato, S. Castiglioni, R. Bagnati and R. Fanelli. 2003. Strategic survey of therapeutic drugs in the rivers po and lambro in northern Italy. Environ. Sci. Technol. 37: 1241–1248. Doi:10.1021/es020158e.

Calisto, V., A. Bahlmann, R.J. Schneider and V.I. Esteves. 2011. Application of an ELISA to the quantification of carbamazepine in ground, surface and wastewaters and validation with LC-MS/MS. Chemosphere. 84: 1708–1715. Doi:10.1016/j.chemosphere.2011.04.072.

Canesi, L., C. Ciacci, L.C. Lorusso, M. Betti, G. Gallo, G. Pojana et al. 2007. Effects of Triclosan on *Mytilus galloprovincialis* hemocyte function and digestive gland enzyme activities: Possible modes of action on non target organisms. Comp. Biochem. Physiol. Part C Toxicol. Pharmacol. 145: 464–472. Doi:10.1016/j.cbpc.2007.02.002.

Canosa, P., I. Rodríguez, E. Rubí, M.H. Bollaín and R. Cela. 2006. Optimisation of a solid-phase microextraction method for the determination of parabens in water samples at the low ng per litre level. J. Chromatogr. A. 1124: 3–10. Doi:10.1016/j.chroma.2006.03.045.

Chai, L., H. Wang, H. Zhao and H. Deng. 2016. Chronic effects of triclosan on embryonic development of Chinese toad, *Bufo gargarizans*. Ecotoxicology. 25: 1600–1608. Doi:10.1007/s10646-016-1715-x.

Chanda, M., M. Paul, J. Maity, G. Dash and S. Sen Gupta. 2011. The use of antibiotics and disinfectants in ornamental fish farms of West Bengal, India. J. Nat. Sci. Biol. Med. 2: 139–40. Doi:10.4103/0976-9668.92311.

Chen, H., J. Zha, X. Liang, J. Li and Z. Wang. 2014. Effects of the human antiepileptic drug carbamazepine on the behavior, biomarkers, and heat shock proteins in the Asian clam *Corbicula fluminea*. Aquat. Toxicol. 155: 1–8. Doi:10.1016/j.aquatox.2014.06.001.

Chen, X., B. Xu, B. Han, Z. Mao, Z. Mao, M. Chen, G. Du et al. 2015. The effects of triclosan on pluripotency factors and development of mouse embryonic stem cells and zebrafish. Arch. Toxicol. 89: 635–646. Doi:10.1007/s00204-014-1270-2.

Chen, X., X. Wang, X. Gu, Y. Jiang and R. Ji. 2017. Oxidative stress responses and insights into the sensitivity of the earthworms *Metaphire guillelmi* and *Eisenia fetida* to soil cadmium. Sci. Total Environ. 574: 300–306. Doi:10.1016/j.scitotenv.2016.09.059.

Cleuvers, M. 2003. Aquatic ecotoxicity of pharmaceuticals including the assessment of combination effects. Toxicol. Lett. 142: 185–194. Doi:10.1016/S0378-4274(03)00068-7.

Colborn, T., F.S. Vom Saal and A.M. Soto. 1993. Developmental effects of endocrine-disrupting chemicals in wildlife and humans. Environ. Health Perspect. 101: 378–384. Doi:10.1016/0195-9255(94)90014-0.

Crofton, K.M., K.B. Paul, M.J. DeVito and J.M. Hedge. 2007. Short-term *in vivo* exposure to the water contaminant triclosan: Evidence for disruption of thyroxine. Environmental Toxicology and Pharmacology. Doi:10.1016/j.etap.2007.04.008.

Darbre, P.D., J.R. Byford, L.E. Shaw, R.A. Horton, G.S. Pope and M.J. Sauer. 2002. Oestrogenic activity of isobutylparaben *in vitro* and *in vivo*. J. Appl. Toxicol. 22: 219–226. Doi:10.1002/jat.860.

Daughton, C.G. and T.A. Ternes. 1999. Pharmaceuticals and personal care products in the environment: agents of subtle changes. Environ. Health Perspect. 107: 907. Doi:10.2307/3434573.

David, A. and K. Pancharatna. 2009. Developmental anomalies induced by a non-selective COX inhibitor (ibuprofen) in zebrafish (*Danio rerio*). Environ. Toxicol. Pharmacol. 27: 390–395. Doi:10.1016/j.etap.2009.01.002.

Dayan, A.D. 2007. Risk assessment of triclosan [Irgasan®] in human breast milk. Food Chem. Toxicol. 45: 125–129. Doi:10.1016/j.fct.2006.08.009.

De Lange, H.J., W. Noordoven, A.J. Murk, M. Lürling and E.T.H.M. Peeters. 2006. Behavioural responses of *Gammarus pulex* (Crustacea, Amphipoda) to low concentrations of pharmaceuticals. Aquat. Toxicol. 78: 209–216. Doi:10.1016/j.aquatox.2006.03.002.

Delorenzo, M.E. and J. Fleming. 2007. Individual and mixture effects of selected pharmaceuticals and personal care products on the marine phytoplankton species *Dunaliella tertiolecta*. Doi:10.1007/s00244-007-9032-2.

Desbrow, C., E.J. Routledge, G.C. Brighty, J.P. Sumpter and M. Waldock. 1998. Identification of estrogenic chemicals in STW effluent. 1. Chemical fractionation and *in vitro* biological screening. Environ. Sci. Technol. 32: 1549–1558. Doi:10.1021/es9707973.

Dietrich, S., F. Ploessl, F. Bracher and C. Laforsch. 2010. Single and combined toxicity of pharmaceuticals at environmentally relevant concentrations in *Daphnia magna*—A multigenerational study. Chemosphere. 79: 60–66. Doi:10.1016/j.chemosphere.2009.12.069.

Directive, W.F. 2011. Priority substances under the water framework directive on environmental quality standards directive. 1–2.

Dobbins, L.L., S. Usenko, R.A. Brain and B.W. Brooks. 2009. Probabilistic ecological hazard assessment of parabens using *Daphnia magna* and *Pimephales promelas*. Environ. Toxicol. Chem. 28: 2744–2753. Doi:10.1897/08-523.1.

Dodds, E.C., L. Golderberg, W. Lawson and R. Robinson. 1938. Nature Publishing Group. Nat. Publ. Gr. 141: 247–248.

Dong, D., L. Zhang, S. Liu, Z. Guo and X. Hua. 2016a. Antibiotics in water and sediments from Liao River in Jilin Province, China: occurrence, distribution, and risk assessment. Environ. Earth Sci. 75: 1202. Doi:10.1007/s12665-016-6008-4.

Dong, H., X. Yuan, W. Wang and Z. Qiang. 2016b. Occurrence and removal of antibiotics in ecological and conventional wastewater treatment processes: A field study. J. Environ. Manage. 178: 11–19. Doi:10.1016/j.jenvman.2016.04.037.

Drewes, J.E., J. Hemming, S.J. Ladenburger, J. Schauer and W. Sonzogni. 2003. An assessment of endocrine disrupting activity changes during wastewater treatment through the use of bioassays and chemical measurements. Water Environ. Res. 77: 12–23. Doi:10.2175/106143005X41573.

Duong, C.N., J.S. Ra, J. Cho, S.D. Kim, H.K. Choi, J.H. Park et al. 2010. Estrogenic chemicals and estrogenicity in river waters of South Korea and seven Asian countries. Chemosphere. 78: 286–293. Doi:10.1016/j.chemosphere.2009.10.048.

Dussault, È.B., V.K. Balakrishnan, E. Sverko, K.R. Solomon and P.K. Sibley. 2008. Toxicity of human pharmaceuticals and personal care products to benthic invertebrates. Environ. Toxicol. Chem. 27: 425. Doi:10.1897/07-354R.1.

Esposito, A., L. Fabrizi, D. Lucchetti, L. Marvasi, E. Coni and E. Guandalini. 2007. Orally administered erythromycin in rainbow trout (*Oncorhynchus mykiss*): residues in edible tissues and withdrawal time. Antimicrob. Agents Chemother. 51: 1043–7. Doi:10.1128/AAC.01002-06.

Fairbairn, D.J., M.E. Karpuzcu, W.A. Arnold, B.L. Barber, E.F. Kaufenberg, W.C. Koskinen et al. 2016. Sources and transport of contaminants of emerging concern: A two-year study of occurrence and spatiotemporal variation in a mixed land use watershed. Sci. Total Environ. 551: 605–613. Doi:10.1016/j.scitotenv.2016.02.056.

Farré, M., D. Asperger, L. Kantiani, S. González, M. Petrovic and D. Barceló. 2008. Assessment of the acute toxicity of triclosan and methyl triclosan in wastewater based on the bioluminescence inhibition of *Vibrio fischeri*. Anal. Bioanal. Chem. 390: 1999–2007. Doi:10.1007/s00216-007-1779-9.

Fent, K., A. Weston and D. Caminada. 2006. Ecotoxicology of human pharmaceuticals. Aquat. Toxicol. 76: 122–159. Doi:10.1016/j.aquatox.2005.09.009.

Flippin, J.L., D. Huggett and C.M. Foran. 2007. Changes in the timing of reproduction following chronic exposure to ibuprofen in Japanese medaka, *Oryzias latipes*. Aquat. Toxicol. 81: 73–78. Doi:10.1016/j.aquatox.2006.11.002.

Focazio, M.J., D.W. Kolpin, K.K. Barnes, E.T. Furlong, M.T. Meyer, S.D. Zaugg et al. 2008. A national reconnaissance for pharmaceuticals and other organic wastewater contaminants in the United States—II. Untreated drinking water sources. Sci. Total Environ. 402: 201–216. Doi:10.1016/j.scitotenv.2008.02.021.

Folmar, L.C., M.J. Hemmer, N.D. Denslow, K. Kroll, J. Chen, A. Cheek et al. 2002. A comparison of the estrogenic potencies of estradiol, ethynylestradiol, diethylstilbestrol, nonylphenol and methoxychlor *in vivo* and *in vitro*. Aquat. Toxicol. 60: 101–110. Doi:10.1016/S0166-445X(01)00276-4.

Freitas, R., A.C.V. Almeida, C. Velez, A. Moreira, R.J. Schneider, V.I. Esteves et al. 2016. The impacts of pharmaceutical drugs under ocean acidification: New data on single and combined long-term effects of carbamazepine on Scrobicularia plana. Sci. Total Environ. 541: 977–985. Doi:10.1016/j.scitotenv.2015.09.138.

Gagnaire, B., H. Thomas-Guyon and T. Renault. 2004. *In vitro* effects of cadmium and mercury on Pacific oyster, *Crassostrea gigas* (Thunberg), haemocytes. Fish Shellfish Immunol. 16: 501–512. Doi:10.1016/j.fsi.2003.08.007.

Gagné, F., C. Blaise and C. André. 2006. Occurrence of pharmaceutical products in a municipal effluent and toxicity to rainbow trout (*Oncorhynchus mykiss*) hepatocytes. Ecotoxicol. Environ. Saf. 64: 329–336. Doi:10.1016/j.ecoenv.2005.04.004.

Gilbert, N. 2012. Drug-pollution law all washed up. Nature. 491: 503–504. Doi:10.1038/491503a.

Gimeno, S., H. Komen, A.G.M. Gerritsen and T. Bowmer. 1998. Feminisation of young males of the common carp, *Cyprinus carpio*, exposed to 4-tert-pentylphenol during sexual differentiation. Aquat. Toxicol. 43: 77–92. Doi:10.1016/S0166-445X(98)00056-3.

Gómez-Oliván, L.M., N. Neri-Cruz, M. Galar-Martínez, H. Islas-Flores and S. García-Medina. 2014. Binary mixtures of diclofenac with paracetamol, ibuprofen, naproxen, and acetylsalicylic acid and these pharmaceuticals in isolated form induce oxidative stress on Hyalella azteca. Environ. Monit. Assess. 186: 7259–7271. Doi:10.1007/s10661-014-3925-0.

González, O., B. Bayarri, J. Aceña, S. Pérez and D. Barceló. 2016. Treatment technologies for wastewater reuse: fate of contaminants of emerging concerns. *In*: Fatta-Kassinos, D., D. Dionysiou and K. Kümmerer (eds). The Handbook of Environmental Chemistry 45: Advanced Treatment Technologies for Urban Wastewater Reuse. Springer, Cham-Heidelberg-NewYork-Dordrecht-London, p. 305.

González-Pleiter, M., S. Gonzalo, I. Rodea-Palomares, F. Leganés, R. Rosal, K. Boltes et al. 2013. Toxicity of five antibiotics and their mixtures towards photosynthetic aquatic organisms: Implications for environmental risk assessment. Water Res. 47: 2050–2064. Doi:10.1016/j.watres.2013.01.020.

Gonzalez-Rey, M. and M.J. Bebianno. 2012. Does non-steroidal anti-inflammatory (NSAID) ibuprofen induce antioxidant stress and endocrine disruption in mussel *Mytilus galloprovincialis*? Environ. Toxicol. Pharmacol. 33: 361–371. Doi:10.1016/j.etap.2011.12.017.

Gonzalez-Rey, M., J.J. Mattos, C.E. Piazza, A.C.D. Bainy and M.J. Bebianno. 2014. Effects of active pharmaceutical ingredients mixtures in mussel *Mytilus galloprovincialis*. Aquat. Toxicol. 153: 12–26. Doi:10.1016/j.aquatox.2014.02.006.

Guo, L.-W., Q. Wu, B. Green, G. Nolen, L. Shi, J. LoSurdo et al. 2012. Cytotoxicity and inhibitory effects of low-concentration triclosan on adipogenic differentiation of human mesenchymal stem cells. Toxicol. Appl. Pharmacol. 262: 117–123. Doi:10.1016/j.taap.2012.04.024.

Gyllenhammar, I., L. Holm, R. Eklund and C. Berg. 2009. Reproductive toxicity in *Xenopus tropicalis* after developmental exposure to environmental concentrations of ethynylestradiol. Aquat. Toxicol. 91: 171–178. Doi:10.1016/j.aquatox.2008.06.019.

Hampel, M., J.E. Bron, J.B. Taggart and M.J. Leaver. 2014. The antidepressant drug Carbamazepine induces differential transcriptome expression in the brain of Atlantic salmon, *Salmo salar*. Aquat. Toxicol. 151: 114–23. Doi:10.1016/j.aquatox.2013.12.018.

Han, S., K. Choi, J. Kim, K. Ji, S. Kim, B. Ahn et al. 2010. Endocrine disruption and consequences of chronic exposure to ibuprofen in Japanese medaka (*Oryzias latipes*) and freshwater cladocerans *Daphnia magna* and *Moina macrocopa*. Aquat. Toxicol. 98: 256–264. Doi:10.1016/j.aquatox.2010.02.013.

Hano, T., Y. Oshima, T. Oe, M. Kinoshita, M. Tanaka, Y. Wakamatsu et al. 2005. Quantitative bio-imaging analysis for evaluation of sexual differentiation in germ cells of olvas-GFP/ST-II YI medaka (*Oryzias latipes*) nanoinjected *in ovo* with ethinylestradiol. Environ. Toxicol. Chem. 24: 70–7.

Harada, A., K. Komori, N. Nakada, K. Kitamura and Y. Suzuki. 2008. Biological effects of PPCPs on aquatic lives and evaluation of river waters affected by different wastewater treatment levels. Water Sci. Technol. 58: 1541. Doi:10.2166/wst.2008.742.

Hayashi, Y., L.H. Heckmann, A. Callaghan and R.M. Sibly. 2008. Reproduction recovery of the crustacean *Daphnia magna* after chronic exposure to ibuprofen. Ecotoxicology. 17: 246–251. Doi:10.1007/s10646-008-0191-3.

Heberer, T., K. Reddersen and A. Mechlinski. 2002. From municipal sewage to drinking water: fate and removal of pharmaceutical residues in the aquatic environment in urban areas. Water Sci. Technol. 46: 81–88.

Heckmann, L.-H., R. Connon, T.H. Hutchinson, S.J. Maund, R.M. Sibly and A. Callaghan. 2006. Expression of target and reference genes in *Daphnia magna* exposed to ibuprofen. BMC Genomics. 7: 175. Doi:10.1186/1471-2164-7-175.

Heckmann, L.-H., A. Callaghan, H.L. Hooper, R. Connon, T.H. Hutchinson, S.J. Maund et al. 2007. Chronic toxicity of ibuprofen to *Daphnia magna*: Effects on life history traits and population dynamics. Toxicol. Lett. 172: 137–145. Doi:10.1016/j.toxlet.2007.06.001.

Ho, J.C.H., C.D. Hsiao, K. Kawakami and W.K.F. Tse. 2016. Triclosan (TCS) exposure impairs lipid metabolism in zebrafish embryos. Aquat. Toxicol. 173: 29–35. Doi:10.1016/j.aquatox.2016.01.001.

Hobara, T., S. Uchida, K. Otsuki, T. Matsubara, H. Funato, K. Matsuo et al. 2010. Altered gene expression of histone deacetylases in mood disorder patients. J. Psychiatr. Res. 44: 263–270. Doi:10.1016/j.jpsychires.2009.08.015.

Hu, S., H. Zhang, G. Shen, Z. Yuan, T. Xu and R. Ji. 2017. Effects of 17β-estradiol and 17α-ethinylestradiol on the embryonic development of the clearhead icefish (*Protosalanx hyalocranius*). Chemosphere. 176: 18–24. Doi:10.1016/j.chemosphere.2017.02.094.

Hutt, A.J. and J. Caldwell. 1983. The metabolic chiral inversion of 2-arylpropionic acids—a novel route with pharmacological consequences. J. Pharm. Pharmacol. 35: 693–704.

Isidori, M., M. Lavorgna, A. Nardelli, L. Pascarella and A. Parrella. 2005. Toxic and genotoxic evaluation of six antibiotics on non-target organisms. Sci. Total Environ. 346: 87–98. Doi:10.1016/j.scitotenv.2004.11.017.

Janex-Habibi, M.L., A. Huyard, M. Esperanza and A. Bruchet. 2009. Reduction of endocrine disruptor emissions in the environment: The benefit of wastewater treatment. Water Res. 43: 1565–1576. Doi:10.1016/j.watres.2008.12.051.

Jarvis, A.L., M.J. Bernot and R.J. Bernot. 2014. The effects of the pharmaceutical carbamazepine on life history characteristics of flat-headed mayflies (Heptageniidae) and aquatic resource interactions. Ecotoxicology. 23: 1701–1712. Doi:10.1007/s10646-014-1309-4.

Jobling, S., M. Nolan, C.R. Tyler, G. Brighty and J.P. Sumpter. 1998. Widespread sexual disruption in wild fish. Environ. Sci. Technol. 32: 2498–2506. Doi:10.1021/es9710870.

Johnson, A.C., A. Belfroid and A. Di Corcia. 2000. Estimating steroid oestrogen inputs into activated sludge treatment works and observations on their removal from the effluent. Sci. Total Environ. 256: 163–173. Doi:10.1016/S0048-9697(00)00481-2.

Johnson, A.C. and J.P. Sumpter. 2001. Removal of endocrine-disrupting chemicals in activated sludge treatment works. Environ. Sci. Technol. 35: 4697–4703. Doi:10.1021/es010171j.

Johnson, A.C. and R.J. Williams. 2004. A model to estimate influent and effluent concentrations of estradiol sewage treatment works. Environ. Sci. Technol. 38: 3649–3658. Doi:10.1021/es035342u.

Jos, A., G. Repetto, J.C. Rios, M.J. Hazen, M.L. Molero, A. Del Peso et al. 2003. Ecotoxicological evaluation of carbamazepine using six different model systems with eighteen endpoints. Toxicol. Vitr. 17: 525–532. Doi:10.1016/S0887-2333(03)00119-X.

Kim, H.-Y., I.-S. Lee and J.-E. Oh. 2017. Human and veterinary pharmaceuticals in the marine environment including fish farms in Korea. Sci. Total Environ. 579: 940–949. Doi:10.1016/j. scitotenv.2016.10.039.

Kim, J.-W., H. Ishibashi, R. Yamauchi, N. Ichikawa, Y. Takao, M. Hirano et al. 2009. Acute toxicity of pharmaceutical and personal care products on freshwater crustacean (*Thamnocephalus platyurus*) and fish (*Oryzias latipes*). J. Toxicol. Sci. 34: 227–32.

Kim, S.D., J. Cho, I.S. Kim, B.J. Vanderford and S.A. Snyder. 2007. Occurrence and removal of pharmaceuticals and endocrine disruptors in South Korean surface, drinking, and waste waters. Water Res. 41: 1013–21. Doi:10.1016/j.watres.2006.06.034.

Kjærstad, M.B., C. Taxvig, H.R. Andersen and C. Nellemann. 2010. Mixture effects of endocrine disrupting compounds *in vitro*. Int. J. Androl. 33: 425–433. Doi:10.1111/j.1365-2605.2009.01034.x.

Kolpin, D.W., E.T. Furlong, M.T. Meyer, E.M. Thurman, S.D. Zaugg, L.B. Barber et al. 2002. Pharmaceuticals, hormones, and other organic wastewater contaminants in U.S. streams, 1999–2000: A national reconnaissance. Environ. Sci. Technol. 36: 1202–1211. Doi:10.1021/es011055j.

Kouzarides, T. 2007. Chromatin modifications and their function. Cell. 128: 693–705. Doi:10.1016/j. cell.2007.02.005.

Kovacevic, V., A.J. Simpson and M.J. Simpson. 2016. 1H NMR-based metabolomics of *Daphnia magna* responses after sub-lethal exposure to triclosan, carbamazepine and ibuprofen. Comp. Biochem. Physiol.—Part D Genomics Proteomics. 19: 199–210. Doi:10.1016/j.cbd.2016.01.004.

Ku, P., X. Wu, X. Nie, R. Ou, L. Wang, T. Su et al. 2014. Effects of triclosan on the detoxification system in the yellow catfish (*Pelteobagrus fulvidraco*): Expressions of CYP and GST genes and corresponding enzyme activity in phase I, II and antioxidant system. Comp. Biochem. Physiol. Part C Toxicol. Pharmacol. 166: 105–114. Doi:10.1016/j.cbpc.2014.07.006.

Kümmerer, K. 2009. The presence of pharmaceuticals in the environment due to human use— present knowledge and future challenges. J. Environ. Manage. 90: 2354–2366. Doi:10.1016/j. jenvman.2009.01.023.

Kwong, T.C. 2002. Organophosphate pesticides: Biochemistry and clinical toxicology. Ther. Drug Monit. 24: 144–149. Doi:10.1097/00007691-200202000-00022.

Lacaze, E., J. Pédelucq, M. Fortier, P. Brousseau, M. Auffret, H. Budzinski et al. 2015. Genotoxic and immunotoxic potential effects of selected psychotropic drugs and antibiotics on blue mussel (*Mytilus edulis*) hemocytes. Environ. Pollut. 202: 177–186. Doi:10.1016/j.envpol.2015.03.025.

Laizure, C.S., V. Herring, Z. Hu, K. Witbrodt and R.B. Parker. 2013. The role of human carboxylesterases in drug metabolism: Have we overlooked their importance? Pharmacother. J. Hum. Pharmacol. Drug Ther. 33: 210–222. Doi:10.1002/phar.1194.

Lamichhane, K., S.N. Garcia, D.B. Huggett, D.L. Deangelis and T.W. La Point. 2013. Chronic effects of carbamazepine on life-history strategies of *Ceriodaphnia dubia* in three successive generations. Arch. Environ. Contam. Toxicol. 64: 427–438. Doi:10.1007/s00244-012-9845-5.

Laville, N., S. Aït-Ässa, E. Gomez, C. Casellas and J.M. Porcher. 2004. Effects of human pharmaceuticals on cytotoxicity, EROD activity and ROS production in fish hepatocytes. Toxicology. 196: 41–55. Doi:10.1016/j.tox.2003.11.002.

Legler, J., M. Dennekamp, A.D. Vethaak, A. Brouwera, J.H. Koeman, B. Van der Burg et al. 2002. Detection of estrogenic activity in sediment-associated compounds using *in vitro* reporter gene assays. Sci. Total Environ. 293: 69–83. Doi:10.1016/S0048-9697(01)01146-9.

Lemini, C., a. Hernández, R. Jaimez, Y. Franco, M.E. Avila and a. Castell. 2004. Morphometric analysis of mice uteri treated with the preservatives methyl, ethyl, propyl, and butylparaben. Toxicol. Ind. Health. 20: 123–132. Doi:10.1191/0748233704th202oa.

Li, W.C. 2014. Occurrence, sources, and fate of pharmaceuticals in aquatic environment and soil. Environ. Pollut. 187: 193–201. Doi:10.1016/j.envpol.2014.01.015.

Li, Z.H., P. Li, M. Rodina and T. Randak. 2010. Effect of human pharmaceutical Carbamazepine on the quality parameters and oxidative stress in common carp (*Cyprinus carpio* L.) spermatozoa. Chemosphere. 80: 530–534. Doi:10.1016/j.chemosphere.2010.04.046.

Li, Z.H., V. Zlabek, J. Velisek, R. Grabic, J. Machova, J. Kolarova et al. 2011. Acute toxicity of carbamazepine to juvenile rainbow trout (*Oncorhynchus mykiss*): Effects on antioxidant responses, hematological parameters and hepatic EROD. Ecotoxicol. Environ. Saf. 74: 319–327. Doi:10.1016/j. ecoenv.2010.09.008.

Lin, A.Y.-C. and Y.-T. Tsai. 2009. Occurrence of pharmaceuticals in Taiwan's surface waters: impact of waste streams from hospitals and pharmaceutical production facilities. Sci. Total Environ. 407: 3793–802. Doi:10.1016/j.scitotenv.2009.03.009.

Lin, D., Q. Zhou, X. Xie and Y. Liu. 2010. Potential biochemical and genetic toxicity of triclosan as an emerging pollutant on earthworms (*Eisenia fetida*). Chemosphere. 81: 1328–1333. Doi:10.1016/j. chemosphere.2010.08.027.

Lin, D., X. Xie, Q. Zhou and Y. Liu. 2012. Biochemical and genotoxic effect of triclosan on earthworms (*Eisenia fetida*) using contact and soil tests. Environ. Toxicol. 27: 385–392. Doi:10.1002/tox.20651.

Lin, D., Y. Li, Q. Zhou, Y. Xu and D. Wang. 2014. Effect of triclosan on reproduction, DNA damage and heat shock protein gene expression of the earthworm Eisenia fetida. Ecotoxicology. 23: 1826–1832. Doi:10.1007/s10646-014-1320-9.

Liu, B., X. Nie, W. Liu, P. Snoeijs, C. Guan and M.T.K. Tsui. 2011. Toxic effects of erythromycin, ciprofloxacin and sulfamethoxazole on photosynthetic apparatus in Selenastrum capricornutum. Ecotoxicol. Environ. Saf. 74: 1027–1035. Doi:10.1016/j.ecoenv.2011.01.022.

Liu, J., G. Lu, Z. Xie, Z. Zhang, S. Li and Z. Yan. 2015. Occurrence, bioaccumulation and risk assessment of lipophilic pharmaceutically active compounds in the downstream rivers of sewage treatment plants. Sci. Total Environ. 511: 54–62. Doi:10.1016/j.scitotenv.2014.12.033.

Liu, J.-L. and M.-H. Wong. 2013. Pharmaceuticals and personal care products (PPCPs): A review on environmental contamination in China. Environ. Int. 59: 208–224. Doi:10.1016/j.envint.2013.06.012.

Liu, X., J. Lee, K. Ji, S. Takeda and K. Choi. 2012. Potentials and mechanisms of genotoxicity of six pharmaceuticals frequently detected in freshwater environment. Toxicol. Lett. 211: 70–76. Doi:10.1016/j.toxlet.2012.03.003.

Louvet, J.N., C. Giammarino, O. Potier and M.N. Pons. 2010. Adverse effects of erythromycin on the structure and chemistry of activated sludge. Environ. Pollut. 158: 688–693. Doi:10.1016/j. envpol.2009.10.021.

Luo, Y., W. Guo, H.H. Ngo, L.D. Nghiem, F.I. Hai, J. Zhang et al. 2014. A review on the occurrence of micropollutants in the aquatic environment and their fate and removal during wastewater treatment. Sci. Total Environ. 473-474: 619–641. Doi:10.1016/j.scitotenv.2013.12.065.

Lürling, M., E. Sargant and I. Roessink. 2006. Life-history consequences for *Daphnia pulex* exposed to pharmaceutical carbamazepine. Environ. Toxicol. 21: 172–180. Doi:10.1002/tox.20171.

Malarvizhi, A., C. Kavitha, M. Saravanan and M. Ramesh. 2012. Carbamazepine (CBZ) induced enzymatic stress in gill, liver and muscle of a common carp, *Cyprinus carpio*. J. King Saud Univ. Sci. 24: 179–186. Doi:10.1016/j.jksus.2011.01.001.

Martín, J., D. Camacho-Muñoz, J.L. Santos, I. Aparicio and E. Alonso. 2012. Occurrence of pharmaceutical compounds in wastewater and sludge from wastewater treatment plants: Removal and ecotoxicological impact of wastewater discharges and sludge disposal. J. Hazard. Mater. 239-240: 40–47. Doi:10.1016/j.jhazmat.2012.04.068.

Matés, J.M., C. Pérez-Gómez and I. Núñez de Castro. 1999. Antioxidant enzymes and human diseases. Clin. Biochem. 32: 595–603. Doi:10.1016/S0009-9120(99)00075-2.

McAvoy, D.C., B. Schatowitz, M. Jacob, A. Hauk and W.S. Eckhoff. 2002. Measurement of triclosan in wastewater treatment systems. Environ. Toxicol. Chem. 21: 1323–1329. Doi:10.1002/ etc.5620210701.

MEPs reject restricting pharmaceuticals in water—POLITICO [WWW Document], n.d. URL http://www. politico.eu/article/meps-reject-restricting-pharmaceuticals-in-water/ (accessed 5.11.17).

Metcalfe, C.D., X.-S. Miao, B.G. Koenig and J. Struger. 2003. Distribution of acidic and neutral drugs in surface waters near sewage treatment plants in the lower great lakes, Canada. Environ. Toxicol. Chem. 22: 2881. Doi:10.1897/02-627.

Miller, D., B.B. Wheals, N. Beresford and J.P. Sumpter. 2001. Estrogenic activity of phenolic additives determined by an *in vitro* yeast bioassay. Environ. Health Perspect. 109: 133–138. Doi:sc271_5_1835 [pii].

Mohapatra, D.P., S.K. Brar, R.D. Tyagi, P. Picard and R.Y. Surampalli. 2014. Analysis and advanced oxidation treatment of a persistent pharmaceutical compound in wastewater and wastewater sludge-carbamazepine. Sci. Total Environ. 470-471: 58–75. Doi:10.1016/j.scitotenv.2013.09.034.

Morisseau, C., O. Merzlikin, A. Lin, G. He, W. Feng, I. Padilla et al. 2009. Toxicology in the fast lane: Application of high-throughput bioassays to detect modulation of key enzymes and receptors. Environ. Health Perspect. 117: 1867–1872. Doi:10.1289/ehp.0900834.

Moss, T., D. Howes and F. Williams. 2000. Percutaneous penetration and dermal metabolism of triclosan (2,4,4′-trichloro-2′-hydroxydiphenyl ether). Food Chem. Toxicol. 38: 361–370. Doi:10.1016/S0278-6915(99)00164-7.

Nakada, N., T. Tanishima, H. Shinohara, K. Kiri and H. Takada. 2006. Pharmaceutical chemicals and endocrine disrupters in municipal wastewater in Tokyo and their removal during activated sludge treatment. Water Res. 40: 3297–3303. Doi:10.1016/j.watres.2006.06.039.

Nannou, C.I., C.I. Kosma and T.A. Albanis. 2015. Occurrence of pharmaceuticals in surface waters: analytical method development and environmental risk assessment. Int. J. Environ. Anal. Chem. 95: 1242–1262. Doi:10.1080/03067319.2015.1085520.

Nassef, M., S.G. Kim, M. Seki, I.J. Kang, T. Hano, Y. Shimasaki et al. 2010a. *In ovo* nanoinjection of triclosan, diclofenac and carbamazepine affects embryonic development of medaka fish (*Oryzias latipes*). Chemosphere. 79: 966–973. Doi:10.1016/j.chemosphere.2010.02.002.

Nassef, M., S. Matsumoto, M. Seki, F. Khalil, I.J. Kang, Y. Shimasaki et al. 2010b. Acute effects of triclosan, diclofenac and carbamazepine on feeding performance of Japanese medaka fish (*Oryzias latipes*). Chemosphere. 80: 1095–1100. Doi:10.1016/j.chemosphere.2010.04.073.

Nawaz, M., C. Manzl and G. Krumschnabel. 2005. *In Vitro* toxicity of copper, cadmium, and chromium to isolated hepatocytes from carp, *Cyprinus carpio* L. Bull. Environ. Contam. Toxicol. 75: 652–661. Doi:10.1007/s00128-005-0802-0.

Nie, X.-P., B.-Y. Liu, H.-J. Yu, W.-Q. Liu and Y.-F. Yang. 2013. Toxic effects of erythromycin, ciprofloxacin and sulfamethoxazole exposure to the antioxidant system in *Pseudokirchneriella subcapitata*. Environ. Pollut. 172: 23–32. Doi:10.1016/j.envpol.2012.08.013.

Nilsson, M.F. and W.S. Webster. 2014. Effects of macrolide antibiotics on rat embryonic heart function *in vitro*. Birth Defects Res. Part B Dev. Reprod. Toxicol. 101: 189–198. Doi:10.1002/bdrb.21107.

Okubo, T., Y. Yokoyama, K. Kano and I. Kano. 2001. ER-dependent estrogenic activity of parabens assessed by proliferation of human breast cancer MCF-7 cells and expression of ER and PR. Food Chem. Toxicol. 39: 1225–1232. Doi:10.1016/S0278-6915(01)00073-4.

Oliveira, R., I. Domingues, C. Koppe Grisolia and A.M.V.M. Soares. 2009. Effects of triclosan on zebrafish early-life stages and adults. Environ. Sci. Pollut. Res. 16: 679–688. Doi:10.1007/s11356-009-0119-3.

Owen, R. and S. Jobling. 2012. Environmental science: The hidden costs of flexible fertility. Nature. 485: 441–441. Doi:10.1038/485441a.

Paíga, P., L.H.M.L.M. Santos, C.G. Amorim, A.N. Araújo, M.C.B.S.M. Montenegro, A. Pena et al. 2013. Pilot monitoring study of ibuprofen in surface waters of north of Portugal. Environ. Sci. Pollut. Res. 20: 2410–2420. Doi:10.1007/s11356-012-1128-1.

Pan, M. and L.M. Chu. 2016. Phytotoxicity of veterinary antibiotics to seed germination and root elongation of crops. Ecotoxicol. Environ. Saf. 126: 228–237. Doi:10.1016/j.ecoenv.2015.12.027.

Parolini, M., A. Binelli, D. Cogni, C. Riva and A. Provini. 2009. An *in vitro* biomarker approach for the evaluation of the ecotoxicity of non-steroidal anti-inflammatory drugs (NSAIDs). Toxicol. Vitr. 23: 935–942. Doi:10.1016/j.tiv.2009.04.014.

Parolini, M., A. Binelli and A. Provini. 2011a. Chronic effects induced by ibuprofen on the freshwater bivalve *Dreissena polymorpha*. Ecotoxicol. Environ. Saf. 74: 1586–1594. Doi:10.1016/j.ecoenv.2011.04.025.

Parolini, M., B. Quinn, A. Binelli and A. Provini. 2011b. Cytotoxicity assessment of four pharmaceutical compounds on the zebra mussel (*Dreissena polymorpha*) haemocytes, gill and digestive gland primary cell cultures. Chemosphere. 84: 91–100. Doi:10.1016/j.chemosphere.2011.02.049.

Patil, H.J., A. Benet-Perelberg, A. Naor, M. Smirnov, T. Ofek, A. Nasser et al. 2016. Evidence of increased antibiotic resistance in phylogenetically-diverse aeromonas isolates from semi-intensive fish ponds treated with antibiotics. Front. Microbiol. 7: 1875. Doi:10.3389/fmicb.2016.01875.

Paul, K.B., J.M. Hedge, M.J. DeVito and K.M. Crofton. 2010. Short-term exposure to triclosan decreases thyroxine *in vivo* via upregulation of hepatic catabolism in Young Long-Evans rats. Toxicol. Sci. 113: 367–79. Doi:10.1093/toxsci/kfp271.

Pedersen, K.L., S.N. Pedersen, L.B. Christiansen, B. Korsgaard and P. Bjerregaard. 2000. The preservatives ethyl-, propyl- and butylparaben are oestrogenic in an *in vivo* fish assay. Pharmacol. Toxicol. 86: 110–113. Doi:10.1034/j.1600-0773.2000.pto860303.x.

Pessoa, G.P., N.C. de Souza, C.B. Vidal, J.A.C. Alves, P.I.M. Firmino, R.F. Nascimento et al. 2014. Occurrence and removal of estrogens in Brazilian wastewater treatment plants. Sci. Total Environ. 490: 288–295. Doi:10.1016/j.scitotenv.2014.05.008.

Pires, A., A.C.V. Almeida, R.J. Schneider, V.I. Esteves, F.J. Wrona, A.M.V.M. Soares et al. 2016. Hediste diversicolor as bioindicator of pharmaceutical pollution: Results from single and combined exposure to carbamazepine and caffeine. Comp. Biochem. Physiol. Part—C Toxicol. Pharmacol. 188: 30–38. Doi:10.1016/j.cbpc.2016.06.003.

Pruden, A., R.T. Pei, H. Storteboom and K. Carlson. 2006. Antibiotic resistance genes as emerging contaminants: Studies in northern Colorado. Environ. Sci. Technol. 40: 7445–7450. Doi:10.1021/es0604131.

Purdom, C.E., P.A. Hardiman, V.V.J. Bye, N.C. Eno, C.R. Tyler and J.P. Sumpter. 1994. Estrogenic effects of effluents from sewage treatment works. Chem. Ecol. 8: 275–285. Doi:10.1080/02757549408038554.

Quinn, B., F. Gagné and C. Blaise. 2008. An investigation into the acute and chronic toxicity of eleven pharmaceuticals (and their solvents) found in wastewater effluent on the cnidarian, Hydra attenuata. Sci. Total Environ. 389: 306–314. Doi:10.1016/j.scitotenv.2007.08.038.

Raftery, T.D., N. Jayasundara and R.T. Di Giulio. 2017. A bioenergetics assay for studying the effects of environmental stressors on mitochondrial function *in vivo* in zebrafish larvae. Comp. Biochem. Physiol. Part C Toxicol. Pharmacol. 192: 23–32. Doi:10.1016/j.cbpc.2016.12.001.

Rajapakse, N., E. Silva and A. Kortenkamp. 2002. Combining xenoestrogens at levels below individual no-observed-effect concentrations dramatically enhances steroid hormone action. Environ. Health Perspect. 110: 917–921. Doi:10.1289/ehp.02110917.

Reyhanian, N., K. Volkova, S. Hallgren, T. Bollner, P.E. Olsson, H. Olsén et al. 2011. 17α-Ethinyl estradiol affects anxiety and shoaling behavior in adult male zebra fish (*Danio rerio*). Aquat. Toxicol. 105: 41–48. Doi:10.1016/j.aquatox.2011.05.009.

Rhee, J.S., B.M. Kim, C.B. Jeong, H.G. Park, K.M.Y. Leung, Y.M. Lee et al. 2013. Effect of pharmaceuticals exposure on acetylcholinesterase (AchE) activity and on the expression of AchE gene in the monogonont rotifer, *Brachionus koreanus*. Comp. Biochem. Physiol. -C Toxicol. Pharmacol. 158: 216–224. Doi:10.1016/j.cbpc.2013.08.005.

Riva, C., S. Cristoni and A. Binelli. 2012. Effects of triclosan in the freshwater mussel *Dreissena polymorpha*: A proteomic investigation. Aquat. Toxicol. 118: 62–71. Doi:10.1016/j.aquatox.2012.03.013.

Rocco, L., G. Frenzilli, D. Fusco, C. Peluso and V. Stingo. 2010. Evaluation of zebrafish DNA integrity after exposure to pharmacological agents present in aquatic environments. Ecotoxicol. Environ. Saf. 73: 1530–1536. Doi:10.1016/j.ecoenv.2010.07.032.

Rodgers-Gray, T.P., S. Jobling, C. Kelly, S. Morris, G. Brighty, M.J. Waldock et al. 2001. Exposure of Juvenile roach (*Rutilus rutilus*) to treated sewage effluent induces dose-dependent and persistent disruption in gonadal duct development. Environ. Sci. Technol. 35: 462–470. Doi:10.1021/es001225c.

Rodrigues, F., M. Lehmann, V.S. do Amaral, M.L. Reguly and H.H.R. de Andrade. 2007. Genotoxicity of three mouthwash products, Cepacol®, Periogard®, and Plax®, in the Drosophila wing-spot test. Environ. Mol. Mutagen. 48: 644–649. Doi:10.1002/em.20332.

Rodríguez, P.E.A. and M.S. Sanchez. 2010. Maternal exposure to triclosan impairs thyroid homeostasis and female pubertal development in wistar rat offspring. J. Toxicol. Environ. Heal. Part A. 73: 1678–1688. Doi:10.1080/15287394.2010.516241.

Routledge, E.J., J. Parker, J. Odum, J. Ashby and J.P. Sumpter. 1998a. Some alkyl hydroxy benzoate preservatives (parabens) are estrogenic. Toxicol. Appl. Pharmacol. 153: 12–9. Doi:10.1006/taap.1998.8544.

Routledge, E.J., D. Sheahan, C. Desbrow, G.C. Brighty, M. Waldock and J.P. Sumpter. 1998b. Identification of estrogenic chemicals in STW effluent. 2. *In vivo* responses in trout and roach. Environ. Sci. Technol. 32: 1559–1565. Doi:10.1021/es970796a.

Russell, L.B. and C.S. Montgomery. 1980. Use of the mouse spot test to investigate the mutagenic potential of triclosan (Irgasan®DP300). Mutat. Res. Toxicol. 79: 7–12. Doi:10.1016/0165-1218(80)90142-1.

Saggioro, E.M., A.S. Oliveira, T. Pavesi, M.J. Tototzintle, M.I. Maldonado, F.V. Correia et al. 2014. Solar CPC pilot plant photocatalytic degradation of bisphenol A in waters and wastewaters using suspended and supported-TiO_2. Influence of photogenerated species. Environ. Sci. Pollut. Res. 21: 12112–12121. Doi:10.1007/s11356-014-2723-0.

Saley, A., M. Hess, K. Miller, D. Howard and T.C. King-Heiden. 2016. Cardiac toxicity of triclosan in developing zebrafish. Zebrafish. 13: 399–404. Doi:10.1089/zeb.2016.1257.

Salimi, A., S. Eybagi, E. Seydi, P. Naserzadeh, N.P. Kazerouni and J. Pourahmad. 2016. Toxicity of macrolide antibiotics on isolated heart mitochondria: a justification for their cardiotoxic adverse effect. Xenobiotica. 46: 82–93. Doi:10.3109/00498254.2015.1046975.

Schmid, T., J. Gonzalez-Valero, H. Rufli and D.R. Dietrich. 2002. Determination of vitellogenin kinetics in male fathead minnows (*Pimephales promelas*). Toxicol. Lett. 131: 65–74. Doi:10.1016/S0378-4274(02)00043-7.

Shim, J., L.M. Weatherly, R.H. Luc, M.T. Dorman, A. Neilson, R. Ng et al. 2016. Triclosan is a mitochondrial uncoupler in live zebrafish. J. Appl. Toxicol. 36: 1662–1667. Doi:10.1002/jat.3311.

Siddiqui, W.H. and H.S. Buttar. 1979. Pharmacokinetics of triclosan in rat after intravenous and intravaginal administration. J. Environ. Pathol. Toxicol. 2: 861–71.

Singer, H., S. Müller, C. Tixier and L. Pillonel. 2002. Triclosan: Occurrence and fate of a widely used biocide in the aquatic environment: Field measurements in wastewater treatment plants, surface waters, and lake sediments. Environ. Sci. Technol. 36: 4998–5004. Doi:10.1021/es025750i.

Soares, J., A.M. Coimbra, M.A. Reis-Henriques, N.M. Monteiro, M.N. Vieira, J.M.A. Oliveira et al. 2009. Disruption of zebrafish (*Danio rerio*) embryonic development after full life-cycle parental exposure to low levels of ethinylestradiol. Aquat. Toxicol. 95: 330–338. Doi:10.1016/j.aquatox.2009.07.021.

Söffker, M., J.R. Stevens and C.R. Tyler. 2012. Comparative breeding and behavioral responses to ethinylestradiol exposure in wild and laboratory maintained zebrafish (*Danio rerio*) populations. Environ. Sci. Technol. 46: 11377–11383. Doi:10.1021/es302416w.

Solé, M., D. Raldua, F. Piferrer, D. Barceló and C. Porte. 2003. Feminization of wild carp, *Cyprinus carpio*, in a polluted environment: Plasma steroid hormones, gonadal morphology and xenobiotic metabolizing system. Comp. Biochem. Physiol.—C Toxicol. Pharmacol. 136: 145–156. Doi:10.1016/S1532-0456(03)00192-3.

Soni, M.G., G.A. Budrdok and S.L. Taylor. 2001. Safety assesment of propyl paraben: a review of the published literature. Food Chem. Toxicol. 39: 513–532.

Soni, M.G., I.G. Carabin and G.A. Burdock. 2005. Safety assessment of esters of p-hydroxybenzoic acid (parabens). Food Chem. Toxicol. 43: 985–1015. Doi:10.1016/j.fct.2005.01.020.

Tamura, I., M. Saito, Y. Nishimura, M. Satoh, H. Yamamoto and Y. Oyama. 2011. Elevation of intracellular Ca^{2+} level by triclosan in rat thymic lymphocytes: Increase in membrane Ca^{2+} permeability and induction of intracellular Ca^{2+} release. J. Heal. Sci. 57: 540–546. Doi:10.1248/jhs.57.540.

Terasaki, M., M. Makino and N. Tatarazako. 2009. Acute toxicity of parabens and their chlorinated by-products with *Daphnia magna* and *Vibrio fischeri* bioassays. J. Appl. Toxicol. 29: 242–247. Doi:10.1002/jat.1402.

Ternes, T.A. 1998. Occurrence of drugs in German sewage treatment plants and rivers. Water Res. 32: 3245–3260. Doi:10.1016/S0043-1354(98)00099-2.

Ternes, T.A., M. Stumpf, J. Mueller, K. Haberer, R.D. Wilken and M. Servos. 1999. Behavior and occurrence of estrogens in municipal sewage treatment plants—I. Investigations in Germany, Canada and Brazil. Sci. Total Environ. 225: 81–90. Doi:10.1016/S0048-9697(98)00334-9.

Thibaut, R. and C. Porte. 2008. Effects of fibrates, anti-inflammatory drugs and antidepressants in the fish hepatoma cell line PLHC-1: Cytotoxicity and interactions with cytochrome P450 1A. Toxicol. Vitr. 22: 1128–1135. Doi:10.1016/j.tiv.2008.02.020.

Thorpe, K.L., R.I. Cummings, T.H. Hutchinson, M. Scholze, G. Brighty, J.P. Sumpter et al. 2003. Relative potencies and combination effects of steroidal estrogens in fish. Environ. Sci. Technol. 37: 1142–1149. Doi:10.1021/es0201348.

Thorpe, K.L., M. Gross-Sorokin, I. Johnson, G. Brighty and C.R. Tyler. 2006. An assessment of the model of concentration addition for predicting the estrogenic activity of chemical mixtures in wastewater treatment works effluents. Environ. Health Perspect. 114: 90–97. Doi:10.1289/ehp.8059.

Tixier, C., H.P. Singer, S. Oellers and S.R. Müller. 2003. Occurrence and fate of carbamazepine, clofibric acid, diclofenac, ibuprofen, ketoprofen, and naproxen in surface waters. Environ. Sci. Technol. 37: 1061–1068. Doi:10.1021/es025834r.

Tsiaka, P., V. Tsarpali, I. Ntaikou, M.N. Kostopoulou, G. Lyberatos and S. Dailianis. 2013. Carbamazepine-mediated pro-oxidant effects on the unicellular marine algal species Dunaliella tertiolecta and the hemocytes of mussel *Mytilus galloprovincialis*. Ecotoxicology. 22: 1208–1220. Doi:10.1007/s10646-013-1108-3.

USFDA, U.S.F. and D.A. 2008. Nomination Profile Triclosan [CAS 3380-34-5] Supporting Information for Toxicological Evaluation by the National Toxicology Program July 2008.

Van Den Belt, K., P. Berckmans, C. Vangenechten, R. Verheyen and H. Witters. 2004. Comparative study on the *in vitro/in vivo* estrogenic potencies of 17β-estradiol, estrone, 17α-ethynylestradiol and nonylphenol. Aquat. Toxicol. 66: 183–195. Doi:10.1016/j.aquatox.2003.09.004.

van den Brandhof, E.J. and M. Montforts. 2010. Fish embryo toxicity of carbamazepine, diclofenac and metoprolol. Ecotoxicol. Environ. Saf. 73: 1862–1866. Doi:10.1016/j.ecoenv.2010.08.031.

Vernouillet, G., P. Eullaffroy, A. Lajeunesse, C. Blaise, F. Gagné and P. Juneau. 2010. Toxic effects and bioaccumulation of carbamazepine evaluated by biomarkers measured in organisms of different trophic levels. Chemosphere. 80: 1062–1068. Doi:10.1016/j.chemosphere.2010.05.010.

Voisin, A.S., A. Fellous, R.L. Earley and F. Silvestre. 2016. Delayed impacts of developmental exposure to 17α-ethinylestradiol in the self-fertilizing fish *Kryptolebias marmoratus*. Aquat. Toxicol. 180: 247–257. Doi:10.1016/j.aquatox.2016.10.003.

Volkova, K., N. Reyhanian Caspillo, T. Porseryd, S. Hallgren, P. Dinnétz and I. Porsch-Hällström. 2015. Developmental exposure of zebrafish (*Danio rerio*) to 17α-ethinylestradiol affects non-reproductive behavior and fertility as adults, and increases anxiety in unexposed progeny. Horm. Behav. 73: 30–38. Doi:10.1016/j.yhbeh.2015.05.014.

Wan, J., P. Guo, X. Peng and K. Wen. 2015. Effect of erythromycin exposure on the growth, antioxidant system and photosynthesis of Microcystis flos-aquae. J. Hazard. Mater. 283: 778–786. Doi:10.1016/j.jhazmat.2014.10.026.

Wang, L., Y. Peng, X. Nie, B. Pan, P. Ku and S. Bao. 2016. Gene response of CYP360A, CYP314, and GST and whole-organism changes in *Daphnia magna* exposed to ibuprofen. Comp. Biochem. Physiol. Part—C Toxicol. Pharmacol. 179: 49–56. Doi:10.1016/j.cbpc.2015.08.010.

Welk, A., M. Rosin, C. Lüdtke, C. Schwahn, A. Kramer and G. Daeschlein. 2007. The peritoneal explant test for evaluating tissue tolerance to mouthrinses. Skin Pharmacol. Physiol. 20: 162–166. Doi:10.1159/000098703.

Woo, P.T.K. and D.W. Bruno. (eds.). 2011. Fish diseases and disorders. Volume 3: viral, bacterial and fungal infections. CABI, Wallingford. Doi:10.1079/9781845935542.0000.

Xiu-Sheng, M., B. Farida, M. Chen and C.D. Metcalfe. 2004. Occurrence of Antimicrobials in the Final Effluents of Wastewater Treatment Plants in Canada. Doi:10.1021/ES030653Q.

Xuereb, B., E. Lefèvre, J. Garric and O. Geffard. 2009. Acetylcholinesterase activity in *Gammarus fossarum* (Crustacea Amphipoda): Linking AChE inhibition and behavioural alteration. Aquat. Toxicol. 94: 114–122. Doi:10.1016/j.aquatox.2009.06.010.

Yamamoto, H., Y. Nakamura, Y. Nakamura, C. Kitani, T. Imari, J. Sekizawa et al. 2007. Initial ecological risk assessment of eight selected human pharmaceuticals in Japan. Environ. Sci. 14: 177–93.

Yamamoto, H., I. Tamura, Y. Hirata, J. Kato, K. Kagota, S. Katsuki et al. 2011. Aquatic toxicity and ecological risk assessment of seven parabens: Individual and additive approach. Sci. Total Environ. 410-411: 102–111. Doi:10.1016/j.scitotenv.2011.09.040.

Yang, L.-H., G.-G. Ying, H.-C. Su, J.L. Stauber, M.S. Adams and M.T. Binet. 2008. Growth-inhibiting effects of 12 antibacterial agents and their mixtures on the freshwater microalga *Pseudokirchneriella subcapitata*. Environ. Toxicol. Chem. 27: 1201. Doi:10.1897/07-471.1.

Yao, L., Y. Wang, L. Tong, Y. Deng, Y. Li, Y. Gan et al. 2017. Occurrence and risk assessment of antibiotics in surface water and groundwater from different depths of aquifers: A case study at Jianghan Plain, central China. Ecotoxicol. Environ. Saf. 135: 236–242. Doi:10.1016/j.ecoenv.2016.10.006.

Ye, X., X. Guo, X. Cui, X. Zhang, H. Zhang, M.K. Wang, L. Qiu and S. Chen. 2012. Occurrence and removal of endocrine-disrupting chemicals in wastewater treatment plants in the three Gorges Reservoir area, Chongqing, China. J. Environ. Monit. 14: 2204. Doi:10.1039/c2em30258f.

Yueh, M.-F., K. Taniguchi, S. Chen, R.M. Evans, B.D. Hammock, M. Karin et al. 2014. The commonly used antimicrobial additive triclosan is a liver tumor promoter. Source Proc. Natl. Acad. Sci. United States Am. 111: 17200–17205.

Zacharewski, T. 1997. *In vitro* bioassays for assessing estrogenic substances. Environ. Sci. Technol. 31: 613–623. Doi:10.1021/es960530o.

Zhang, W., M. Zhang, K. Lin, W. Sun, B. Xiong, M. Guo et al. 2012. Eco-toxicological effect of Carbamazepine on *Scenedesmus obliquus* and *Chlorella pyrenoidosa*. Environ. Toxicol. Pharmacol. 33: 344–352. Doi:10.1016/j.etap.2011.12.024.

Zhang, Y., S.-U. Geißen and C. Gal. 2008. Carbamazepine and diclofenac: Removal in wastewater treatment plants and occurrence in water bodies. Chemosphere. 73: 1151–1161. Doi:10.1016/j.chemosphere.2008.07.086.

Zorrilla, L.M., E.K. Gibson, S.C. Jeffay, K.M. Crofton, W.R. Setzer, R.L. Cooper et al. 2009. The effects of triclosan on puberty and thyroid hormones in male wistar rats. Toxicol. Sci. 107: 56–64. Doi:10.1093/toxsci/kfn225.

6

Risk Assessment of Organic UV Filters in Aquatic Ecosystems

M. Silvia Díaz-Cruz* and *Daniel Molins-Delgado*

Introduction

In the beginning of this decade, 22% of the world population was over 50 years old; by 2020, this will increase up to 25% (Persistence Market Research 2015). Of all demographic changes, the ageing population has had the strongest impact on beauty and personal care product (PCPs). As a consequence, greater importance to fighting the ageing process than other areas of beauty and personal care has been recorded. In another plain, we find that especially in developing countries, the growing urban population and the increasing per capita spending power is boosting the growth in PCPs industry, as more people work together and the awareness of personal appearance and hygiene becomes important.

The PCPs' global market in 2015 was US$ 465 billion, and it is expected to increase over the next years, with an estimate of US$ 500 billion by 2020 (Persistence Market Research 2015).

Asia Pacific represents the largest share, with 29% of the global PCPs market (EuroPlat 2015), followed by Europe (Premium Beauty News 2015) and by North America (TechSci Research 2014). Within the Asian region, China still is the largest market for PCPs. For the next five years, sales are expected to grow over 8%, with estimated income at US$ 28.2 billion (Gentlemen Marketing Agency 2014). Additionally, the recent introduction of the two-child policy is expected to boost the baby and child-specific care and hygiene products' market (Euromonitor International 2016).

Institute of Environmental Assessment and Water Research (IDÆA), Spanish Council of Scientific Research (CSIC), Jordi Girona 18-26, 08034, Barcelona, Spain.
E-mail: danielmolinsdelgado@gmail.com
* Corresponding author: sdcqam@cid.csic.es

Personal beauty and hygiene products' market is evidently an expanding and increasingly diverse market. Product categories include skin, dental, hair and nail care products, cosmetics, fragrances, bathing and shaving creams and lotions, among others. The chemical ingredients of these products involve many different compounds, such as surfactants, emulsifiers, emollients, pigments and UV filters, among others (Gago-Ferrero et al. 2011a, Transparency Market Research 2015, Molins-Delgado et al. 2016a). The ingredients in PCPs market are growing in parallel; with US$ 7.46 billion in 2014, it is expected to reach US$ 11.76 billion in the next ten years (Transparency Market Research 2015). In terms of quantity produced, global annual PCPs production in 2008 was over one million tons, and is just expected to increase (Champagne 2008).

The increasing use of these ingredients also increases the concern for their introduction into the environment (Molins-Delgado et al. 2015a). As a consequence of their constant use and release, these compounds are classified as pseudo-persistent emerging contaminants irrespective of their features as persistent, bio-accumulative and toxic substances. As to other chemicals of this kind, a lack of regulations regarding their presence in the environment is still observed. This may be troublesome as the eco-toxicological effects that PCPs may display in short (acute) and long term (chronic) are mostly unknown. Besides, there is still a lack of data on their occurrence, fate and impacts on the environment (Zenker et al. 2014).

Within PCPs, UV filters (UVFs), also known as sunscreens, are a popular group of photo-chemical compounds able to absorb, reflect or scatter the damaging solar UV radiation. Their extended use relays mostly in the increased public awareness about the detrimental effects of UV sunlight. We must not forget that controlled sun exposure has beneficial effects, such as the production of vitamin D, which favors calcium absorption, especially important in children and old people. However, over-exposition to sun leads to severe skin and eye damage. Thus, the addition of UVFs to PCPs seeks to protect our skin, hair and nails from sunburns, photoaging, photocarcirogenesis, and photoinmunosupression (Whitmore and Morison 1995, Seité et al. 2000, Liardet et al. 2001).

UVFs can be classified into two groups: inorganic, such as TiO_2 and ZnO, and organic, which encompasses a wide range of molecules (benzophenones, benzotriazoles, crylenes, camphors, etc.). In organic UVFs, their UV absorption properties (UVA: 400–320 nm and UVB: 320–280 nm) are the result of their high conjugation with carbonyl groups in the chemical structure, along with the presence of aromatic benzyl rings and chromophore groups. UVFs are generally lipophilic substances having a wide spectrum of octanol-water partition coefficients (K_{ow}) (Li et al. 2007, Zenker et al. 2008). Given their properties, UVFs are also widely applied in different industrial sectors; they are common additives in plastics and textiles to avoid photo-degradation (preventing yellowing and polymers' degradation). Furthermore, ink, paint, and photography industries use them extensively to avoid decoloration (Zenker et al. 2008).

With some UVF agents reaching production above 1,000 tons per year, they are considered High Production Volume Chemicals (HPVC). The bulk of production of UVFs in the world is estimated to be over 10,000 tons per year (Danovaro et al. 2008), with North America and Europe as the biggest markets. However, its market share is increasing year after year, and is expected to be over $ 672 million by 2021. One of the most cited reasons for the huge increase in demand for UVFs is the extensive use of anti-aging products, as aforementioned (Lucintel 2016).

Legislation exists in some countries, although these regulations only take into consideration the security of the consumers, rather than the environmental risk. Taking as an example the biggest markets for UVFs, in the European Union, UVFs are regulated by the regulation 1223/2009/EC on cosmetic products (The European Parliament and the Council of the European Union 2009), whereas in the USA, it is done through the Cosmetic Act and Title 21 of the Federal Regulations (21 CFR) (The Congress of the United States 1938), both rules focusing on maximum levels allowed and banned compounds in consumer goods. At an environmental level, the Water Framework Watch List has included, in recent years, the sunscreen agent ethylhexyl methoxycinamate (EHMC) for review and future potential regulation (Tavazzi et al. 2016).

Due to their continuous use, release into the environment, and the wide range of physicochemical properties that UVFs possess, they tend to end, retained not only in environmental matrixes such as sediments and suspended particulate matter (Zhang et al. 2011, Gago-Ferrero et al. 2011a), but also in living organisms (Rodil and Moeder 2008, Gago-Ferrero et al. 2013a). The concern about the potential adverse effects that UVFs and their transformation products (TPs) may pose to living organisms has been on the rise during the last years and some efforts have been made in order to characterise them. Some *in vitro* (Morohoshi et al. 2005, Kunz et al. 2006, Danovaro et al. 2008) and *in vivo* (Kunz et al. 2006, Weisbrod et al. 2007, Danovaro et al. 2008) bioassays have been performed in order to determine the potential hormonal effects of some of these compounds, as well as their acute and chronic eco-toxicity (Seeland et al. 2012, Molins-Delgado et al. 2016a). Because of their continuous emissions into the environment, poor biodegradability and physicochemical properties, the estimation of the potential risk posed by these compounds has gained interest. Environmental risk assessment (ERA) attempts to examine those risks from a quantitative view point (Molins-Delgado et al. 2015b).

In this chapter, we address organic UV filters by reviewing and compiling the literature available on their occurrence, eco-toxicity and risk assessment in the aquatic environment.

Occurrence of UV Filters in the Aquatic Environment

With the advances in science and technology, thousands of new chemical compounds have been developed in order to improve the yields of crops, the production of animal farms and forestry, and to improve, in general terms, our quality of life (Edinger et al. 1998, Bainbridge et al. 2009, Wang et al. 2011). This has fuelled the introduction of anthropogenic chemical compounds into the environment, a widespread occurrence that reaches nearly all the planet, from urban and rural areas (Gago-Ferrero et al. 2011a, Serra-Roig et al. 2016), to remote places like Antarctica (Emnet et al. 2015). Like other emerging organic pollutants, UVFs are no exception, and can be found almost everywhere.

The fate and distribution of these chemicals into the different environmental compartments are governed by their physicochemical properties. UVFs are soluble in water; they mostly show water solubility constants in the mg L^{-1} range (Díaz-Cruz et al. 2008, Rodil et al. 2009a). Dissociation in water phase under environmental pH conditions of UVFs is not likely to happen as their acid dissociation constant, pKa, is generally higher than six. In solid phases, sorption is the driving force that determines their mobility. As aforementioned, generally these compounds have log K_{ow} values higher than three which make them sorb onto sewage sludge, soil, sediments, and suspended particulate matter, and to accumulate in tissues of living organisms. The high soil organic-water partition coefficient (K_{oc}) for UVFs, with values usually far above 2,000, make them tend to be retained rather than to pass through the solid phase. Similarly, the bio-concentration factor (BCF) for most of these chemicals is extremely high, with values exceeding 600,000. Accordingly, they can readily bio-accumulate in the living organisms. In contrast, volatilization from the water surface or from sediment and soil is a phenomenon rather unlikely as their low Henry's constants (10^{-6}–10^{-8} atm m^3 mol^{-1}) show.

UVFs reach the environment both directly and indirectly. The direct entry is through recreational activities such as bathing in natural waters. The American Dermatology Association (ADA 2016) estimates that beachgoers spend 4 h on the beach and use over 72 g of sunscreen in that time. More than 25% of the sunscreen applied on the skin washes off when entering the water (Danovaro et al. 2008), and taking into account that between 5–20% of the product, depending on the different regulations worldwide, are UV filters (Sánchez-Quiles and Tovar-Sánchez 2015), the quantity released into the water is of concern. Other important pathway on the rise is cruise travel in marine water. Cruises represent 2% of the total leisure travel market. The United Nations World Tourism Organization (UNWTO 2016) estimates that the growth of this holiday sector in the decade 2004 to 2014 has reached 20% (UNWTO 2016). The Cruise Lines International Association (CLIA) announced that throughout 2015, 23.2 million people cruised. This figure exceeded by 4% that registered in the previous year (CLIA 2017).

UVFs indirect entry pathways to the environment include run-offs and domestic and industrial discharges. Pollutants released through indirect pathways generally end up in wastewater treatment plants (WWTPs) where they will be removed with more or less efficiency depending on their physicochemical properties. Most lipophilic compounds will be adsorbed onto the sludge, whereas the more polar ones, when not biodegraded, will be released back into natural waters through the WWTP effluent. The use of the sewage sludge as fertilizer in agriculture is a common practice, but it may also end up dumped in landfills. Both ends extend the potential impact of the recalcitrant UVFs on surface and groundwater. Moreover, pollutants released into the aquatic environment by the WWTPs may be retained in the sediment and the suspended particulate matter of the water bodies, and a fraction of it may be accumulated in the ecosystems' living organisms (Molins-Delgado et al. 2015a).

Table 1. Worldwide UVF concentrations in natural, swimming pool and spa waters.

Location	Compounds	Concentrations	Matrix	Reference
Natural Waters				
Antarctica	BP1, BP3, 4MBC, EHMC	0.5–7 ng l⁻¹	Seawater and ice water	Emnet et al. 2015
China	BP3, OC	0.1–547 ng l⁻¹	River and estuarine water	Min et al. 2014
Germany	BP3, BP4, 4MBC, OC, EHMC, ODPABA, BD-DBM, EHS, HMS	40–4,381 ng l⁻¹	Lake water	Rodil et al. 2009b
Greece	BP3, 4MBC, EHMC	1.8–6.9 ng l⁻¹	Seawater and bathing water	Giokas et al. 2004
Italy	BP3, OC, EHMC	3.–122 ng l⁻¹	River and seawater	Magi et al. 2012
Japan	BP3, 4MBC, ODPABA, OC, EHMC, HMS, UV120, UV234, UV326, UV327, UV328, UV329, UV1577	6–4,780 ng l⁻¹	River water	Kameda et al. 2011
Slovenia	BP3, OC, EHMC, ODPABA, HMS	35–345 ng l⁻¹	River water	Cuderman and Heath 2007
Spain	BP1, BP3, BP3, 4DHB, 4MBC, EtPABA	24.9–73.1 ng l⁻¹	River water and groundwater	Serra-Roig et al. 2016
Switzerland	BP3, BP4, 4MBC, EHMC	6–68 ng l⁻¹	River water	Fent et al. 2010
UK	BP1, BP2, BP3, BP4	0.3–1,293 ng l⁻¹	River water	Kasprzyk-Hordern et al. 2008
Swimming pool and spa water				
Greece	BP3, 4MBC, EHMC	3–6.9 ng l⁻¹	Swimming pool water	Giokas et al. 2004
Greece	BP3, ODPABA	2.4–3.3 µg l⁻¹	Swimming pool water	Lambropoulou et al. 2002
Slovenia	BP3, 4MBC, OC, EHMC, ODPABA, HMS	27–266 ng l⁻¹	Swimming pool water	Cuderman and Heath 2007
Spain	BP1, BP2, BP3, DHMB, THB, 4DHB, 4MBC, ODPABA, BZT, MeBZT, DMeBZT	1.2–69.3 ng l⁻¹	Swimming pool and spa water	Ekowati et al. 2016

Additionally, even more recalcitrant UVFs may end up in the drinking water supply, impacting the general population (Díaz-Cruz et al. 2012, Rodil et al. 2012).

Sparse data exist on the concentrations of UVFs in the environment. An overview of UVFs' reported concentrations in different matrices is presented in Tables 1 to 4. UVFs, especially those whose Log K_{ow} are low, such as benzophenone derivatives,

Table 2. Worldwide UVF concentrations in sediment.

Location	Compounds	Concentrations	Matrix	Reference
Sediment				
Chile Colombia	BP3, 4MBC, EHMC	1.05–47.1 ng g^{-1} dw	River and coastal sediment	Barón et al. 2013
China	UV326, UV327, UV328, TBHPBT	0.4–3.8 ng g^{-1} dw	River sediment	Zhang et al. 2011
Japan	BP3, 4MBC, ODPABA, OC, EHMC, HMS, UV120, UV234, UV326, UV327, UV328, UV329, UV1577	0.1–1,266 ng g^{-1} dw	River sediment	Kameda et al. 2011
Norway	BP3, EHMC, OC, UV324, UV327, UV328, UV329	5–25.1 ng g^{-1} dw	Marine sediment	Langford et al. 2015
Spain	BP3, 4DHB, 4MBC, OC, ODPABA	0.8–570 ng g^{-1} dw	River sediments	Gago-Ferrero et al. 2011a

have impacted all sort of water bodies across the world, as can be seen in Table 1. Reported concentrations are: seawater 0.5–7 ng l^{-1} (Emnet et al. 2015), lake water 40–4,381 ng l^{-1} (Rodil et al. 2009b), river water 0.3–1,293 ng l^{-1} (Kasprzyk-Hordern et al. 2008), groundwater 25–73 ng l^{-1} (Serra-Roig et al. 2016), and swimming pool and spa water 1.2–266 ng l^{-1} (Lambropoulou et al. 2002, Giokas et al. 2004, Cuderman and Heath 2007, Ekowati et al. 2016).

Sediments show concentrations of UVFs whose LogK$_{ow}$ is higher, such as 4-methylbenzylidene-camphor (4MBC), octocrylene (OC), and benzotriazole derivatives, in the range 0.1–1,266 ng g^{-1} dry weight (dw) (Kameda et al. 2011, Zhang et al. 2011, Gago-Ferrero et al. 2011a, Barón et al. 2013, Langford et al. 2015) (see Table 1). WWTPs and densely urbanised areas (including increased population by tourism) are pointed out as the major source of this UVF contamination (Kasprzyk-Hordern et al. 2008, Kameda et al. 2011, Emnet et al. 2015).

A number of studies, some of them compiled in Table 3, have shown that the removal of UVFs is incomplete, being able to detect UVFs in both influent and effluent wastewaters. Reported concentrations in the range 66–5,322 ng l^{-1} in influent streams from Germany (Rodil et al. 2009b) were comparable to those observed in effluent wastewaters from Norway (5–6,969 ng l^{-1}) (Langford et al. 2015). In sewage sludge from Switzerland, higher levels of more lipophilic UVFs were reported (Plagellat et al. 2006), reaching up to 27,700 µg g^{-1} dw.

Aquatic organisms are readily exposed to these pollutants, UVFs having been already reported in diverse species, as listed in Table 4. UVFs' residues bioaccumulate in fish and invertebrates from Norway (1–11,875 ng g^{-1} dw) (Langford et al. 2015) and the Antarctic ocean (0.9–1,450 ng g^{-1} lipid weight (lw)) (Emnet et al. 2015), in

Table 3. Worldwide UVF concentrations in wastewaters and sewage sludge.

Location	Compounds	Concentrations	Matrix	Reference
Wastewaters				
Antarctica	BP1, BP3, 4MBC, EHMC	30–11,700 ng l⁻¹	Effluent wastewaters	Emnet et al. 2015
Australia	BP3	32.7 ng l⁻¹	Effluent wastewaters	Liu et al. 2011
Germany	BP3, BP4, 4MBC, OC, EHMC, ODPABA, BD-DBM, EHS, HMS	66–5,322 ng l⁻¹; 3–179 ng l⁻¹	Influent wastewaters; Effluent wastewaters	Rodil et al. 2009b
Italy	BP3, OC, EHMC	23–551 ng l⁻¹; 5–21 ng l⁻¹	Influent wastewaters; Effluents wastewaters	Magi et al. 2012
Japan	BP3, 4MBC, ODPABA, OC, EHMC, HMS, UV120, UV234, UV326, UV327, UV328, UV329, UV1577	3–169 ng l⁻¹	Effluent wastewaters	Kameda et al. 2011
Norway	BP3, EHMC, OC, UV324, UV327, UV328, UV329	5–6,969 ng l⁻¹	Effluent wastewaters	Langford et al. 2015
USA	BP3, EHMC	0.1–10.4 µg l⁻¹; 0.6–1.3 µg l⁻¹	Influent wastewaters; Effluents wastewaters	Loraine and Pettigrove 2006
Sewage sludge				
Australia	BP3, 4MBC, OC, EHMC, UV326, UV329	32.9–250 ng g⁻¹ dw	Biosolids	Liu et al. 2011
China	UV234, UV329, UV326, UV328, UVP	20.6–67.8 ng g⁻¹ dw	Biosolids	Zhang et al. 2011
Norway	BP3, EHMC, OC, UV324, UV327, UV328, UV329	4–41,910 ng g⁻¹ dw	Biosolids	Langford et al. 2015
Spain	BP3, 4HB, 4DHB, 4MBC, OC, EHMC	0.1–9.2 µg g⁻¹ dw	Biosolids	Gago-Ferrero et al. 2011b
Switzerland	4MBC, OC, EHMC, OT	10–27,700 µg g⁻¹ dw	Biosolids	Plagellat et al. 2006

dolphin mother and foetus from Brazil (8.5–11,130 ng g⁻¹ lw) (Alonso et al. 2015, Gago-Ferrero et al. 2013b), revealing maternal transfer of UVFs, and in aquatic birds from Switzerland (340 ng g⁻¹ lw) (Fent et al. 2010), suggesting that biomagnification across the food web might be taking place (Fent et al. 2010).

Table 4. Worldwide UVF concentrations in freshwater and marine biota.

Matrix	Location	Species	Tissue	Compounds	Concentration	Reference
Fish	Antarctica	*Trematomus bernachii*	Muscle Liver	BP3	235–1,450 ng g^{-1} lw 1,690 ng g^{-1} lw	Emnet et al. 2015
	Norway	*Coregonus lavaretrus; Gadus morthua; Lota lota; Perca fluviatilis*	Muscle	BP3, EHMC, OC, UV324, UV327, UV328, UV329	2–11,875 ng g^{-1}	Langford et al. 2015
	Spain	*Anguilla anguilla; Barbus graellsii; Cyprinus carpio; Gobio lozanoi; Luciobarbus sclateri; Micropterus salmoides Salmo trutta; Silurus glanis*	Bulk	BP3, 4MBC, EHMC, OC	2.2–241.7 ng g^{-1} dw	Gago-Ferrero et al. 2015
	Switzerland	*Anguilla anguilla; Barbus barbus; Gammarus* sp.; *Leuciscus cephalus; Salmo trutta*	Muscle and adipose tissue	EHMC	49.2–172.5 ng g^{-1} lw	Fent et al. 2010
Mussel	Antarctica	*Laternula elliptica*	Muscle	BP3	1,690 ng g^{-1} lw	Emnet et al. 2015
	France	*Mytilus edulis; Mytilus galloprovincialis*	Soft tissue	EHMC, OC, ODPABA	2–7,122 ng g^{-1} dw	Bachelot et al. 2012
	Switzerland	*Dreissena polymorpha*	Muscle	EHMC	84.2 ng g^{-1} lw	Fent et al. 2010
Echinoidea	Antarctica	*Sterichinus neumayeri*	Bulk	BP3	0.9 ng g^{-1} ww	Emnet et al. 2015
Invertebrate	Norway	*Carcinus meanas; Pandalus borealis*	Bulk	BP3, EHMC, OC, UV324, UV327, UV328, UV329	10–68.9 ng g^{-1}	Langford et al. 2015
Dolphin	Brazil	*Franciscana*	Liver	OC	79–782 ng g^{-1} lw	Gago-Ferrero et al. 2013b
Dolphin pairs mother-foetus	Brazil	*Franciscana & Guiana*	Blubber Muscle Milk	4MBC, EHMC, OC, ODPABA	35.5–205 ng g^{-1} lw 45–11,130 ng g^{-1} lw 8.5–120 ng g^{-1} lw	Alonso et al. 2015
Aquatic bird	Switzerland	*Phalacrocoracidae* sp.	Muscle	EHMC	340 ng g^{-1} lw	Fent et al. 2010

Environmental Risk Assessment of UV Filters

So far, the potential risk of UVFs filter residues reaching the aquatic ecosystems has been poorly quantified. The minimum requirements for assessing ecological risk by UVFs are the accurate documentation of hazards and the realistic identification of the corresponding exposures that may exist. Despite the fact that in recent years, there has been an increase in data essential to estimate UVFs' environmental risk, it is still very limited and greatly fragmented. Available eco-toxicological information, because of the experimental test and analytical methods followed, is expressed in different concepts, i.e., concentration in lipid weight, in dry weight or wet weight. Moreover, as it is well known that the environmental prevalence of UVFs is season-dependent, with higher levels observed during the summer, the data obtained in different species, different seasons, bulk or different tissues, makes difficult the direct comparison among them. A consequence of this lack of harmonized information prevents the comprehensive understanding of their toxic mode of action and to perform reliable screening and prioritization of UVFs' environmental risk. Moreover, taking into account the continuous release of these chemicals into the water bodies, effects upon long-term exposure of aquatic organisms is still unknown as very few studies have addressed chronic toxicity (Sieratowicz et al. 2011).

When we mention UVFs' residues, we are referring to parent compounds, but also to their biotic (metabolites) and abiotic TPs. Nowadays, biotransformation processes are able to resemble liver metabolism and, thus, to produce derivatives of the parent compound with the same structural formula than those of the species metabolites. These commercial metabolites and TPs facilitate the environmental occurrence survey of these compounds. However, as these derivatives can exhibit even greater eco-toxicity than the corresponding parent compound, they should also be included in future environmental risk assessments for reliable outcomes.

Another issue also ignored is the bio-accumulative potential of most UVFs. Although a chemical is characterized by its low toxicity and low concentration in aquatic ecosystems, due to its strong lipophilicity, it can be present at high level in the living aquatic organisms, which makes it far more dangerous than could be considered based only on its toxicity and prevalence. So far, few studies have reported BCFs for a number of aquatic species. In this case, BCFs inform about the differential distribution of a certain UVF between the organism and the surrounding media. Depending on the tendency of a compound to accumulate in water or sediment, BCFs are estimated in relation to the environmental compartment in which it is mainly found. That is, for very polar UVFs, the relationship between UVF's concentration in the organism with respect to its concentration in water will be calculated; consequently, for the most apolar ones, it will be estimated considering its concentration in the sediment. In general, quite high BCFs are reported showing the strong tendency of these chemicals to be retained in the organisms' tissues, especially in the fatty ones. Available data shows BCFs, mostly with respect to water, above 1 and up to $6 \cdot 10^5$ (Giokas et al. 2007, HSDB 2011, USEPA 2012).

The number of studies on marine ecological risk assessment is far below the estimations performed on freshwater aquatic ecosystems. According to the European Commission Guidelines on risk assessment (European Commission 2003), the risk estimation in marine water is pretty similar to that in freshwater, with the exception of applying an assessment factor that can be from 10 to 10,000. Nevertheless, the toxicity information specific to marine species is very limited. As a consequence, the available toxicity data from fresh water organisms must be used. Nevertheless, at least one study exists documenting that this approach, most probably, may underestimate the risk of UVFs in the marine environment when using the same measured environmental concentrations (MEC) with freshwater-based parameters (Sang and Leung 2016).

In general, risk assessment is evaluated through the estimation of the hazard quotient (HQ), according to EMEA guideline (EMEA 2006). HQ represents the ratio between the MEC or predicted (PEC) concentrations of a certain substance and the predicted no-effect concentration (PNEC). When PNEC is not available, it is usually estimated by dividing reported no-observed effect concentration (NOEC) by a safety factor (Sanderson et al. 2003). Risk classification considers that HQ values above one represents high risk and values between 0.5 and 1.0, medium risk that might evolve to a future risk scenario. HQ ratios below 0.5 are associated to low risk (Molins-Delgado et al. 2015b, Gago-Ferrero et al. 2016). Usually, the worst-case scenario is set up by using maximum MECs or PECs and minimum PNECs or NOECs.

The data in Table 5 indicates that UVFs pose several ecological risks to the aquatic ecosystems. These risks involve coral bleaching, hindered reproduction in fish, and growth inhibition in algae.

As aforementioned, eco-toxicological data considered for risk estimation is quite fragmented and sparse. Therefore, the comparison among risk assessment for different compounds and/or different scenarios must be taken with caution. Bioassays conducted to estimate required information such as PNEC or NOEC values, usually differ in time of exposure, the species assayed, and the endpoint selected. Moreover, in general, mixtures of different UVFs are reported to exist; cumulative risk should be estimated for more accurate risk classification. Thus, cumulative HQs (CHQs) are calculated as the addition of individual HQs where more than one UVF is measured. Despite the simplicity of the approach, to the author's knowledge, only one study has reported cumulative HQs for a set of UVFs (Serra-Roig et al. 2016). In river water, CHQs (at 48 h exposure) for *Daphnia magna* were in the range $3E^{-2}$ and $1.3E^{-2}$, for *Pimephales promelea* $7.6E^{-2}$, and between $2.6E^{-2}$ and $1.5E^{-2}$ for *Ceriodaphnia dubia*. In the light of these preliminary results, mixture eco-toxicity should be considered in next environmental risk assessments.

In view of these results, marine environments are at risk and would be threatened mainly by BP3, 4-MBC and EHMC residues. Inland ecosystems appear to be at moderate risk by the occurrence of BP3, EHMC, and MeBZT, most likely due to discharge of effluents. At any rate, the fragmented information so far available makes us to not rule out major current and future risks for the environment.

Table 5. Hazard Quotients (HQs) from different aquatic organisms of organic UVFs.

Country	Water Source	UVF	HQ	Reference
Norway	Effluent	BP3	0.00004	Langford et al. 2015
		OC	0.00003	
	Surface water-Effluent	BP3	0.06	
		OC	0.01	
	Surface water-Leach	BP3	0.03	
		OC	0.002	
Switzerland	Surface water	BP3	0.09	Kim and Choi 2014
USA	Influent		**5.20**	
USA	Influent		**7.88**	
Spain	Influent	BP4	0.01–0.04	Molins-Delgado et al. 2016b
	Effluent		0.01–0.02	
	Influent		0.08–0.30*	
	Effluent		0.02–0.22*	
Spain	Influent	BZT	0.01–**5.49**	Molins-Delgado et al. 2015b
	Effluent		0.01–0.04	
	Influent	MeBZT	0.01–**5.42**	
	Effluent		0.01–**1.23**	
Spain	Groundwater	BP1	4.9×10^{-4}–1×10^{-2}	Molins-Delgado et al. 2016a
		BP3	3.6×10^{-4}–6.5×10^{-3}	
		4HB	1.4×10^{-4}–1.8×10^{-4}	
		BP4	1.1×10^{-4}–1.2×10^{-3}	
		4MBC	1.2×10^{-3}–2.2×10^{-3}	
Spain	Marine water	BP3	0.1–**6.6**	Sánchez-Rodríguez et al. 2015
		4-MBC	0.1–**10.4**	
		EHMC	0.4–**18.9**	
Spain	River water	4DHB	1.6×10^{-4}	Serra-Roig et al. 2016
		BP1	1.2×10^{-3}–3×10^{-3}	
		BP3	1.3×10^{-2}–3×10^{-2}	
		4-MBC	2×10^{-3}	
		BZT	1.5×10^{-2}–7.3×10^{-3}	
		MeBZT	6×10^{-2}–7.9×10^{-3}	
		BP1	5.8×10^{-4}	
	Groundwater	BP3	1.7×10^{-3}–2.3×10^{-3}	
		4-MBC	1.2×10^{-3}–4.8×10^{-3}	
		BZT	2.3×10^{-3}–2.1×10^{-2}	
		MeBZT	7.1×10^{-3}–9×10^{-2}	
China	River water impacted by effluents	EHMC	0.02–**23**	Tsui et al. 2014a
		BP3	0.02–**3.4**	
		4-MBC	0.02	
China	Surface water	BP1	0.001–0.06	Tsui et al. 2014b
USA		BP4	0.001–0.19	
		ODPABA	0.18	
China	Freshwater	BP3	0.04	Sang and Leung 2016
		4-MBC	0.07	
		EHMC	0.48	
		OC	< 0.001	
	Marine water	BP3	**5.94**	
		4-MBC	0.75	
		EHMC	**4.79**	
		OC	< 0.001	

*chronic toxicity values

Conclusions and Outlook

Environmental chemical pollution studies have shifted the focus in the last two decades from the well-known priority pollutants to the so-called emerging contaminants. Among them, organic UVFs constitute a group of current concern. Considering the continuous demand of toiletries and cosmetics, plastics and textiles products along with other industrial commodities containing UVFs, the volume of production and scope of application of these chemicals will increase in the coming years.

The lack of environmental regulation along with the scattered and scarce data available on their occurrence, fate and effects in the aquatic environment have led, in recent years, to the emergence of a number of works dealing with their ultimate impact on aquatic ecosystems. Despite the fact that it has become a hot topic in the scientific community, there is still knowledge gaps to be filled about this class of contaminants in the aquatic environment.

Summarising existing knowledge, organic UVFs are continuously released into the aquatic environment either directly or indirectly through recreational activities and WWTPs effluents after incomplete degradation, respectively. This makes UVFs to be pseudo-persistent pollutants, which invade all aquatic compartments worldwide.

The data on the environmental risk posed for UVFs is scattered and difficult to extrapolate from one scenario to another, from fresh water to marine water, from summer studies to winter assessments, from one species and another. Somehow, a harmonization of bioassays in time and species addressed, as well as the availability of occurrence data covering all the environmental compartments, would help to carry out a more comprehensive and truthful ecological risk assessment. Furthermore, as most likely under natural and technical waterways conditions, organic pollutants may undergo transformation processes; the TPs produced and emitted to the waters should be part of the different factors to judge the environmental hazard posed.

Additionally, due to the bio-magnification potential of some UVFs, these risks could be magnified through the marine and terrestrial food webs and ecological cycle. Thus, for a proper estimation of the hazards, the bioaccumulation potential of contaminants should be integrated within ecological risk assessment.

An approach to minimize such dramatic situation with no ending would be to improve source contamination control by both appropriate labelling on the products, which would include the hazard for the environment and proper use and disposal guidance, and by improving wastewater treatment technologies. Being more radical but still realistic, the ban on those substances of documented ecological risk should be set. These economic and political decisions are costly, time-consuming as well as require the general acceptance by consumers but also by hygiene and toiletry industries. New sunscreen active agents can be developed on the basis of an improved green/natural and environmental-friendly consumer practices.

Finally, further research on the eco-toxic potential of mixtures of UVFs is imperative. Moreover, given the large number of organic UV filters released into the aquatic ecosystems and time and cost restrictions, it is necessary to prioritize UVFs for worldwide monitoring and ecological risk assessment in the framework of the different water directives of each country. Progress on these topics should facilitate a scientific basis for suitable and rational regulation of organic UV filters and their TPs along with their release into aquatic ecosystems.

List of Abbreviations

ADA: American Dermatology Association; BCF: Bio-concentration factor; BD-DBM: Butylmethoxy-dibenzoylmethane; BP1: Benzophenone 1; BP2: Benzophenone 2; BP3: Benzophenone 3 (oxybenzone); BP4: Benzophenone 4; BZT: Benzotriazole; CHQs: Cumulative hazard quotients; CLIA: Cruise Lines International Association; 4DHB: 4,4'-Dihydroxybenzophenone; DHMB: 2,2'-dihydroxy-4-methoxybenzophenone; DMeBZT: Dimethyl benzotriazole; dw: Dry weight; EHMC: Ethylhexyl methoxycinamate; EHS: Ethylhexyl salicylate; ERA: Environmental risk assessment; EtPABA: Ethyl-p-aminobenzoic acid; 4HB: 4-Hydroxybenzophenone; HMS: Homosalate; HPVC: High production volume chemical; K_{oc}: Soil organic-water partition coefficient; K_{ow}: Partition coefficient octanol-water; lw: Lipid weight; 4MBC: 4-Methylbenzylidene-camphor; MeBZT: Methyl benzotriazole

Acknowledgements

SDC is grateful to the Spanish Ministry of Economy and Competitiveness (SOLAR Project Ref. 2015801004).

References

Alonso, M., M.L. Feo, C. Corcellas, P. Gago-Ferrero, C.P. Bertozzi, J. Marigo et al. 2015. Toxic heritage: Maternal transfer of pyrethroid insecticides and sunscreen agents in dolphins from Brazil. Environ. Pollut. 207: 391–402.

American Dermatology Association. 2016. Available from https://www.aad.org/about.

Bachelot, M., Z. Li, D. Munaron, P. Le Gall, C. Casellas, H. Fenet et al. 2012. Organic UV filter concentrations in marine mussels from French coastal regions. Sci. Total Environ. 420: 273–279.

Bainbridge, Z.T., J.E. Brodie, J.W. Faithful, D.A. Sydes and S.E. Lewis. 2009. Identifying the land-based sources of suspended sediments, nutrients and pesticides discharged to the Great Barrier Reef from the Tully—Murray Basin, Queensland, Australia. Mar. Freshw. Res. 60: 1081–1090.

Barón, E., P. Gago-Ferrero, M. Gorga, I. Rudolph, G. Mendoza, A.M. Zapata et al. 2013. Occurrence of hydrophobic organic pollutants (BFRs and UV-filters) in sediments from South America. Chemosphere. 92: 309–316.

Champagne, P. 2008. Personal care products. pp. 86–140. *In*: Bhandari, A., R. Surampalli and C. Adams (eds.). Contam. Emerg. Environ. Concern. Reston, Virginia: American Society of Civil Engineers.

CLIA. 2017. Cruise Lines International Asociation in Spain. Available from: http://www.cliaspain.com/.

Cuderman, P. and E. Heath. 2007. Determination of UV filters and antimicrobial agents in environmental water samples. Anal. Bioanal. Chem. 387: 1343–1350.

Danovaro, R.L.B., C. Corinaldesi, D. Giocannelli, E. Damiani, P. Astolfi, L. Greci et al. 2008. Sunscreens cause coral bleaching by prmoting viral infections. Front. Ecol. Environ. 116: 441–447.

Díaz-Cruz, M.S., M. Llorca and D. Barceló. 2008. Organic UV filters and their photodegradates, metabolites and disinfection by-products in the aquatic environment. TrAC—Trends Anal. Chem. 27: 873–887.

Díaz-Cruz, M.S., P. Gago-Ferrero, M. Llorca and D. Barceló. 2012. Analysis of UV filters in tap water and other clean waters in Spain. Anal. Bioanal. Chem. 402: 2325–2333.

Edinger, E.N., J. Jompa, G.V. Limmon, W. Widjatmoko and M.J. Risk. 1998. Reef degradation and coral biodiveersity in Indonesia: Effects of land-bassed pollution, destructive fishing pratices and changes oveer time. Mar. Pollut. Bull. 36: 617–630.

Ekowati, Y., G. Buttiglieri, G. Ferrero, J. Valle-Sistac, M.S. Díaz-Cruz, D. Barceló et al. 2016. Occurrence of pharmaceuticals and UV filters in swimming pools and spas. Environ. Sci. Pollut. Res. 23: 14431–14441.

Emnet, P., S. Gaw, G. Northcott, B. Storey and L. Graham. 2015. Personal care products and steroid hormones in the Antarctic coastal environment associated with two Antarctic research stations, McMurdo Station and Scott Base. Environ. Res. 136: 331–342.

Euromonitor International. 2016. Beauty and Personal Care in China. Available from: http://www.euromonitor.com/beauty-and-personal-care-in-china/report.

European Commission. 2003. Technical Guidance Document on Risk Assessment in Support of Commission Directive 93/67/EEC on Risk Assessment for New Notified Substances, Commission Regulation (EC) N1488/94 on Risk Assessment for Existing Substances. Joint Research Centre, EUR20418 EN/.

EuroPlat. 2015. Asia Pacific to Continue Personal Care Ingredients Market Dominance, Global Market to Reach US$11.76 bn by 2023. Available from: http://www.europlat.org/asia-pacific-to-continue-personal-care-ingredients-market-dominance-global-market-to-reach-us11-76-bn-by-2023.htm.

Fent, K., A. Zenker and M. Rapp. 2010. Widespread occurrence of estrogenic UV-filters in aquatic ecosystems in Switzerland. Environ. Pollut. 158: 1817–1824.

Gago-Ferrero, P., M.S. Díaz-Cruz and D. Barceló. 2011a. Fast pressurized liquid extraction with in-cell purification and analysis by liquid chromatography tandem mass spectrometry for the determination of UV filters and their degradation products in sediments. Anal. Bioanal. Chem. 400: 2195–2204.

Gago-Ferrero, P., M. Díaz-Cruz and D. Barceló. 2011b. Occurrence of multiclass UV filters in treated sewage sludge from wastewater treatment plants. Chemosphere. 84: 1158–1165.

Gago-Ferrero, P., M.S. Díaz-Cruz and D. Barceló. 2013a. Multi-residue method for trace level determination of UV filters in fish based on pressurized liquid extraction and liquid chromatography—quadrupole-linear ion trap-mass spectrometry. J. Chromatogr. A. 1286: 93–101.

Gago-Ferrero, P., M.B. Alonso, C.P. Bertozzi, J. Marigo, M.L. Barbosa, M. Cremer et al. 2013b. First determination of UV filters in marine mammals. octocrylene levels in Franciscana dolphins. Environ. Sci. Technol. 47: 5619–5625.

Gago-Ferrero, P., M.S. Díaz-Cruz and D. Barceló. 2015. UV filters bioaccumulation in fish from Iberian river basins. Sci. Total Env. 518: 518–525.

Gentlemen Marketing Agency. 2014. The 2014 Personal and Beauty Care Market in China.

Giokas, D.L., V.A. Sakkas and T.A. Albanis. 2004. Determination of residues of UV filters in natural waters by solid-phase extraction coupled to liquid chromatography–photodiode array detection and gas chromatography–mass spectrometry. J. Chromatogr. A. 1026: 289–293.

Giokas, D.L., A. Salvador and A. Chisvert. 2007. UV filters: Fron sunscreens to human body and the environment. Trends Food Sci. Technol. 26: 360–374.

HSDB. 2011. Hazardous Substances Data Bank (HSDB) Fact Sheet. Bethesda, Maryland.

Kameda, Y., K. Kimura and M. Miyazaki. 2011. Occurrence and profiles of organic sun-blocking agents in surface waters and sediments in Japanese rivers and lakes. Environ. Pollut. 159: 1570–1576.

Kasprzyk-Hordern, B., R.M. Dinsdale and A.J. Guwy. 2008. The occurrence of pharmaceuticals, personal care products, endocrine disruptors and illicit drugs in surface water in South Wales, UK. Water Res. 42: 3498–3518.

Kim, S. and K. Choi. 2014. Occurrences, toxicities, and ecological risks of benzophenone-3, a common component of organic sunscreen products: A mini-review. Environ. Int. 70: 143–157.

Kunz, P.Y., H.F. Galicia and K. Fent. 2006. Comparison of *in vitro* and *in vivo* estrogenic activity of UV filters in fish. Toxicol. Sci. 90: 349–361.

Lambropoulou, D., D.L. Giokas, V. Sakkas, T. Albanis and M.I. Karayannis. 2002. Gas chromatographic determination of 2-hydroxy-4-methoxybenzophenone and octyldimethyl-p-aminobenzoic acid sunscreen agents in swimming pool and bathing waters by solid-phase microextraction. J. Chromatogr. A. 967: 243–253.

Langford, K.H., M.J. Reid, E. Fjeld, S. Øxnevad and K.V. Thomas. 2015. Environmental occurrence and risk of organic UV filters and stabilizers in multiple matrices in Norway. Environ. Int. 80: 1–7.

Li, W., Y. Ma, C. Guo, W. Hu, K. Liu, Y. Wang et al. 2007. Occurrence and behavior of four of the most used sunscreen UV filters in a wastewater reclamation plant. Water Res. 41: 3506–3512.

Liardet, S., C. Scaletta, R. Panizzon, P. Hohlfeld and L. Laurent-Applegate. 2001. Protection against pyrimidine dimers, p53, and 8-hydroxy-2'-deoxyguanosine expression in ultraviolet-irradiated human skin by sunscreens: Difference between UVB + UVA and UVB alone sunscreens. J. Invest. Dermatol. 117: 1437–1441.

Liu, Y.S., G.G. Ying, A. Shareef and R.S. Kookana. 2011. Simultaneous determination of benzotriazoles and ultraviolet filters in ground water, effluent and biosolid samples using gas chromatography-tandem mass spectrometry. J. Chromatogr. A. 1218: 5328–5335.

Loraine, G.A. and M.E. Pettigrove. 2006. Seasonal variations in concentrations of pharmaceuticals and personal care products in drinking water and reclaimed wastewater in Southern California. Environ. Sci. Technol. 40: 687–695.

Lucintel. 2016. Global UV Filter Market for Personal Care Products. Irving, TX. Available from: http://www. prnewswire.com/news-releases/global-uv-filter-market-for-personal-care-products-300376893. html.

Magi, E., M. Di Carro, C. Scapolla and K.T.N. Nguyen. 2012. Stir bar sorptive extraction and LC-MS/MS for trace analysis of UV filters in different water matrices. Chromatographia. 75: 973–982.

Min, L., Q. Sun, A. Hu, L. Hou, J. Li, X. Cai et al. 2014. Pharmaceuticals and personal care products in a mesoscale subtropical watershed and their application as chemical markers. J. Hazard. Mater. 280C: 696–705.

Molins-Delgado, D., M. Díaz-Cruz and D. Barceló. 2015a. Introduction: Personal care products in the aquatic environment. pp. 1–34. *In*: Díaz-Cruz, M. and D. Barceló (eds.). Pers. Care. Prod. Aquat. Environ. Handb. Environ. Chem. Berlin, Germany: Springer-Verlag.

Molins-Delgado, D., M. Díaz-Cruz and D. Barceló. 2015b. Removal of polar UV stabilizers in biological wastewater treatments and ecotoxicological implications. Chemosphere. 119: S51–S57.

Molins-Delgado, D., P. Gago-Ferrero, M. Díaz-Cruz and D. Barceló. 2016a. Single and joint ecotoxicity data estimation of organic UV filters and nanomaterials toward selected aquatic organisms. Urban groundwater risk assessment. Environ. Res. 145: 126–134.

Molins-Delgado, D., M. Díaz-Cruz and D. Barceló. 2016b. Ecological risk assessment associated to the removal of endocrine-disrupting parabens and benzophenone-4 in wastewater treatment. J. Hazard. Mater. 310: 143–151.

Morohoshi, K., H. Yamamoto, R. Kamata, F. Shiraishi, T. Koda and M. Morita. 2005. Estrogenic activity of 37 components of commercial sunscreen lotions evaluated by *in vitro* assays. Toxicol. Vitr. 19: 457–469.

Persistence Market Research. 2015. The Future of Personal Care in the Globe Asia Pacific, Persistence Market Research, Personal Care Chemicals and Ingredients Market: Global Industry Analysis and Forecast to 2020.

Plagellat, C., T. Kupper, R. Furrer, L.F. De Alencastro, D. Grandjean and J. Tarradellas. 2006. Concentrations and specific loads of UV filters in sewage sludge originating from a monitoring network in Switzerland. Chemosphere. 62: 915–925.

Premium Beauty News. 2015. The European cosmetics and personal care market shows signs of recovery. Available from: http://www.premiumbeautynews.com/en/the-european-cosmetics.

Rodil, R. and M. Moeder. 2008. Development of a simultaneous pressurised-liquid extraction and clean-up procedure for the determination of UV filters in sediments. Anal. Chim. Acta. 612: 152–159.

Rodil, R., M. Moeder, R. Altenburger and M. Schmitt-Jansen. 2009a. Photostability and phytotoxicity of selected sunscreen agents and their degradation mixtures in water. Anal. Bioanal. Chem. 395: 1513–1524.

Rodil, R., S. Schrader and M. Moeder. 2009b. Non-porous membrane-assisted liquid-liquid extraction of UV filter compounds from water samples. J. Chromatogr. A. 1216: 4887–4894.

Rodil, R., J.B. Quintana, E. Concha-Graña, P. López-Mahía, S. Muniategui-Lorenzo and D. Prada-Rodríguez. 2012. Emerging pollutants in sewage, surface and drinking water in Galicia (NW Spain). Chemosphere. 86: 1040–1049.

Sánchez-Quiles, D. and A. Tovar-Sánchez. 2015. Are sunscreens a new environmental risk associated with coastal tourism? Environ. Int. 83: 158–170.

Sánchez-Rodríguez, A., M. Rodrigo-Sanz and J.R. Betancort-Rodríguez. 2015. Occurrence of eight UV filters in beaches of Gran Canaria (Canary Islands). An approach to environmental risk assessment. Chemosphere. 131: 85–90.

Sanderson, H., D. Johnson, C. Wilson, R. Brain and K. Solomon. 2003. Probabilistic hazard assessment of environmentally occurring pharmaceuticals toxicity to fish, daphnids, and algae by ECOSAR screening. Toxicol. Lett. 144: 383–395.

Sang, Z. and K.S.Y. Leung. 2016. Environmental occurrence and ecological risk assessment of organic UV filters in marine organisms from Hong Kong coastal waters. Sci. Total Environ. 566-567: 489–498.

Seeland, A., M. Oetken, A. Kiss, E. Fries and J. Oehlmann. 2012. Acute and chronic toxicity of benzotriazoles to aquatic organisms. Environ. Sci. Pollut. Res. 19: 1781–1790.

Seité, S., A. Colige, P. Piquemal-Vivenot, C. Montastier, A. Fourtanier, C. Lapière et al. 2000. A full-UV spectrum absorbing daily use cream protects human skin against biological changes occurring in photoaging. Photodermatol. Photoimmunol. Photomed. 16: 147–155.

Serra-Roig, M.P., A. Jurado, M.S. Díaz-Cruz, E. Vázquez-Suñé, E. Pujades and D. Barceló. 2016. Occurrence, fate and risk assessment of personal care products in river-groundwater interface. Sci. Total Environ. 568: 829–837.

Sieratowicz, A., D. Kaiser, M. Behr, M. Oetken and J. Oehlmann. 2011. Acute and chronic toxicity of four frequently used UV filter substances for *Desmodesmus subspicatus* and *Daphnia magna*. J. Environ. Sci. Health A Tox Hazard. Subst. Environ. Eng. 46: 1311–9.

Tavazzi, S., G. Mariani, S. Comero, M. Ricci, B. Paracchini, H. Skejo et al. 2016. Analytical method for the determination of compounds selected for the first Surface water watch list.

TechSci Research. 2014. US Cosmetic Chemicals Market to Grow due to Increasing Demand for Personal Care Products. Available from: http://www.techsciresearch.com/news/186-us-cosmetic-chemicals-market-to-grow-due-to-increasing-demand-for-personal-care-products.html.

The Congress of the United States. 1938. Federal Food, Drugs and Cosmetic Act.

The European Parliament and the Council of the European Union. 2009. Regulation of the European Parliament and of the Council of 30 November 2009 on cosmetic products. EC No. 1223/2009.

Transparency Market Research. 2015. Global Organic Personal Care Products Market to Grow at CAGR of 9.30% from 2014 to 2020 due to Rising Preference for Natural Products.

Tsui, M., H. Leung, P. Lam and M. Murphy. 2014a. Seasonal occurrence, removal efficiencies and risk assessment of multiple classes of organic UV filters in wastewater treatment plants. Water Res. 53: 1–30.

Tsui, M., H. Leung, T.-C. Wai, N. Yamashita, S. Taniyasu, W. Liu et al. 2014b. Occurrence, distribution and ecological risk assessment of multiple classes of UV filters in surface waters from different countries. Water Res. 67: 55–65.

UNWTO. 2016. United Nations World Tourism Organization.

USEPA. 2012. Toxics Release Inventory (TRI) Program. Persistent Bioaccumulative Toxic (PBT) Chemicals Rules Under the TRI Program. Available from: https://www.epa.gov/toxics-release-inventory-tri-program/persistent-bioaccumulative-toxic-pbt-chemicals-rules-under-tri.

Wang, C., W. Wang, S. He, J. Du and Z. Sun. 2011. Sources and distribution of aliphatic and polycyclic aromatic hydrocarbons in Yellow River Delta Nature Reserve, China. Appl. Geochemistry. 26: 1330–1336.

Weisbrod, C.J., P.Y. Kunz, A.K. Zenker and K. Fent. 2007. Effects of the UV filter benzophenone-2 on reproduction in fish. Toxicol. Appl. Pharmacol. 225: 255–266.

Whitmore, S.E. and W.L. Morison. 1995. Prevention of UVB-induced immunosuppression in humans by a high sun protection factor sunscreen. Arch. Dermatol. 131: 1128–1133.

Zenker, A., H. Schmutz and K. Fent. 2008. Simultaneous trace determination of nine organic UV-absorbing compounds (UV filters) in environmental samples. J. Chromatogr. A. 1202: 64–74.

Zenker, A., M. Rita, F. Prestinaci, P. Bottoni and M. Carere. 2014. Bioaccumulation and biomagnification potential of pharmaceuticals with a focus to the aquatic environment. J. Environ. Manage. 133: 378–387.

Zhang, Z., N. Ren, Y.F. Li, T. Kunisue, D. Gao and K. Kannan. 2011. Determination of benzotriazole and benzophenone UV filters in sediment and sewage sludge. Environ. Sci. Technol. 45: 3909–3916.

7

Persistence of Organic Pollutants

Half Life or Mineralization and their Factors of Influence

IIIIIIIIIIIIIIIIIIIIIIIIIIIIIIIIIIIIIIIIIIIIIIIIIIIIIIIIIIIIIIIIIIIIIIIIIIIIIIIIIIIIIIIIIIIIIIIIIIIIIIIIIIIIIIIIIIIIIIIIIIIIIIIIIIIIIIIII

Fábio Veríssimo Correia,[1,*] *Tomaz Langenbach,*[2]
Simone Tieme Taketa Bicalho,[3] *Daniele Alves Marinho*[4]
and *Patrícia Silva Ferreira*[5]

Introduction

The processes in which the organic molecules are completely biodegraded down to their mineral constituents is called **mineralization** and is promoted mainly by microorganisms that use these catabolism as energy source and nutrients (Moreira and Siqueira 2002). **Biodegradation** is one of the most fundamental processes in life necessary to maintain an equilibrium with continuous biosynthesis of organic molecules. The cell catabolism is essential to produce precursors for producing

---

[1] Universidade Federal do Estado do Rio de Janeiro - UNIRIO, Av. Pasteur, 458, Urca, Rio de Janeiro, RJ, CEP: 22290-240.
[2] Pontifícia Universidade Católica do Rio de Janeiro – Puc-Rio, Rua Marquês de São Vicente, 225, Gávea, Rio de Janeiro, RJ, CEP: 22451-900.
E-mail: tomazlange@yahoo.com.br
[3] Centro De Tecnologia Paula Souza. Faculdade De Tecnologia De Inadaiatuba "Dr. Archimedes Lammoglia" - Fatecid, R. Dom Pedro I, 65 - Cidade Nova I, Indaiatuba, São Paulo, CEP: 13334-100.
E-mail: simonetaketa@gmail.com
[4] Instituto Federal de Educação, Ciência e Tecnologia do Espírito Santo, Av. Rio Branco, 50, Santa Lucia, Vitória, ES, CEP: 29056-255.
E-mail: daniele.marinho@ifes.edu.br
[5] Instituto Federal de Educação, Ciência e Tecnologia do Rio de Janeiro (IFRJ), Campus São Gonçalo, Rua Oliveira Botelho s/n, Neves, São Gonçalo, RJ, CEP: 24425-005.
E-mail: patricia.ferreira@ifrj.edu.br
* Corresponding author: fabiovcorreia@hotmail.com

organic compounds, as well for biochemical interconversion and "*de novo*" synthesis to maintain living cells. When a plant or animal feeds another animal, their organic molecules are catabolized in smaller molecules that, guided by the genetic code, form new molecules of the predator.

Nowadays, new artificial pesticides are produced to attend to industrial demands in high amounts. However, when introduced into the environment, many of these molecules are not easily biodegraded. Ideally, a pesticide should effectively control the target organism for a critical period of time during its growth and then be degraded to products harmless to man and other organisms. In practice, certain pesticides are termed **"persistent organic pollutants"** (POPs), and some uses may lead to continued existence of the parent compound and/or biologically active metabolites over prolonged periods. For POP's bioremediation or any other remediation, techniques are expensive but useful for small areas but are not economically feasible for large agriculture areas.

Thus, these chemical substances are deemed **"persistent"** when they remain untransformed into the environment for a very long time (Tang 2013). This disturbs the equilibrium between **biodegradation** and biosynthesis resulting in a gradual accumulation of these molecules in the environment with enhanced nonstop deleterious effects. The term **persistence** was introduced into the pesticide scientific literature to describe the continuing existence of certain insecticides in the environment and is now applied to any organic chemical.

The term **persistence** is employed by scientists in many disciplines. An agronomist must consider whether a pesticide will survive long enough to control a plague, be it weed or insect, and also whether it will leave toxic residues that may adversely affect other lifeforms. The environmental chemist determines the measurable presence of a substance in a medium at a specific period of time, regardless of its bioavailability or effect. The toxicologist examines the effects of food-stuffs containing residues of the parent compound or relevant metabolic products for human safety. The ecologist is interested in the even wider environmental problems caused by pesticide dispersal such as adverse effects in nontarget organisms.

Measurements of **persistence** of organic compounds in soils are usually conducted under controlled conditions where samples are under contained conditions with the use of radioactive (^{14}C) or non-radioactive (^{13}C) isotopes in order to follow the carbon backbone degradation through intermediate metabolites to the end-result of **mineralization** into CO_2 (US-EPA 1982(83), SETAC 1995, OECD 2002). The data obtained from these experiments can measure the time needed to degrade 50% of all carbons applied up to CO_2.

The concept of **environmental half-life** has been commonly measured in open systems as field or lisimeter under environmental conditions. However, the **half-life** in this context only expresses the disappearance of the residue under field conditions (EPPO 1993). The data obtained using this methodology represent biodegradation as well losses by volatilization, leaching, run-off, biosphere uptake/bioaccumulation, and residues bound to the soil matrix. In fact, this data represents the fate of the pollutant but it is different from environmental degradation of the molecules. **Persistent organic chemicals** need to be destroyed and not just disappear from the soil moving from one environmental compartment into another one and continue polluting waters, air and biosphere with deleterious effects. The displacement of the substance implies the recalculation of the **half-life** to another environmental compartment, water or atmosphere. Comparing **mineralization** with **half-life** can also result in an ambiguity, since with regard to first order kinetics, which considers a constant equation, independent of concentration.

The concept of **biological half-life** $(T_{1/2})$ used intensively in toxicology is different and indicates the absorption, transformation and excretion of molecules from the organism (IUPAC 1997). Biological half-life $(T_{1/2})$ is a pharmacokinetic parameter important to characterize detoxification procedures. This concept is different from **mineralization** and **the fate** of residues in the environment.

The wide spread pollution caused by pesticides and some other molecules of industrial use in the environment makes remediation difficult and the sustainable alternative is to restrict or ban the use of persistent molecules. Therefore, the criteria for the registration of these products are of the highest priority (Table 1).

Hence, **persistence** does not denote an absolute characteristic of a chemical, but is a variable which is a function of many interactions. Persistence is defined by chemical properties of a molecule as susceptibility to oxidation, reduction, hydrolysis, photolysis, the fate in the environment with movement trough soil, leaching and volatilization with physical-chemical parameters of vapor pressure, solubility, dissociation constant, partition coefficient and sorption to soil, and finally, the characteristics of environment such as water content, organic matter, pH, microbial biomass and temperature. Experimental methodologies employed also have an influence on mineralization and half-life measurements.

The first question of this work is to demonstrate that half-life is not a synonymous of persistence and mineralization. A second question of why occurs the high variation of biodegradation data of a given molecule such as atrazine, was highlighted in this work. An investigation of the importance of different parameters, as well as distinct measuring methodologies to explain this, is discussed.

Three types of soils were subjected to four different approaches to determine the mineralization after application of atrazine. Field and laboratory experiments were performed comparing disturbed and undisturbed soils, as well as cultivated and uncultivated in different systems. Soils were chosen for experimentation considering that pesticides are used mainly in an agricultural context, either directly applied to the soil or to plants. However, soil is always the final destination, since rain washes down molecules from the plants, while plant senescence also causes these compounds to be directed to the soil. In addition, large amounts of theses POPs are discarded in this environmental compartment where microbe population density with potential capacity of biodegradation is much higher

Table 1. Criterion for pesticide persistence definition (IBAMA 1990).

Level of persistence	Mineralization at 28 days (%)	Half-life $(T_{1/2})$ days
High	0–1	> 180
Medium	1–10	90–180
Low	10–25	30–90
No-persistence	> 25	< 30

with 10^8–10^9 cells.g^1 compared to water and air environments, with less than 10^6 cells.g^{-1} and 10^3 cells.m^{-3} respectively. Two approaches will be considered: one regarding soil parameters, such as organic matter content, pH, mineral composition, texture, microbial population with and without the presence of plants. The other approach is the experimental methodology used to measure biodegradation in the field or under controlled laboratory conditions. In this case, we need to point out that generally humidity and temperature conditions in the laboratory are more constant than under field conditions.

Atrazine was chosen due to the high amount of scientific information available in the literature and the fact that our group had intensively worked with this molecule under tropical environmental conditions. This work demonstrates that quite different results can be obtained with the same molecule under different experimental conditions, making the definition of the grade of persistence more complicated when discussing banning or restricting the use of this molecule.

Materials and Methods

In the above-presented experiments, many parameters and different aspects are considered. Experiments use three different soils with distinct structures as red yellow Ultisol, dark latosol and red yellow latosol. The experimental conditions of each soil consider forest soil, conventional tilled soil and soil with no tillage when soil is covered by straw of stubble of the last cultivation occur enhancement of organic matter, microbial population and other forms of life in the soil. One important variation that was introduced was to treat soil with atrazine a given time before making experiments with new addition of the same herbicide. The applied methodologies were field experiments, while assays conducted in microcosms, erlenmeyers or volumetric flasks were used to follow the final microbial degradation up to mineralization with ^{14}C-atrazine. By field experiments, residue/metabolites were extracted and analyzed by HPLC and in mineralization experiments, with the use of radio labeled molecules, ^{14}C-CO$_2$ was captured during the experiment and radioactivity was measured in a scintillation counter system.

Atrazine

All experiments received the same dose of atrazine to simulate the agricultural practice of 3 kg a.i. ha in the field, the atrazine commercial product Gesaprim 500 was applied and in laboratory experiments, 14C-atrazine was diluted in a commercial atrazine product. The 14C-atrazine, which contains 14C in all the atoms of the atrazine ring, was donated by Syngenta Chemical Company. Purification was performed by thin layer chromatography TLC using dichloromethane/methanol (95:5 v/v) up to 99% purity.

Soils used in experiment

Three of the most widespread agricultural soils in tropical regions were used in the experiments, as follows:

Soil 1. An Ultisol soil known as Red-Yellow, sampled from the experimental area of the Department of Phytotechnology, Universidade Federal Rural do Rio de Janeiro, Seropédica (RJ); (22° 49' S, 43° 38' W). The soil characteristics are: 66% sand, 10% silt, 24% clay, 2.8% organic matter and pH 6.5 (EMBRAPA 1997).

Soil 2. A dark red Latosol (Oxisol), collected at the experimental area of Embrapa field located in Dourados, Mato Grosso do Sul, Brazil (22° 14' S, 54° 49' W). Soil samples from this area were collected under four distinct conditions: natural forest (NF); conventional tillage (CT); no tillage management (NT); one soil samples where atrazine (Gesaprim 500) had been applied one year before mineralization no tillage management (NTa) and one soil sample with no tillage (without atrazine application in filed) (NT). The soil characteristics were: 10% sand, 11% silt, 79% clay, 3.2% organic matter and pH 6.0 (EMBRAPA 1997).

Soil 3. A Red-Yellow Latosol (Oxisol), collected at the campus of the Pontifical Catholic University of Rio de Janeiro, Gávea (RJ) located at 22° 97' 74.01" S and 43° 23' 24.61" W. Soil characteristics are 40% sand, 16% silt, 44% clay, 3.6% organic matter and pH 5.2 (EMBRAPA 1997).

Methodological approaches

Four distinct approaches were used to characterize mineralization after the application of atrazine, described below.

Field experiments

Field experiments were performed to determine the half-life of atrazine under different conditions. For this were used the soil 1 (Ultisol) with conventional management and soil 2 (Oxisol) with conventional (CT) and no tillage management (NT), which were tilled, fertilized and sown with maize. Field experiments were performed with Ultisol and Oxisol soils with different managements (CT and NT).

After 30 days, when the maize seedlings were 3–5 cm high, Gesaprim 500, the commercial product of atrazine and the most specific herbicide for maize, was applied over the cultivated field. Soil samples of (200 g) were randomly collected in triplicate before and at 2, 7, 15, 30, 60 and 90 days after Gesaprim 500 application. The sampled soil layers were 5 cm thick and were collected in plastic bags from the surface down to a depth of 50 cm (Correia et al. 2007). The samples were stored at 4°C for later analysis.

Atrazine analysis in soil

The extraction and purification method was adapted from Huang and Pignatello (1990) and Balinova and Balinov (1991). Atrazine was extracted from 50 g of soil samples with 100 mL of acetone. A mixture of soil-acetone was mixed for 20 minutes and then sonicated (Elma transonic digital) for 10 minutes. Subsequently, this suspension was filtered through a Whatman n° 4 filter. The residue was dried, resuspended in 100 ml of a methanol:water solution (85:15 v v^{-1}) and transferred into a separation funnel with 30 ml of dichloromethane. After vigorous shaking, the dichloromethane phase with residues was collected. This process was repeated three times. The collected phases of residues were mixed, dried in a rotating evaporator and resuspended in 10 ml of methanol. Then, 2 ml of this aliquot was pipetted into an octadecyl C18 (40 lm APD, 60A") reverse phase column, previously washed with 5 ml methanol. The sample in the column was rinsed with 5–10 ml of water and discarded. Afterwards, the columns were eluted with 5.0 ml of dichloromethane:methanol (7:3 v v^{-1}), and collected in a volumetric flask, dried and suspended in 5.0 ml of acetonitrile:water (8:2 v v^{-1}). Aliquots of the samples were filtered using a Millipore GV Millex/polyethylene membrane (0.22 nm) and 20 µl of the solution was injected into an HPLC (Waters 600 Controller) equipped with a reverse phase column RP18 (250 mm–4.6 mm i.d.), preceded by a guard column (10–3.0 mm i.d.). Absorption was measured by an UV detector at 254 nm. The mobile phase was a methanol:water solution (60:40 v v^{-1}). The operational temperature of the column was 26°C and the flow speed was 0.5 ml min^{-1}. Atrazine detections were confirmed in different mobile phases of the acetonitrile:water solution with gradients (50:50 v v^{-1}, 65:35 v v^{-1}), under the same conditions as described above, to avoid the coincidence of other molecules with atrazine. The recovery average efficiency of atrazine from soil was 85%. Atrazine concentrations were determined by means of an analytical curve constructed with standard atrazine (purity 99%). The half-life in all experiments was calculated by the following equation (Frank et al. 1991):

Half-life = elapsed time × log 2/log (Beginning amount/ending amount) measured.

Mineralization of atrazine in test flasks

Two types of flasks were used: (A) Erlenmeyer, and (B) Volumetric flasks with temperature and humidity control. In both soil 2 samples, air dried for 24 h at room temperature and then sieved through a 2-mm mesh were used.

A   Erlenmeyer flask

Experiments were performed in dark red latosol (Oxisol) subjected to tillage and not subjected tillage with 20 and 80% WHC. All experiments were carried out with soils treated with atrazine for the first time three years previously. Soil samples of 30 g, one under humidity conditions of 80% water-holding capacity (WHC) and the other under dry stress conditions (20% WHC). This was regularly controlled by weighing the incubation flask and readjusted every week by adding distilled water. Gesaprim 500 was applied to 4 replicate soil samples. These samples were introduced in a 125 mL Erlenmeyer flask connected to another flask containing a trap with 20 mL ethanolamine and diethyleneglycol–monobutylether (1:1 v/v) to absorb the $^{14}CO_2$ from the pesticide. The air flowing through the flask was powered by a pump and bubbled slowly through the trap solution. Incubation was performed at room temperature and samples from the trap solution were collected every day during the first week and then twice a week for 60 days. Radioactivity was measured in 5 ml aliquots from the trap solutions mixed with 10 ml of a liquid scintillation cocktail (4 g PPO, 0.25 g POPOP, 333 ml Triton X.100 in 667 ml toluene) and then counted in a Beckman 4100 (USA) liquid scintillation counter. Erlenmeyer flasks test was applied for two soil samples where atrazine (Gesaprim 500) had been applied previously (Soil 1): no tillage management (NTa) and (Soil 2) conventional tillage (CTa).

B Volumetric flask with temperature and humidity control

From samples of dark red Latosol (Oxisol) of natural forest soil, no tillage and no tillage with previous application of atrazine (one year before), 30 g soil was introduced into a volumetric flask with a double wall to allow a water flow to maintain a constant temperature of 28°C. In addition, a constant air flow was also applied which transported the $^{14}C\text{-}CO_2$ to a trap containing ethanolamine plus monoglycoldiethyl-monobutyl ether (1:1) for $^{14}C\text{-}CO_2$ absorption. The air flow was controlled and powered by a pump system in which the incoming air was passed through an Erlenmeyer flask filled with distilled water to maintain humidity up to saturation. Samples from the trap were collected three times a week and radioactivity was measured, as described above. The volumetric flasks tests were applied for 3 soil samples: natural forest (NF), no tillage management (NT) and no tillage management with previous Gesaprim application (NTa).

Mineralization in a microcosm with undisturbed soil

The mineralization measurements were performed in three soil samples: Ultisol (Soil 1), a dark red Latosol (Soil 2) under no tillage management (NTa) and under a conventional tillage (CTa).

Microcosm apparatus and experimental conditions

Undisturbed soil cores were taken by pressing the stainless-steel columns of the microcosms into the soil up to 30 cm; the cores were then transported to the laboratory. Experiments were carried out with four soil replicates. The collected soil core samples were placed within a laboratory microcosm system at room temperature (15–25°C) (Correia et al. 2007) and connected to an airflow operated by a pump system throughout the experiment. The gas flow meter was set to 17 l h^{-1}. Wind was simulated by a propeller with a speed of 1 m s^{-1} powered by a device outside the microcosm. The microcosm airflow was connected externally to a trap containing 20 ml ethanolamine and diethylenoglycol-monobutylether (1:1 v/v) which were used to absorb $^{14}CO_2$ in order to quantify the mineralization rates. Samples were collected twice a week for the first two weeks and thereafter, on a weekly basis. Rainfall simulation was maintained by watering the microcosms three times a week at a rate corresponding to a 300 mm rainfall month^{-1}, typical for tropical rain in the region (Fig. 1).

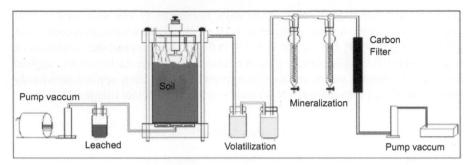

Fig. 1. Microcosm system.

Mineralization in a plant columns system

The soil used was a red yellow latosol (Oxisol) of the superficial layer of 20 cm deep and with 20 to 40 cm deep layer. Experiments were done without plants and with *Cecropia hololeuca* Miq. and *Trema micrantha* (L.) Blum., two common species of the riparian forest, which were both used in soil-plant microcosms. These species are helophytes, grow fast, are commonly found in all riparian forest and are used in reforestation. The apparatus used for mineralization was a microcosm with PVC tube, 40 cm high with 15 cm diameter, in which was introduced red yellow latosol with one plant. Treatments in the superficial soil (0–20 cm) were performed on soil without plants, soil cultivated with imbaúba (*Cecropia hololeuca* Miq. soil cultivated and *Trema micrantha* (L.) Blum.), while treatments in the subsuperficial soil (20–40 cm) were performed on control soil without plants and soil cultivated with *Trema micrantha* (L.) Blum. This soil was sieved with a mesh with diameter < 2 mm and adjusted to pH 7.0 with lime. Thirty grams of NPK (4-14-8) fertilizer were applied to the soil, as per agricultural recommendation (Fig. 2).

Six months old *C. hololeuca* and *T. micrantha* seedlings were transplanted into microcosm individually and acclimatized for one month. The plants were watered daily during acclimatization and afterwards, three times a week. Tap water was added to a plastic dish, commonly used in gardening, placed underneath the microcosm.

The dose recommended by the legislation was used after preliminary tests showed that *C. hololeuca* survive with a tenth of the usual concentration of atrazine without toxic symptoms such as leaf clorosis.

The microcosm was closed in the bottom with nylon screen. Microcosm was filled with 3 cm of sand in the bottom. Seedling was planted in which roots were covered by gentle addition of sieved soil. In each microcosm, 200 mL of water was applied each day, three times a week, and the microcosm remained under acclimatization for 20 days. Watering was stopped 24 hours before applying the solution of Gesaprim 500 plus ^{14}C-labeled atrazine homogeneously on the sand layer, a condition simulating ground water contamination. After 24 h, watering began again. One day after application, microcosm was covered in the superficial surface with polyurethane foam 3 mm thick to capture the volatile products obtained at the end of the experiment. To close the microcosm, plastic foil was used without harming the

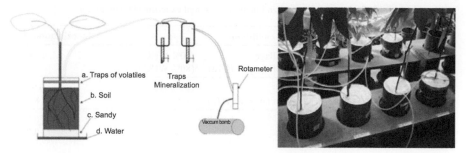

Fig. 2. Plant column system.

aerial part of the plant and, finally, the top layer of plastic was fixed with an adhesive tape. The tube for $^{14}C\text{-}CO_2$ capture was positioned in the space between the soil surface and the polyurethane foam and two chemical traps in sequence, containing 35 mL of a trap solution described above, were connected. The airflow was powered by a pump system and controlled by a gas flow meter at 17 L h^{-1}. To maximize the efficiency, the trap system was kept under refrigeration. The samples of the chemical traps of radioactive CO_2 had been collected after ^{14}C-atrazine application three times per week in the first 15 days, after which twice a week, and a 5 mL aliquot was measured in the scintillation system as described above. During the experiment, temperature variation was between 25°C and 30°C.

At the end of the experiment, the soil profile was sliced from the bottom to the upper layers. First, a sand layer slice was collected, followed by four soil layer slices of 5 cm each and then, a 3 cm surface layer was collected. Roots were collected from each layer; the bulk soil was separated by manual agitation and the rhizosphere was then removed. Roots of each layer were separated into diameter of > 1 mm and fine diameter with thickness bigger than < 1 mm roots and cut into small pieces, dried at room temperature for 24 h after which they were weighed and stored at 4°C. The rhizosphere and bulk soil of each layer were air-dried at room temperature and carefully homogenized by maceration. The measurements taken from the upper part of the plants were: height of the plants, number of leaves, and the dry weight of stems and leaves. The stems were homogenized by milling and the leaves were carefully cut into small pieces and both were dried at room temperature for 24 h. Triplicates of 1.0 g of bulk soil, rhizosphere, fine and thick roots, stem, and leaves, were weighed and burnt in a Zinsser Oxidizer (Oximat 500, Germany) in which the $^{14}CO_2$ liberated was measured in a scintillation system as previously described.

Results

Mineralization

The results obtained for atrazine mineralization under different experimental conditions of natural soil, no tillage and no tillage with previous application of atrazine are summarized in Table 2. The dry soils (20% WHC) show low mineralization with

Table 2. Atrazine Mineralization under different experimental conditions.

Method	Soils	Experimental conditions			Mineralization (%)
Erlenmeyer flasks	Dark red Latosol	Conventional tillage pre-treatment of atrazine (CTa)	(20% WHC)		0.002
			(80% WHC)		2.5
		No tillage pre-treatment of atrazine (NTa)	(20% WHC)		0.002
			(80% WHC)		8.9
Volumetric flasks	Dark red Latosol	Natural Soil No tillage (NT)			0.8
					0.7
		No tillage pre-treatment of atrazine (NTa)	(90% WHC)		45
Microcosm system	Ultisol		7–8 Kg		0.12
Plant column system	Red yellow Latosol	Superficial soil	0–20 cm	Without plants	1.2
				C. hololeuca	10.2
				T. micrantha	10.2
		Subsuperficial soil	20–40 cm	Without plants	1.3
				T. micrantha	1.9

WHC—water holding capacity

only 0.002% of applied radioactivity compared to the humid soils (80% WHC) with values of 2.5%. Soil with pre-treatment of atrazine after three years of the first application showed an increase of mineralization with 8.9% compared to the conventional management samples. Mineralization of the one year pretreated "no tillage" soil samples measured by the volumetric flasks method show much higher values with 45%.

Half-life

The determined half-life of atrazine in Table 3, ranges from 13 to 1,730 (133-fold variation). The half-life of atrazine in field experiment presented in Table 3 was of 13 and 21 days, in CT and NT, respectively. In the plant column system of superficial soil (0–20 cm), atrazine half-life without plants is 1,730 days with *C. holoeuca* 76 days and by *T. micrantha*, 132 days. The half-life values in the surface soil without plant (1,730 days) was approximately three times higher than on the subsurface soil (20–40 cm) with 697 days under the same conditions. The half-life in subsuperficial soil without plant (697 days) was increased 5.3 fold compared to subsuperficial soil cultivated with *T. micrantha* (131 days). The half-life in aerobic conditions in surface soil is 49 and subsoil 119 days are lower than in anaerobiosis (surface soil 124 and subsoil 407).

Table 3 presents the half-life results determined herein in comparison with some other authors of the literature.

Table 4 shows that plants display radioactive atrazine/metabolites uptake beginning by the roots, mainly fine roots (14.1, 8.9, 12.6%), and moving upwards

Table 3. Atrazine half-life under different environmental conditions and experimental approaches.

Methods	Soils	Experimental conditions		Half-life (days)	Reference
Field	Ultisol	Conventional tillage		15	Correia et al. 2007
	Dark red Latosol	Conventional tillage		13	Correia et al. 2010
		No tillage		21	
Plant columns system	Red yellow Latosol	Surface $_{(0-20 cm)}$	Without plants	1,730	Bicalho and Langenbach 2012
			C. Hololeuca	76	
			T. micrantha	132	
		Subsoil $_{(20-40 cm)}$	Without plants	697	Not published
			T. micrantha	131	
Microcosm Field	Clay soil			21	Winkelmann and Klaine 1991
				14	
Field	Clay soil		in summer	37	Frank et al. 1991
			in winter	125	
Laboratory	Clay soil	Surface $_{(0-20 cm)}$	Aerobic condition	49	Accinelli et al. 2001
		Subsoil $_{(80-110 cm)}$		119	
		Surface $_{(0-20 cm)}$	Anaerobic conditions	124	
		Subsoil $_{(80-110 cm)}$		407	

Table 4. ^{14}C-Atrazine distribution in microcosm with and without plant (% Bc).

^{14}C-Atrazine (%Bc)	Superficial soil (0–20 cm)			Sub-superficial soil (20–40 cm)	
	T. micrantha	C. hololeuca	Without plants	T. micrantha	Without plants
Volatilization	0.02	0.01	0.0	0.0	0.0
Mineralization (CO_2)	10.2	10.2	1.3	1.9	1.3
Leaves	5.4	19.6	–	24.9	–
Steams	8.6	5.5	–	3.6	–
Fine roots	14.1	8.9	–	12.6	–
Thick roots	4.5	5.9	–	0.7	–
Rhizosphere	4.7	7.4	–	3.3	–
Bulk soil	56.2	47.1	96.8	45.7	91.1
Bottom mesh	N.D.	N.D.	N.D.	0.0	0.1
Bottom dish	N.D.	N.D.	N.D.	0.0	0.2
Mass Balance	103.72	104.61	98.1	92.7	92.7

N.D. = non-detectable

to the leaves, arriving at concentrations between 5.6 and 24.9%. About half of the residues are incorporated in different plant tissues compared to bulk soil without plants. The calculated mass balance ranges between 92.5 and 104.6%.

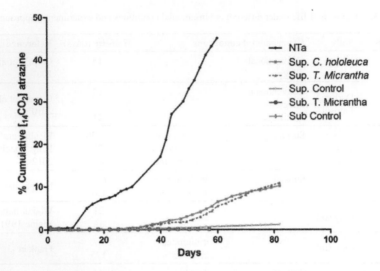

Fig. 3. Mineralization of non-tilled soils with previous atrazine treatment, in soil with *C. hololeuca*, in soil with *T. micrantha* and soil control.

Figure 3 displays the mineralization curves of non-tillage with previous atrazine treatment and soils from surface and sub-surface layers with different plants.

Discussion

The challenge for sustainability is to ensure environmental cleaning after pesticide application by degradation after a certain period. Restrictions on or banning of certain compounds are defined in the compounds registration process, based on scientific information. The main contributing factor for the environmental cleaning is biodegradation and microorganisms are the most important players in this process. When microorganism use molecules as energy and nutrient source, the degradation occurs up to CO_2 that is an inorganic molecule and this process is called mineralization. As a result, microorganisms are inactive under dry conditions (20% WHC), and similar mineralization values were observed in tilled and non-tilled soils, with values close to zero (Table 2). Issa and Wood (2005) demonstrated low mineralization by low humidity, and increase by higher humidity but under very humid conditions soil become anaerobic and the herbicide isoproturon mineralization is decreased. In the environment, soils are exposed to different rain amounts, as well as intense evaporation by sun irradiation which can promote strong dryness. Comparing the data of natural soil without agricultural use and no tillage soil, both have quite low mineralization values of atrazine (0.7 to 0.8%), probably due to dryness, despite other factors that will be discussed further.

Mineralization in no tillage soils pretreated with atrazine showed much higher values, ranging from 8.95 to 45%, compared to conventional tillage, with 0.8 to 2.5%. These results need to be addressed, once to the presence of straw on the soil by no tillage management and second, to atrazine application after the first application several years ago (pre-treatment). In the composition of straw, about 18% is lignin that will be released in the soil. Experiments have shown that brown coals (lignite) induce white rod fungi to produce nonspecific lignolytic enzymes, such as Mn peroxidase, lignin peroxidase and laccase (Klein et al. 2014). These enzymes have demonstrated a biodegradation capacity regarding atrazine (Gorbatova et al. 2006, Nwachukiwu and Osuji 2007) and many other persistent organic pollutants, as compiled in the review by Maqbool et al. (2016). These enzymes are extracellular, without cell control (Glen and Gold 1983) that makes it easy to get reactions with pollutants and generally occur in microbial consortium, resulting in efficient biodegradation process. The results obtained herein show higher mineralization under no tillage soil management, probably influenced by nonspecific lignolytic enzymes excreted by microorganisms, which can act as a co-metabolism for atrazine.

The application of a pesticide for the first time can introduce a new selection pressure for soil microbiota, allowing biodegradation genes expression for these molecules (Devers et al. 2004). In a second application of the pesticide, a kind of memory happens, in which microbiota with atrazine degradation enzymes are still active and do not need a lag phase and after some repeated applications, generally results in an enhanced biodegradation (Racke and Coats 1990). At the initial period in which atrazine is mainly bioavailable, the molecules are easy targets for the enzyme action and, therefore, mineralization could be highly efficient.

The results with soil without pre-treatment with atrazine showed a low mineralization rate, similar to that observed by Jablonowski et al. (2009) of 1.1% ± 0.22%, after 139 days of incubation. By the first atrazine use, mineralization observed by these authors arrive to 13.41% ± 0.3%, similar to the present study (Table 2), but by continuous exposure, resulted in a mineralization increase up to about 82% (Martinazzo et al. 2010). The continuous use of atrazine makes the population with biodegradation genes very active and this molecule will be degraded so fast that it has no time to adsorb molecules efficiently, conditions in which many biodegradation enzymes could not be active (Langenbach 2013).

The results obtained by Correia (2007) of 8.95% of mineralization under quite similar conditions and as observed in other data presented in Table 2 with 45% indicate that experimental conditions could be very important. In this case, the room temperature variation without agitation (Correia 2007) is different, as continuous temperature and constant agitation with a much higher exposure to oxygen (Hussain 2007) could be the reason for this great difference. The curve observed in Fig. 1 indicates that during the first month, mineralization was about 10% but after the 40th day, a strong increase occurred, arriving 45% by day 60. Mineralization measured using the volumetric flask method with high constant humidity (80% WHC) and temperature is much higher (45%), suggesting that these conditions are quite near the optimal microbial activity. However, these conditions are not normally constant in the environment. The results obtained herein agree with Issa and Wood (2005), in which case the rate of degradation was the highest in samples maintained at a moisture content of 90% WHC compared with lower soil moisture as well under saturation conditions. For the observed high mineralization of 45%, many factors would come together. First, atrazine biodegradation enzymes induced by lignin; second, pretreatment with atrazine with selection of microbes with efficient biodegradation enzymes for atrazine; third, the more constant conditions of temperature, humidity and last, the enhanced oxygenation by agitation. Recent findings point out that nitrogen could be limited by atrazine catabolism or transport gene expression (Garcia-González et al. 2003), mechanism regulated by a complex circuit (Govantes et al. 2009). This effect probably does not occur in this case while the soil management uses nitrogen fixation capacity instead of nitrogen fertilizer.

Plants enhance biodegradation as shown in (Table 2) and probably root exudation is responsible for the stimulation effect on microorganism activities. In soils, several parameters influence the rate of biological processes (microbial growth and degradation rates), including environmental factors such as moisture (Issa and Wood 2005), temperature, physicochemical properties of the soil carbon source, nitrogen (Guillen Garces et al. 2007), microbial population, microbial adaptation, and aerobic or anaerobic conditions which are important in mineralization intensity. Nevertheless, the differences of the mineralization rates in experiments with plants at the surface and sub-surface soils suggest that the amount of available carbon source/organic matter in the soil is very determinant, as observed by others (Desitti et al. 2017). Experiments with atrazine in pretreated soil have a fast and intense mineralization at the beginning with gradual reduction, suggesting the combination of high bioavailable atrazine with an intense enzymatic activity. The other set of experiments with plants shows a period of low biodegradation followed by a period of increased degradation activity. In the meantime, adsorption of atrazine in the soil is in progress and reduces the bioavailable amount of residues that can be biodegraded. Therefore, the calculations in the tables did not consider the adsorption constant Kd and the introduction of error with a higher biodegradation rate occurred in the environment.

Surface soil shows a much higher mineralization amount with plants than sub-surface soil. The main difference is the higher carbon content in surface soils compared to subsurface soils. Atrazine biodegradation was described when it was the only carbon source or by microbial consortium activity but in sewage treatment plants where atrazine was added, the molecule was released to liquid effluent without biodegradation despite a large biodiversity of microorganisms in the sludge. Therefore, when a high carbon source is offered to microbiota, they use molecules easy to degrade, avoiding difficult to degrade molecules such as atrazine (Oliveira et al. 2013). Studies pertaining to molecular signaling mechanism for biodegradation are still scarce in literature (Bisht et al. 2015). Nevertheless, some information is available and is important in this context. Root exudate comprises about 35% of plant photosynthates and is not only an important source of carbon, but also produces certain molecules that attract specific microorganisms with biodegradation capacity. Plant-microbial interactions can release flavonoids, salicylic acid and other compounds which can stimulate growth and activity of polyaromatic hydrocarbons (PAH) degrading bacteria (Thomas et al. 2003, Leight et al. 2006, Bish et al. 2015). Phenolic plant products such as catechin and coumarin may serve as co-metabolites for PCB degrading bacteria (Kuiper et al. 2004). Vegetation could enhance the magnitude of rhizosphere microbial communities, microbial biomass content, and heterotrophic bacterial community, but did little to influence those community components.

The colonization movement of microorganism in the soil and the root growth are important in the biodegradation process. Root growth in the soil introduces nutrients in the different soil layers attractive for microorganism. Plant roots can act to incorporate nutrients and improve aeration (Kuiper et al. 2004). Chemotaxis of *P. fluorescens* WC365 toward organic acids and amino acids (but not to sugar) play an important role during root colonization (Kuiper et al. 2004). Variovorax paradoxus is an aerobic soil bacterium frequently associated with important biodegradative processes in nature. Swarming movement of this microorganism has been related to both carbon and nitrogen sources, as well as mineral salts base (Jamielson et al. 2009). Studies about molecular communication between plants and microbes can promote the catabolic pathways in polluted soils, enhancing rhizoremediation efficiency (Singh et al. 2004).

Degradation of atrazine in soil samples collected at two different soil depths (0–20 and 80–110 cm) and incubated under aerobic and anaerobic conditions was also studied by Accinelli et al. (2001). Under aerobic conditions, the half-life of atrazine in surface soil was 49 days, while in subsoil, the half-life was 119 days. Under anaerobic conditions, atrazine degradation was markedly slower than under aerobic conditions, with a half-life of 124 and 407 days in surface soil and subsoil, respectively, and in lower temperatures, the half-life is even higher. Frank et al. (1991) reported that sandy soils with more leaching have much lower half-life than clay-soils. The lower mineralization in experiments with sub-surface soil may be due to the lower density of microbial biomass and consequently, enzyme activities within the soil profile, indicating that the decrease in microbial activity with depth depends on organic matter content and microbial biomass.

Atrazine declined rapidly over the summer months with a half-life disappearance of 37 days. When the dissipation period was extended to cover the winter months, the half-life disappearance increased to 125 days (Frank et al. 1991).

The data presented in Table 2 indicate that mineralization values in soils with conventional management are lower than in soils with no tillage, which is opposite of the half-life measurements (Table 3) that show 18 days for soils with conventional management compared with 21 days with "no tillage". Therefore, it is quite clear that mineralization and half-life that characterize persistence of molecules are based on different processes. Mineralization is due to microbial biodegradation and was influenced by all parameters that influence microorganism and half-life is the fate of the molecules in the environment including leaching, volatilization, non-extractable residues, plant uptake as well as biodegradation down to mineralization (Correia et al. 2009). Table 4 shows that plant mineralization is increased up to 10.2%, at the same time, the opposite is observed regarding half-life, of 697 days, due to the lack of leaching while the water supply was added on the bottom (Table 3). To know if a molecule is persistent or not, the criteria must be based on mineralization while half-life is a sum of many other processes as leachate, volatilization adsorption and mineralization. Half-life in general is measured in the environment and contributes to an overall information and mineralization with radiolabeled molecules that are performed in contained experiments as microcosm or flasks that works under controlled conditions, making possible to draw conclusions of how each parameter functions. Experiments with small samples in contained conditions can optimize mineralization and can result in higher values than experiments in the environment.

In the registration process, experimental conditions are previously defined to avoid manipulation but with the purpose of obtaining the best results, a given chemical half life is sometimes chosen by the producer instead of mineralization. Different experimental conditions for a molecule can show very different results, as shown in Tables 3 and 4. For example, mineralization with null values, as observed for tebuthiuron (Lourencetti et al. 2008, Bicalho and Lagenbach 2013), with no metabolite identification, makes banning the best choice, as observed in Europe, but not in most countries. However, for atrazine, there is much different mineralization data available and most of it, with low biodegradation performance, although, nowadays, in some cases, a good biodegradation performance up to 89% could be observed (Table 2). To ban a molecule with variable biodegradation, as shown here, is much more difficult and in this case, other parameters get very important to take a decision. The contamination frequency of wells in Europe and US shows that this molecule is the most polluting, championing ground water pesticide pollution (Jablonowski et al. 2011) and therefore, this information should be sufficient to ban this herbicide considering that there are better products with similar effects on the market. Modernity is not defined only by the new technologies or scientific advances, but also needs to be tracked by the exclusion of hazardous technologies, a prerequisite for sustainable agriculture.

Conclusions

Atrazine mineralization traced by ^{14}C-CO_2 shows different results as those measured by half-life that represent the disappearance resulting from the fate of the molecule in the environment. Half-life is the residue amount in the soil with the exception of molecules strongly adsorbed to the soil, leached to ground water or run-off, volatilized and incorporated in plants and biota, and also includes biodegradation and mineralization processes. For the registration process, it is advisable to use both measurements but never to substitute mineralization with half-life in the environment to characterize persistence.

The main influences that increase mineralization are those that contribute to energy and nutrient sources as plant exudation and straw of no tillage soil management.

The regular application of a given molecule on the soil can select microorganism/consortiums with high biodegradation ability. In this case known as memory, biodegradation is enhanced.

Temperature and humidity have high variation in the environment but when constantly maintained with optimized values in a controlled apparatus, mineralization could show very high values not occurring in the environment.

Acknowledgments

The authors are grateful for the financial support from CNPQ, FAPERJ and PRONEX.

References

Accinelli, C., G. Dinelli, A. Vicari and P. Catizone. 2001. Atrazine and metolachlor degradation in subsoils. Biol. Fertil. Soils. 33: 495–500.

Balinova, A. and I. Balinov. 1991. Determination of herbicide residues in soil in the presence of persistent organochlorine insecticides. Fresenius J. Anal. Chem. 339: 409–412.

Bicalho, S. and T. Langenbach. 2012. Distribution of the herbicide atrazine in a microcosm with ri-arian forest plants. J. Env. Sci. and Health, part B: Pest. 47: 505–511.

Bicalho, S.T.T. and T. Langenbach. 2013. The fate of tebuthiuron in microcosm with riparian forest seedlings. Geoderma. 207: 66–70.

Bisht, S., P. Pandey, B. Bhargava, S. Sharma, V. Kumar and K.D. Sharma. 2015. Bioremediation of polyaromatic hydrocarbons (PAHs) using rhizosphere technology. Braz. J. Microbiol. 46(1).

Correia, F.V., A. Macrae, L.R.G. Guilherme and T. Langenbach. 2007. Atrazine sorption and fate in a Ultisol from humid tropical Brazil. Chemosphere. 67: 847–854.

Correia, F.V., T. Langenbach and T. Campos. 2010. Avaliação do transporte de atrazina em solos sob diferentes condições de manejo agrícola. Rev. Bras. Ciênc. Solo, v. 34: 525–534.

Desitti, C., M. Beliavski, S. Tarre and M. Green. 2017. Stability of a mixed microbial population in a biological reactor during long term atrazine degradation under carbon limiting conditions. Int. Biodeterior. Biodegradation. 123: 311–319.

Devers, M., G. Soulas and F. Martin-Laurent. 2004. Real-time reverse transcription PCR analysis of expression of atrazine catabolism genes in two bacterial strains isolated from soil. J. Microbiol. Methods. 56(1): 3–15.

EMBRAPA. 1997. Centro Nacional de Pesquisa de Solos. Manual de métodos de análise de solos. 2sd ed. rev. e atual. Rio de Janeiro: EMBRAPA. 212 p.

EPPO-European Mediterranean Plant Protection Organization. 1993. Decision making scheme for the environmental risk assessment of plant protection products. EPPO Bulletin 23, Chapter 3.

Frank, R., B.S. Clegg and N.K. Patni. 1991. Dissipation of atrazine on a clay loam soil, Ontario, Canada, 1986–90. Arch. Environ. Contam. Toxicol. 21: 41–50.

García-González, V., F. Govantes, L.J. Shaw, R.G. Burns and E. Santero. 2003. Nitrogen control of atrazine utilization in *Pseudomonas* sp. strain ADP. Appl. Environ. Microbiol. 69: 6987–6993.

Glenn, J.K. and M.H. Gold. 1983. Decolorization of several polymeric dyes by the lignin degrading basidiomycete *Phanerochaete chrysosporium*. Appl. Environ. Microbiol. 45: 1741–1747.

Gorbatova, O.N., O.V. Kololeva, E.O. Landesman, E.V. Stepanova and A.V. Zerdev. 2006. Increase of the detoxification potential of basidiomycetes by induction of laccase biosynthesis. Appl. Biochem. Microbiol. 42(4): 414–419.

Govantes, F., O. Porrúa, V. García-González and E. Santero. 2009. Atrazine biodegradation in the lab and in the field: enzymatic activities and gene regulation. Microb. Biotechnol. 2(2): 178–185.

Govantes, F., O. Porrúa, V. García´González and E. Santero. 2009. Minireview: Atrazine biodegradation in the lab and in the field: enzymatic activities and gene regulation. Microbial. Biotec. 2(2): 178–185.

Guillen Garces, R.A., A.M. Hansen and M. Van Afferden. 2007. Mineralization of atrazine in agricultural soil: inhibition by nitrogen. Environ. Toxicol. Chem. 26: 844–850.

Huang, L. and J. Pignatello. 1990. Improved extraction of atrazine and metolachlor in field soil samples. J. Assoc. Off. Anal. Chem. 73: 443–446.

Hussain, S., M. Arshad, M. Saleem and A. Khalid. 2007. Biodegradation of α- and β-endosulfan by soil bacteria. Biodegradation. 18(6): 731–740.

IBAMA. 1990. Instituto Brasileiro de Meio Ambiente. Manual de testes para avaliação da ecotoxicidade de agentes químicos. 2.ed. Brasília, 351 p.

Issa, S. and M. Wood. 2005. Degradation of atrazine and isoproturon in surface and sub-surface soil materials undergoing different moisture and aeration conditions. Pest Manag. Sci. 61: 126–132.

IUPAC-International Union of Pure and Applied Chemistry. 1997. Compendium of Chemical Terminology, 2nd ed. (the "Gold Book"). Compiled by A. D. McNaught and A. Wilkinson. Blackwell Scientific Publications, Oxford. XML on-line corrected version: http://goldbook.iupac.org (2006-) created by M. Nic, J. Jirat, B. Kosata; updates compiled by A. Jenkins. ISBN 0-9678550-9-8. doi:10.1351/goldbook.

Jablonowski, N.D., S. Köppchen, D. Hofmann, A. Schäffer and P. Burauel. 2009. Persistence of ^{14}C labeled atrazine and its residues in a field lysimeter soil after 22 years. Environ. Pollut. 157(7): 2126–2131.

Jablonowski, N.D., A. Schaeffer and P. Burauel. 2011. Still present after all these years: persistence plus potential toxicity raise questions about the use of atrazine. Environ. Sci. Pollut. Res. 18: 328–331.

Jamieson, D.W., M.J. Pehl, G.A. Gregory and P.M. Orwin. 2009. Coordinated surface activities in *Variovorax paradoxus* EPS. BMC Microbiol. 9: 124.

Klein, O.I., N.A. Kunikova, E.V. Stepanova, O.I. Filippova, T.V. Fedorova, L.G. Maloshenok et al. 2014. Preparation and characterization of bioactive products obtained via the solubilization of brown coal by white rot fungi. Appl. Biochem. Microbiol. 50(10): 730–736.

Kuiper, E.l., G.V. Lagendijk and B. Lugtenberg. 2004. Rizoremediation: A beneficial plant microbe interaction. Mol. Plant Microbe. Interact. 17: 6–15.

Langenbach, T. 2013. Persistence and bioaccumulation of persistent organic pollutants (POP's). pp. 305–329. *In*: Yogesh and Prakash Rao (eds.). Applied Bioremediation Active and Passive Approaches. Intech, Chapter 13.

Leight, M.B., P. Prouzova, M. Mackova, T. Macek, D.P. Nagle and J.S. Fletcher. 2006. Polychlorinated biphenyl (PCB)—degrading bacteria associated with trees in a PCB contaminated site. Appl. Environ. Microbiol. 72: 2331–2342.

Lourencetti, C., M.R.R. Marchi and M.L. Ribeiro. 2008. Determination of sugar cane herbicides in soil and soil treated with sugar cane vinasse by solid-phase extraction and HPLC–UV. Talanta. 77: 701–709.

Martinazzo, R., N.D. Jablonowski, G. Hamacher, D.P. Dick and P. Burauel. 2010. Accelerated degradation of ^{14}C-Atrazine in Brazilian soils from different regions. J. Agric. Food Chem. 58(13): 7864–7870.

Maqbool, Z., S. Hussain, M. Imram, F. Mahmood, T. Shahzad, Z. Ahmed et al. 2016. Perspectives of using fungi as bioresource for bioremediation of pesticides in the environment: a critical review. Environ. Sci. Pollut. Res. 23: 16904–16925.

Moreira, F.M.S. and J.O. Siqueira. 2002. Microbiologia e bioquímica do solo. Lavras: UFLA. 626 p.

Nwachukiwu, E.O. and J.O. Osuji. 2007. Bioremedial degradation of some herbicides by indigenous white rot fungus, *Lentinus subnudus*. J. Plant Sci. 2: 619–624.

OECD-Organization for Economic Co-operation and Development. 2002. Aerobic and Anaerobic Transformation in Soil, OECD Guideline for Testing of Chemicals 307, adopted 24.

Oliveira, J., E. Ferreira, D. Silva, M. Dezotti and T. Langenbach. 2013. Fate of the herbicide atrazine during sewage treatment by lab-scale bioreactor. AMBIAGUA 28(2).

Racke, J. and M.R. Coats. 1990. Enhanced Biodegradation of Pesticides in the Environment. Kenneth, D. (ed.). American Chemical Society ISBN13: 9780841217843 Volume 426.

SETAC-Society of Environ. Toxicol. Chem. 1995. Procedures for Assessing the Environmental Fate and Ecotoxicology of Pesticides. Ed Mark R. Lynch.

Singh, N., M. Megharaj, R.S. Kookana, R. Naidu and N. Sethunathan. 2004. Atrazine and simazine degradation in *Pennisetum rhrizosphere*. Chemosphere. 56: 257–263.

Tang, H.P. 2013. Recent development in analysis of persistent organic pollutants under the Stockholm convention review article. Trends Anal. Chem. 45: 48–66.

Thomas, G.J., T.B. Lam and D.C. Wolf. 2003. A mathematical model of phytoremediation for petroleum contaminated soil: Sensivity analysis. Int. J. Phytoremediation. 5: 125–136.

US-EPA/Environmental Protection Agency U.S. 1982. Pesticide Assessment Guidelines, Subdivision N, Chemistry: Environmental Fate, Series 162-1 Aerobic Soil Metabolism Studies. U.S. EPA Office of Pesticide Programs, Washington, DC.

8

Implementing the Current Knowledge of Uptake and Effects of Nanoparticles in an Adverse Outcome Pathway (AOP) Framework

Nadja Rebecca Brun,[1,]* Willie J.G.M. Peijnenburg,[2] Marinda van Pomeren[1] and Martina G. Vijver[1]

Introduction

Hazard identification of nanoparticles to organisms

Unlike most other environmental pollution issues, safety assessments of nanoparticles (NPs) were meant to be the prime example of how to foresee and tackle predicted environmental concerns. For once, research efforts were ahead of mass production and potential release into environments (Nowack and Bucheli 2007, Handy et al. 2008). Anyhow, these small particles with their inherent reactivity arose as a real challenge in fate and response assessments. Consequently, safety research is still mostly performed under controlled laboratory conditions, focusing on the central question of whether the unique properties of NPs cause fundamentally different effects as compared to their larger counterparts. Subsequently, it is asked: if so, what are the nano-specific induced responses we can expect? Ever since the appearance of

[1] CML - Institute of Environmental Sciences, Department of Conservation Biology, Leiden University, Einsteinweg 2, 2333 CC Leiden, The Netherlands.
E-mail: m.van.pomeren@cml.leidenuniv.nl
E-mail: vijver@cml.leidenuniv.nl
[2] Centre for Safety of Substances and Products, RIVM - National Institute for Public Health and the Environment, PO Box 1, 3720 BA Bilthoven, The Netherlands.
E-mail: willie.peijnenburg@rivm.nl
* Corresponding author: n.r.brun@cml.leidenuniv.nl

NPs and early safety and risk assessments, nanotechnology industry has expanded rapidly due to widespread use of NPs in commercially available products. The global production of engineered NPs was estimated to increase from 10,000 tons in 2011 to 60,000 tons in 2020, reaching a market value of $ 3 trillion by 2020 (Łojkowski et al. 2015, Piccinno et al. 2012). Although concentrations of environmental nanoparticles are currently forecasted to be low (Gottschalk et al. 2013), the continuous use and accumulation of non-degradable or slowly degradable NPs will inevitably impose increasing pressure on our natural environment.

The ecotoxicological profiling of particles in the nano range is specifically challenging due to their various features. NPs are defined as "particles, in an unbound state or as an aggregate or as an agglomerate where, 50% or more of the particles in the number size distribution, in one or more external dimensions, are in the size range 1 nm–100 nm" (EU 2011). Nanosized particles find manifold applications in electronics, medicine, cosmetics and consumer products such as wall paint or sport clothing, only to name a few. NPs are not only manmade, but can come from natural sources such as products from combustion (e.g., forest fires), simple erosions or volcanic dust. In industrial and consumer products, their small particle size brings various desirable properties: NPs have a very large surface area compared to larger materials (from now on referred to as bulk materials), offering a larger surface area for chemical reactions and adsorption capacity (Auffan et al. 2008). The number of atoms located at the surface exponentially increases with the decrease of NP size. Although NPs are routinely defined as having a dimension between 1 and 100 nm, Auffan et al. (2009) point out that many particles undergo dramatic changes in crystalline structure at a size of 30 nm or less, suggesting to focus on this smaller set of NPs when conducting toxicity studies.

Experimental results indicate that metal-based NPs do not necessarily react in the same way as their bulk counterparts, nor as dissolved metals or metal ions (Gomes et al. 2011, Muller et al. 2015). In response to this, ecotoxicological assessments of NPs require input from the disciplines of chemical toxicology as well as colloidal chemistry. The main difficulty in assessing toxicity profiles of NPs is that their sizes and shapes are as manifold as their applications. Every modification in core, size, shape or coating of the NP can affect its fate and response, thus hampering general predictability. In addition, the physicochemical behavior of NPs changes with almost every new medium and is highly dynamic over time, making repeatability and translation between laboratories or test organisms difficult to control. Lastly, the mechanistic pathways of responses remain unclear. Detected biological effects are often related to the nanoparticle's inherent elements, such as metals masking the nanoparticle's effect and thus adding to the challenges in nanoparticle research. Nanospecific modes of actions are to a large extent unknown, but their endocytic uptake mechanism (Zhu et al. 2013) and reactive surface suggest different intracellular effects than soluble compounds.

NPs in the environment

Sediments, either from terrestrial or aquatic environments, are particularly at risk for NP contamination, because they act as sink for many contaminants discharged, including NPs. This chapter will focus on the aquatic environment since 30 times more studies focus on this environment than terrestrial environments (Chen et al. 2015, Selck et al. 2016). Nanoparticles enter the aquatic systems indirectly from wastewater treatment plant (WWTP) runoffs or directly as surface runoffs and by deposition. WWTPs mainly collect NPs originating from medical uses, cosmetics and household products (e.g., TiO_2, ZnO, Ag), whereas surface runoffs mainly transport NPs from fuels (CeO_2), wall paints, sunscreens (TiO_2), anti-microbial coatings (Ag), leachates from landfills and accidentally released NPs at production sites. Unless NPs are released accidentally from the point of manufacturing, they will reach the environment mostly as degraded particles released from consumer goods, medical or industrial applications. Once the NPs have entered the aquatic environment, further transformation processes (e.g., agglomeration, aggregation, dissolution, sulfidation, see Fig. 1) affect the state of the particles. These processes may vary depending on salinity, pH, temperature and content of dissolved organic matter (DOM) of the receiving aquatic environments and finally determine the toxic potential of NPs. Regardless of the transformation processes that occur, NPs show a strong tendency to settle from the water column and are ultimately concentrated in the sediments where benthic organisms, sediment dwellers and microorganisms are at risk. Modeled concentrations of NPs in European lake sediments range from 0.1 to 10,000 μg kg^{-1} (Gottschalk et al. 2013). These complex interactions exemplify the need for NP characterization in exposure media to understand their ecotoxicological potential. Yet, few studies are available regarding how NPs will

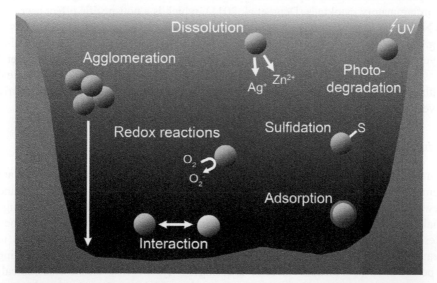

Fig. 1. Schematic overview of dynamic processes in surface waters. NPs can agglomerate into larger particles, which may settle out of the water column. Dissolution processes result in free ions and smaller particles. In the presence of Sulfur (S), NPs (e.g., AgNP or CuNP) are likely to dissolve and are sulfidized, which then decreases dissolution. Redox reactions can affect surface stability, affect dissolution and sulfidation rates. Adsorption of other compounds (e.g., humic acid) and photodegradation of coatings lead to surface modification. Particles may also interact with other particles and biota. (Figure drawn by N.R. Brun, modified from Lowry et al. 2012.)

behave in natural environments. It is challenging to measure NP behavior in a complex system where the presence of a multitude of particles mask the measurement of the target particle.

Uptake routes and effects

When it comes to NP effects on organisms, there are two features which get special attention: size and subsequent reactivity. NPs may be taken up by organisms through common uptake routes such as ingestion, skin lesions or gills in fish and then, due to their small size, be translocated through cell membranes. This could increase internal concentrations of core elements as one particle contains many densely packed elements. Metal-based NPs, for example, can deliver high amounts of free metal ions into the cell (Gilbert et al. 2012). NPs can cross the cell membrane *via* endocytic processes. In some cases, NPs are also reported to interact with membrane proteins such as toll-like receptors (Hu et al. 2016). Once entering the intracellular space, NPs can be translocated or stored in cell organelles which differ from their bulk or ionic counterpart. Due to the enlarged surface-volume ratio, the reactivity of a NP is enormous and hence influences the dissolution behavior of metal-based NPs. Their inherent reactivity is commonly related to generation of reactive oxygen species (ROS) at the target site (Nel et al. 2006). In addition, the reactive surface preferably forms ligands with proteins, which can lead to accelerated protein degradation or denaturation, ultimately leading to disrupted enzyme function. The protein binding can provoke macrophage uptake and complement activation, resulting in the release of inflammatory cytokines (Deng et al. 2011), which is a nonspecific effect ascribed to NPs. Both ROS and inflammatory reactions can lead to adverse effects in exposed organisms. Moreover, dissolution of metal-based NPs, either on the outer epithelial layer or in the intracellular space, results in a mixture of colloids and toxic metal ions, which can potentially lead to synergistic effects. However, how organisms deal with NPs over time as well as threshold values for the environment has been poorly investigated so far.

Adverse outcome pathways

Currently, the various possible biological effects of a large number of NPs are being assessed in laboratories all over the world. Screening every existing and newly designed particle for its potential ecotoxicological outcomes presents a huge challenge. Thus, common mechanistic pathways must be identified and based upon these pathways, high-throughput *in vitro* assays are to be developed. This fits in neatly with the Adverse Outcome Pathway (AOP) conceptual framework, linking a perturbation at molecular level of a biological system with an adverse (apical) outcome at higher levels of biological organization which are of regulatory relevance (e.g., impact on growth, reproduction, or survival; Fig. 2). This approach includes the description of key events (KEs) of responses at molecular, cellular, organ or sub-organismal levels which are measurable and necessary for an adverse outcome to occur. The first KE represents the molecular initiating event (MIE), whereas the last KE represents the adverse outcome (AO). The MIE is the direct site of interaction

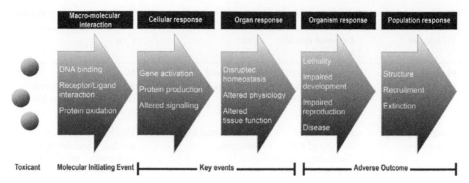

Fig. 2. Schematic overview of the key features of an Adverse Outcome Pathway across biological levels. (Figure adapted from the AOP knowledge base; http://www.aopkb.org/.)

between a toxicant and its molecular target within an organism. This interaction can be either highly specific, such as binding to a specific receptor, or non-specific, such as a reactive chemical that can covalently modify a wide range of proteins. The latter is likely to be the case for NPs, since NP recognition by receptors is rarely observed. The AO should be relevant to regulatory decision-making and thus will most often be an outcome of demographic significance.

In 2012, the OECD together with the EU-Commission's Joint Research Centre, US-EPA and US Army Engineer Research and Development Center, launched a new program to share and discuss the development of AOPs related knowledge. This so called AOP knowledge base brings together four different platforms (AOP-Wiki, Effectopedia, Intermediate Effects DB, and AOP Xplorer), facilitating the sharing of AOP knowledge between the scientific community and stakeholders.

Given the pace of NP development, advancements in understanding ecological effects of NPs are urgently needed. This chapter gives an overview of the present understanding of NP toxicity in aquatic organism. Briefly, state-of-the-art techniques to detect NPs in tissues are summarized and the present understanding of cellular and organismal NP uptake routes is given. The location of NPs in tissues bears several challenges but is the first step in identifying target organs or cells and, thus, is important in the search for mechanisms of action. The evaluation of our current knowledge of cellular and organismal responses when exposed to NPs, ultimately, allows for the identification of key knowledge gaps and foresees research directions and needs to develop Adverse Outcome Pathways for NPs.

Methods to Determine Uptake and Internalization of NPs

Several methods are available to determine uptake and cellular internalization in organisms. While some methods enable an overview of the spatial distribution (e.g., organs) of a contaminant in whole organisms, other methods determine accumulation in different subcellular compartments. In the following table, a summary of state-of-the-art techniques to localize NPs in organs or cells is given (Table 1). Many of the techniques rely on fluorescently labelled NPs, which is a superb technique

Table 1. Pros and cons of a variety of methods currently in use to study the distribution of nanoparticles.

Technique	Detected specific NPs; where?	Pro	Con
Fluorescence microscopy	Fluorescent NP; localization in tissue and whole organism	Can be used in many applications	No single particle detection due to limited resolution of 200 to 500 nm
Autoradiography microscopy	Radioisotopes of selected NP; distribution in cross sections of organs or whole body	High contrast in fine structures	Highly equipped lab needed, laborious sample preparation, strict health safety rules, resolution restricted to grain-size used
Light sheet microscopy (LSM)	Fluorescent and Au NP; live imaging technique, detected in whole organism and organs	Imaging in real time in a non-invasive manner	none
(cryo) Transmission electron microscopy (TEM)	Any NP; intracellular localization	Detailed information on subcellular structures up to 0.2 nm, good penetration depth, low photo-bleaching	Single slices, laborious sample preparation
Scanning electron microscopy (SEM)	Any NP; intracellular localization	Detailed information on subcellular structures with good field of depth	Single slices, laborious sample preparation, samples often need to be coated in conductive material
TEM or SEM in combination with Energy-dispersive X-ray spectroscopy (EDX)	Any NP; intracellular localization, useful for very small NPs	Identification of elemental composition, mapping of additional elements (P, Ca, Fe) may allow conclusions about toxic effects	Single slices, time consuming
Confocal scanning laser microscopy (CSLM)	Fluorescent and Au NP; live imaging technique, detected in whole organism, organs or subcellular fractions	Layer by layer imaging of thick samples, cellular details including circulating blood cells	High sensitivity is obtained by strong excitation light only, causing tissue photodamage and dye bleaching
Multifocal multi-photon microscopy (MPM)	Any NP; live imaging technique	Larger imaging depth than CSLM, high temporal resolution	Only 4 cell layers thick, lower spatial resolution than CSLM

Table 1 contd. ...

...Table 1 contd.

Technique	Detected specific NPs; where?	Pro	Con
Coherent anti-Stokes Raman scattering (CARS)	Any NP; live imaging technique	Detection of intrinsic and specific chemical structures with vibrational spectroscopy, increased depth penetration, low phototoxicity	Difficult to detect low concentrations
Induced coupled plasma mass spectroscopy (ICP-MS) and atomic absorption spectroscopy (AAS)	Metal-based NP; quantifying elements in extracted organs or subcellular fractions	Quantification of the metal present	Dissolved metals not distinct from metal-based NP
Time-resolved ICP-MS	Metal-based NP; detecting NPs in extracted organs or subcellular fractions	Distinction between NPs and dissoluted metals possible	If NPs contain elements with high natural abundance, separation of background difficult, recently developed method (under development)
Laser ablation ICP-MS	Metal-based NP; spatial distribution of elements in fixed tissues and organs	High sensitivity up to ppb with low detection limits	Dissolved metals not distinct from metal-based NP
Scanning micro X-ray fluorescence (µXRF) spectroscopy	Metal-based NP; spatial distribution of elements in fixed tissues and organs	Mapping of additional elements (P, Ca, Fe) may allow conclusions about toxic effects	Low spatial resolution
Flow cytometry	Fluorescent NP; intracellular localization	Analysis of thousands of cells in seconds, measurement of particle size distribution directly in biological fluids	Cannot distinguish between externally attached and fully internalized NP

to study biodistribution. However, fluorescence labeling of NPs always bears the risk of changing NPs bioreactivity. Other disadvantages are their time-dependent photobleaching and potential fluorophore leakage from the NP (Salvati et al. 2011). The use of metal NPs often possesses the risk of free metal dissolution and, thus, a final confirmation of NPs present in tissues is usually not given (Brun et al. 2014). To study subcellular distribution, various microscopic techniques are available. Such techniques can give detailed information on subcellular structure and localization. However, as they rely on single slices with sections of an organ or tissue, only a small volume of 1 to 10 μm³ is analyzed (Ostrowski et al. 2015). Therefore, the overall picture of the NP distribution might be biased as it is "seeking a needle in a hay stack".

Adsorption versus absorption

In practice, bioaccumulation is a summation of the amount of compound adsorbed and absorbed, the relative proportions usually not being quantified. However, not all accumulated NP burden is necessarily absorbed into the body (see Fig. 4). A proportion may remain in association with the external surface, or be bound to extracellular compounds by physicochemical forces (Handy et al. 2008). Adsorption of NPs to the membrane is therefore defined as an extracellular process, and to make it visible, it can even be washed off (Nowack and Bucheli 2007, Van Pomeren et al. 2017). To distinguish between accumulation of particles in the gut and absorption to the gut epithelium, a depuration time after exposure is usually included (Skjolding et al. 2014). Multiple ways to eliminate adsorbed chemicals and particles are reported in literature, many challenges are there and interpretation of data on the quantitative distinction of the two processes is needed.

Uptake Routes

An aquatic environment loaded with man-made NPs undoubtedly leads to exposure of the organisms living in this environmental compartment. Whether the particles are actually incorporated into cells or not is still a topic of scientific debate. NPs must overcome several challenges such as phospholipid membranes, harsh intracellular conditions and, finally, clearing mechanisms which hamper their uptake. Due to their distinct physicochemical properties, NPs interact with a cell in a different way than their soluble counterparts. This affects uptake mechanism, intracellular fate and target organs (and ultimately toxic effects). The current knowledge on cellular uptake mechanisms in aquatic organisms is given in the following section.

A NP reaching an organism will either interact with the outer or with the inner epithelial layer after being ingested. Upon contact with a biological surface, a NP can be adsorbed to the surface or actually be absorbed into the cell (Lesniak et al. 2013). Although an adsorbed NP is of lesser concern, it may act as point source for metal dissolution or for other pollutants adsorbed to the particle. Furthermore, particles adsorbed to the body surface may cause moving hindrance. This is described for particles adsorbed to the antennae and filtering screens of *Daphnia magna*, inhibiting movement and thus increasing mortality (Lewinski et al. 2010).

In general, the outer body surface is not the main route of uptake for NPs. Nevertheless, there are susceptible organs for uptake on the outside such as the gills and the eye. The gills represent a fish specific organ vulnerable to NPs, where aggregates accumulate on the surface of the gill epithelium and potentially increase uptake (Johnston et al. 2010, Scown et al. 2010). However, the fact that NPs aggregate to a large extent on the epithelial surface of the gill, renders the NPs less likely to diffuse across cellular membranes. Recently, it has been shown that NPs can cross the retina of zebrafish embryos (Kim et al. 2013, Van Pomeren et al. 2017). It remains speculative whether the particles are stored in the eye or are further translocated into the brain for example. The predominant uptake route of NPs is ingestion (Skjolding et al. 2017, Fig. 3). In the gut, the NPs can encounter a variation in pH and ionic strength in comparison to the aquatic environment they come from. It is well known that aggregation and disaggregation are pH- and ionic strength-driven (Keller et al. 2010) and, thus, uptake behavior of NPs may change in the gut fluids. As a result, absorption may be favored under gut conditions. Indeed, most studies (Van Pomeren et al. 2017) describing accumulation of NPs in inner organs first observed the particles in the intestine of vertebrates and invertebrate organisms. Similar to food, translocation of NPs from the digestive tract to other organs occurs by uptake into the intestinal epithelium and distribution in the body *via* the bloodstream and lymphatic system in vertebrates or hemolymph in invertebrates. Since the blood vessels can only be reached after bypassing several cell layers, migration of macromolecules and nanoparticles into the bloodstream is not easy and depends on several factors.

Cellular uptake is determined by four main factors: size, shape, charge, and protein corona (Savolainen et al. 2013, Fig. 4). The most important driving factor for NP uptake, whether on the outer epithelium or on the inner, is again its size. Size not only determines whether a particle is taken up or not, but moreover how. Only the smallest NPs, with up to 6 nm and with fitted surface properties, are allowed by the cell to pass the plasma membrane by passive diffusion (Verma et al. 2008). Larger particles require an active transport system through the cell membrane by endocytosis, which is a vesicular transport (Xia et al. 2008). Depending on the particle size, different endocytic uptake mechanisms such as phagocytosis (> 1 μm), macropinocytosis (> 1 μm), clathrin-mediated endocytosis (~ 120 nm), and caveolin-mediated endocytosis (~ 60 nm), as well as clathrin- and caveolin-independent pathways (~ 90 nm) take care of the transport, each having its own dynamics and size rules (Zhu et al. 2013). Some of these uptake mechanisms are more efficient than others: NPs with a diameter of 50 nm are internalized by cells to a higher extent than smaller

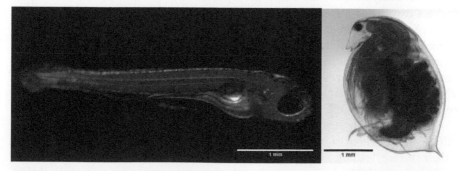

Fig. 3. Ingestion as the major route of uptake for NPs. Red fluorescent polystyrene NPs accumulate in the gut of 5 days old *Danio rerio* embryos (left) and adult *Daphnia magna* (right). (Pictures taken by M. van Pomeren and N.R. Brun.)

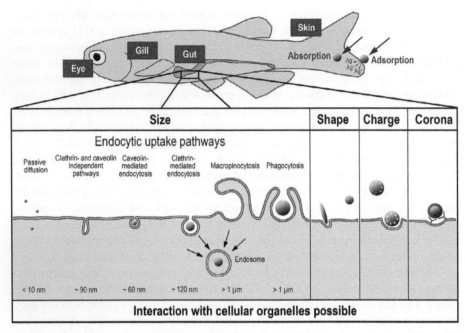

Fig. 4. Uptake routes and factors determining cellular uptake (absorption). Ingestion is likely to be the most important route of uptake. Passage through the cellular membrane is dictated by NP characteristics: NPs are mostly internalized through endocytic uptake mechanism, which are size restrictive; NPs with a higher aspect ratio can exhibit an increased internalization rate compared to spherical shaped NPs; positively charged NPs can be attracted by the negatively charged cell membrane; a protein corona is playing a vital role in defining surface charge and recognition by membrane receptors. (Figure drawn by N.R. Brun, adapted from Monopoli et al. 2012, Thurn et al. 2007, Zhu et al. 2013.)

or larger particles (Chithrani et al. 2006, Lu et al. 2009). In *Daphnia* for instance, nanowires of 40 nm and ZnO NPs of 10–30 nm are more frequently internalized into midgut cells than larger NPs of the same core (Mattsson et al. 2016, Santo et al. 2014). Not solely size, but also shape and aspect ratio determine uptake. Rod-shaped particles experience a facilitated uptake in comparison to spheres. Moreover, the length of the rod has an effect, with an intermediate length (aspect ratio of 2.1–2.5) internalized the fastest (Gratton et al. 2008, Meng et al. 2011, Zhu et al. 2013). Factors affecting NP excretion from the cells are lacking attention so far, but excretion was shown to be a size dependent exocytic event as well (Chithrani and Chan 2007, Fröhlich 2016). Furthermore, exocytosis is less effective than endocytosis, with reported release rates of 15 to 30% (Fang et al. 2011).

In addition to physical properties (size and shape), extrinsic factors that dictate cellular uptake also exist. When NPs enter a biological system, biomolecules adsorb to their surface, leading to the formation of a protein corona (Cedervall et al. 2007, Lundqvist et al. 2008). With this coating, surface properties such as surface charge (tendency to aggregate) and hydrodynamic diameter are altered and the presence of surface proteins usually increases cellular recognition (e.g., by receptors); thus, uptake is likely to be enhanced. The composition of the protein corona varies over time (Cedervall et al. 2007), is dependent on the NPs surface properties (Esmaeili et al. 2008), size (Zhang et al. 2011), shape (Carnovale et al. 2016) and medium (e.g., blood or body fluid; Zhang et al. 2011) around it. Furthermore, the surface charge of NPs, which can be altered by the corona, can be decisive for increased uptake. Due to the slightly negative charged cell membrane, positively charged NPs are suggested to favor adhesion (Arvizo et al. 2010). In coherence with that, positively charged Au NPs induce more ROS in daphnid guts than negatively charged Au NPs (Dominguez et al. 2015). These factors shaping the NP's identity are highly variable and hard to control or determine.

While after vesicular internalization, the NP is enclosed in an endosome and thus coated by a membrane, it is uncoated after diffusion through the membrane. The latter process allows it to directly bind to plasma proteins and other molecules in the cell, nano-specific interactions can thus be expected. In contrast, NPs trapped in endosomes are subjected to acidification due to a drop in pH with increasing stage of the endosome (Zhu et al. 2013). This can be especially fatal in case the NP is metallic. Even though NPs are very small in size, they obviously contain considerably more atoms than their ionic counterpart. For example, a ZnO NPs of 50 nm contains up to 8 million zinc atoms. If diluted in a typical cell volume of approximately 500 femtoliters, it results in a concentration of up to 25 umol L^{-1} zinc, which is already in the cytotoxic range (Krug and Wick 2011). This cytotoxic effect of small amounts of ZnO NPs bypassing the cell membrane has been observed by several authors (George et al. 2010, Xia et al. 2008).

Once in the cell, the NP can be translocated (in their endosomes) to various regions and organelles. While NPs less than 100 nm in diameter have been shown to enter cells, a size of less than 40 nm allows it to enter the cell nucleus, and less than 35 nm to cross the blood-brain barrier (Dawson et al. 2009). Gold nanorod particles remain in their vesicular system and are finally stored in lysosomes (Zhang et al. 2013). Ag NPs were located in the perinuclear region but not in the cell nucleus, endoplasmic reticulum (ER) or Golgi complex (Greulich et al. 2011). Polystyrene, Ti NPs and Si NPs were transported to the nucleus as well as the mitochondria, strengthening the concept of direct interactions with cellular organelles and thus interfering with cellular functions (Hemmerich and von Mikecz 2013, Sun et al. 2011, Xia et al. 2008). When comparing ZnO NPs with soluble zinc, the particles were predominantly found in organelles and cytosol, whereas the metal ions were detected in the cell membrane (Li et al. 2011). NPs that are engulfed by endosomes in the cytosol during mitosis can be inherited by daughter cells (Rees et al. 2011). To this end, it can be concluded that depending on the NP properties, different cellular compartments are targeted and thus toxicological interactions and effects might vary.

In invertebrates, the organ specialized for vesicular uptake is the hepatopancreas, whereas in fish, endocytic transport is of particular importance in the intestinal epithelium (Moore 2006). NPs that were able to adsorb through the gut epithelium are potentially released into the blood stream from where they are distributed in the organism body, accumulate at target sites or are excreted. Due to the large concentration of tissue resident phagocytic macrophages, NPs are often cleared from the blood circulation into the liver and spleen.

Excretion through the kidney is highly dependent on size, as glomerular filtration eliminates NPs with a hydrodynamic diameter of less than 5.5 nm only (Choi et al. 2007). However, classical metabolism is not directly applicable for NPs. Other processes act on NPs such as dissolution, de-agglomeration and chemical degradation, leading to particle degradation. Degradation of Si NPs for example, leads to the formation of soluble silicic acid, which is excreted *via* feces and urine (Park et al. 2009). In contrast, metal oxides are bound and transformed by metallothioneins, which are abundantly expressed in liver and kidney.

Among aquatic organisms, fish is investigated the most regarding target organs of NPs. Indeed, biodistribution of NPs (Au, Ag, CNT, polystyrene) is described and accumulation of NPs is mainly found in liver, but also in the blood, brain, gill, eye, and heart (Kashiwada 2006, Kwok et al. 2012, Scown et al. 2010, Skjolding et al. 2017, Smith et al. 2007). However, the fate of NPs indicates that invertebrates populating the sediment are especially at risk. In most cases, detection of internalization in invertebrates failed, such as for ZnO and Cu NPs in *Daphnia magna* (Adam et al. 2014) as well as for fullerene NPs in the sediment-dwelling larvae *Chironomus riparius* (Waissi-Leinonen et al. 2012). However, recently it was demonstrated that nanowires can be translocated through the gut epithelium in *Daphnia magna* (Mattsson et al. 2016).

Responses at Cellular Level

NPs trespassing the phospholipid membrane may interact with subcellular structures and proteins (Colvin 2003, Service 2004). If engulfed by endosomes, NPs are less prone to intracellular interactions and may manifest as overload of the endosomal or lysosomal system. Such accumulated NPs are often stored in fish liver and hepatopancreas or midgut gland of arthropods, molluscs and fish. If escaping from lysosomes, NPs can damage organelles or DNA (Nel et al. 2009, He et al. 2014). *In vitro* studies show that depending on the target organelle, different mechanistic pathways may be affected (Unfried et al. 2007). There is increasing evidence that NPs disrupt mitochondrial and ER functioning (Xia et al. 2006, Chen et al. 2014, Christen et al. 2014). The former activates the oxidative stress-mediated signaling cascade and the latter interferes with protein folding and maturation as well as mitochondrial perturbation and thus oxidative stress (Xia et al. 2006). A persisting state of oxidative stress induces the production of inflammatory cytokines and if all rescue attempts fail, programmed cell death is initiated (Khanna et al. 2015, Chen et al. 2016). Also, persistent ER stress can promote production of pro-inflammatory cytokines and lead to apoptosis (Chen et al. 2014). Moreover, the protein binding capacity of NPs can result in accelerated protein denaturation or degradation, leading to functional changes (e.g., enzyme function; Gao et al. 2016). Lastly, NPs which are translocated into the nucleus may damage the genetic material (Hemmerich and von Mikecz 2013). These described cellular responses are summarized in Fig. 5. To date, suggested NP-related cellular effects are based on known toxicological pathways. In the near future, high-throughput sequencing could enable the discovery of new NP specific effects.

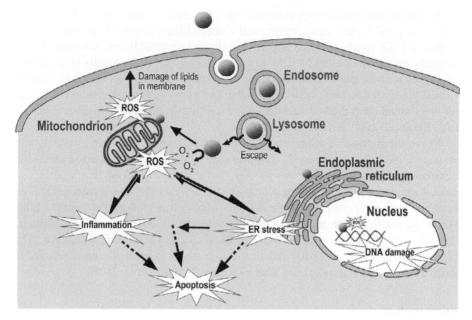

Fig. 5. Intracellular behavior of NPs, its potential translocation to the endoplasmic reticulum (ER), mitochondrion or nucleus and associated responses. (Figure drawn by N.R. Brun, adapted from Shang et al. 2014.)

Reactive Oxygen Species (ROS)

NPs, which are able to penetrate the cell, can induce ROS production and inflict oxidative stress (Xia et al. 2006). The generation of ROS is the key mechanism of NP toxicity and currently the best understood paradigm for NP toxicity. ROS formation can have different causes: (1) redox active surfaces of NPs interact with molecular dioxygen (O_2) and the capture of an electron leads to the formation of superoxide anion (O_2^-) which is a precursor of more reactive ROS such as H_2O_2 and OH (Foucaud et al. 2007), (2) the dissolution of transition metal ions acting as catalysts for ROS formation as they react with H_2O_2 to yield OH and an oxidized metal ion (Limbach et al. 2007), (3) NPs are translocated to the mitochondria where they disturb the balance in the respiratory chain and thereby increase mitochondrial ROS generation (Xia et al. 2006). In addition, organs which are not directly exposed to NPs can still show oxidative stress due to rapid distribution of ROS with blood circulation (Federici et al. 2007).

Under normal conditions, ROS are produced and neutralized in the mitochondrion. ROS at low concentrations play vital roles of controlling cellular processes such as gene expression, apoptosis and as a second messenger in signal transduction pathways (Blokhina et al. 2003, Valavanidis et al. 2006). In excess, ROS can cause severe damage to proteins, lipids and DNA, possibly resulting in deleterious effects on the cell such as apoptosis, lipid peroxidation and cancer initiating processes. Thus, in the presence of excessive ROS, cells activate their antioxidant defense mechanism to restore the redox equilibrium. Upon NP exposure, the cells respond by activating an enzymatic antioxidant system. O_2^- is converted to oxygen or H_2O_2 by the enzyme superoxide dismutase (SOD), and catalase (CAT) catalyzes the transformation of H_2O_2 to water and oxygen (Valavanidis et al. 2006). Activation of these phase I antioxidant enzymes is frequently detected in aquatic organisms exposed to NPs, such as zebrafish embryos, carp, daphnids and mussels, and is an established method to detect NP damage (Brun et al. 2014, Gomes et al. 2011, Hao et al. 2009, Kim et al. 2010).

When the first defense against ROS, antioxidant enzymes, fails to restore the balance, cellular damage proceeds. The presence of free radicals can cause oxidative degradation of lipids in cell membranes, commonly called lipid peroxidation. Malondialdehyde (MDA), an indicator of lipid peroxidation, is recognized as molecular marker for evaluating progressive oxidative stress induced by nanoparticles (Ma et al. 2010). Increased MDA levels were measured in ZnO NPs exposed zebrafish embryos (Zhao et al. 2013), in liver of adult zebrafish where Ag NPs accumulated (Choi et al. 2010) and in the digestive gland of the mussel *Mytilus edulis* where Au NPs accumulated after exposure (Tedesco et al. 2010).

Inflammation

At higher levels of oxidative stress, the antioxidant response is overtaken by inflammation and mitochondrial-mediated apoptosis. Cellular inflammation is a response to tissue damage and/or infection and can, if unresolved, cause chronic conditions. The immune system responds by activating signaling cascades (MAPK and NF-κB) leading to the release of pro-inflammatory cytokines, such as TNFα or interleukins, activating kinases and inhibition of phosphatases. Moreover, there is a feedback loop to increase ROS production, as inflammatory phagocytes (e.g., neutrophils and macrophages) induce oxidative burst. When neutrophils are recruited to the site of injury, the assembly of NADPH oxidase is stimulated. Its activation leads to reduction of O_2 to form superoxide anions (O_2^-) and other ROS. The rapid release of these radicals is important for successful defense against invading bacteria and fungi and is termed oxidative burst. Although ROS production plays an important role in killing microorganisms and degrading particles, it can end in a vicious cycle for the production of free radicals and cause destruction of surrounding tissue (Machlin and Bendich 1987).

Whereas mammalian studies confirm the inflammation reactions and immune responses to NP exposure (Nel et al. 2006, Oh et al. 2010), such reports on aquatic organisms are scarce. Global gene expression analyses in zebrafish embryos exposed to waterborne TiO_2 NPs and Au NPs highlight genes involved in immune response and endocytosis (Park and Yeo 2013, Truong et al. 2013), and nanostructured graphene oxide induced an immune response in adult zebrafish spleen (Chen et al. 2016). Furthermore, when using primary kidney goldfish neutrophils as a model, several metal-oxide NPs increased neutrophil respiratory bursts and mRNA of pro-inflammatory genes (Ortega et al. 2015). Also in mussel (*Mytilus galloprovincialis*) hemocytes, rapid activation of MAPKs was measured after exposure to nanosized carbon black (Canesi et al. 2008). These few studies indicate that the inflammatory processes may be a common response mechanism to NPs among human cells and cells of aquatic invertebrates and vertebrates.

Endoplasmic reticulum (ER) stress

Recent findings indicate inhibition of protein translation by NP aggregation in the ER (Chen et al. 2014, Gao et al. 2016, Han et al. 2014). The ER is the cellular organelle responsible for protein folding and maturation, synthesis of lipids and storage of free calcium. Failure of the ER's function results in accumulation of unfolded proteins and release of calcium and consequently in activation of the unfolded protein response (UPR), which is a protective mechanism to counteract the stress situation. Prolonged ER stress interferes with inflammatory pathways, oxidative stress or apoptosis (Hotamisligil 2010).

This injury pathway is triggered in zebrafish embryos when exposed to Ag NPs, including down-stream activation of inflammatory and apoptotic pathways (Christen et al. 2013). It is suggested that Ag NPs enter the ER of zebrafish embryos, thereby blocking protein synthesis and increase mortality at a later stage of development (Gao et al. 2016). In addition, in human cell lines exposed to ZnO NPs, Au NPs and SiO_2 NPs, ER stress was the predominant response and links to oxidative stress, inflammatory response and apoptosis were demonstrated (Chen et al. 2014, Christen et al. 2014, Noël et al. 2016, Tsai et al. 2011). The interaction of NPs with the ER is certainly underexplored, especially in aquatic organisms. However, this is a promising early marker for nanotoxicology.

If the stress situation is severe or persists for a longer period, the cell can initiate multiple signaling cascades of apoptosis. NPs are likely to activate the mitochondria-dependent caspase cascades and there are three major situations by which it can be triggered: (1) an extreme overload with ROS will result in mitochondrial membrane damage, leading to release of pro-apoptotic factors and ultimately cell death, (2) NPs can also take a short cut by directly targeting the mitochondria and thus trigger mitochondrial perturbation, (3) ER stress leads to calcium release from the ER and this calcium enters the mitochondria where it depolarizes the inner membrane and activates the caspase cascade.

Genotoxicity

Sustained oxidative stress can result in DNA damage through free-radical attack and ultimately abnormal cell growth. Furthermore, especially the smaller NPs may reach the nucleus *via* transportation through the nuclear pore and then directly interact with the DNA. Thus, genotoxicity can represent a particle-specific mechanism.

Genotoxic effects triggered by NPs may manifest as either damage to the genome or some adaptive changes in gene expression or both. Small sized Ag NPs (5 nm to 20 nm) induce high levels of γ-H2AX—a marker for double DNA strand breaks—in the liver of adult zebrafish (Choi et al. 2010). Moreover, an increased level of hepatic oxidative damage shows the role of oxidative damage as a precursor of genetic damage for NP toxicity in fish (Choi et al. 2010). A global transcriptomic analysis in *Daphnia magna* revealed particle specific gene expression profiles for Ag

NPs, including disruption of protein metabolism and DNA damage (Poynton et al. 2012). Biota exposed to genotoxic agents consequently may show long-lasting and profound adverse changes at cellular and organismal level. However, controversial results are found in literature suggesting no genotoxic activity of at least Si NPs (Barnes et al. 2008, Kwon et al. 2014).

In addition to the above described mechanistic pathways where NPs can interact, other forms of injury, such as membrane damage and the formation of foreign body granulomas are possible. It is also possible that NPs can lead to novel mechanisms of toxicity. Most of the effects described herein at the cellular level may not lead to a specific adverse outcome such as impaired reproduction but may generally reduce fitness of target organisms and thus weaken its health and capability of responding to other stressors. For AOP development, more knowledge is needed on the long term effects of these mechanistic pathways in ecotoxicological relevant species.

Responses at Organismal Level

The adverse sub-lethal effects of NPs on aquatic organisms have been the main subject of research in nano-ecotoxicology. Sub-lethal responses assessed for NPs are diverse and thus allow evaluation of NP-related physiological and morphological effects. Of particular interest are adverse effects, which may cause impacts at community and ecosystem levels. The general dose-response model is commonly applied for NPs aiming at defining the threshold for a particular response. These threshold values are often in the mg L^{-1} range for NPs (Adam et al. 2015). Thus, even though environmental concentrations are largely unknown, effective concentrations can be expected to be rather high. However, species sensitivity between laboratory model organisms and free-living organisms can vary substantially and effects on the most sensitive species in an ecosystem may change the community already (Song et al. 2015). Sediment organisms are especially at risk to be exposed to elevated NP levels as they continuously settle out of the water column. Moreover, laboratory assessments often reveal acute effects, whereas chronic effects remain largely unexplored. NPs have the potential of being persistent in the environment (Savolainen et al. 2013) and continuous gradual input may lead to population decline. Whether organisms are able to acclimate to an increasing NP load remains an unanswered question.

Physiological and morphological responses

Morphological changes in response to NP exposure are mainly assessed as acute effects. These give a good indication of which organ or physiological process is targeted by the NPs. However, the vast majority of cases cannot be directly translated to environmental scenarios, as exposure concentrations at laboratory scale are beyond expected environmental concentrations. Increasingly, studies attempt to underpin the morphological response with molecular modes of actions. However, often the adverse outcomes at organism level can originate from several molecular mechanisms and connections are not yet established.

Fish embryos are the best studied organisms in terms of morphological response to NPs. The eye development is targeted by Ag and Au NPs, resulting in decreased width (Asharani et al. 2011, Bar-Ilan et al. 2009, Kim et al. 2013, Lee et al. 2007, Wu et al. 2010). The occurrence of edema is frequently observed in embryos treated with Ag, Au, TiO_2, and ZnO NPs and is an indicator of a defective cardiovascular system (Hao et al. 2009, Wu et al. 2010, Zhu et al. 2009). Slow blood flow or decreased heart rate is likely to be a precursor of edema and is also observed in fish embryos exposed to Ag, Au, and Pt NPs (Kim et al. 2013, Park et al. 2013, Wu et al. 2010). Hatching interference is often observed with metal NPs. The underlying mechanism is the interference of metal ions with the hatching enzyme. However, NPs tend to accumulate on the chorion, resulting in more metal ions released into the perivitelline space compared to ionic exposures (Muller et al. 2015).

In invertebrates, a decrease in growth and reproduction can be measured after exposure to various NP. However, this is a more general response to stress occurring often with chemical exposure as metabolic rates increase under toxic stress while energy resources of organisms are limited.

Disruption of the microbiome

Uptake of NPs occurs mainly *via* ingestion and they are accumulated in the gut. The gastrointestinal tract is a site of complex, symbiotic interactions between host cells and the resident microbiome. There is increasing evidence that NPs change the populations of intestinal microbiota and modulate gut-associated immune response, but it is yet an unexplored field (Bergin and Witzmann 2013, Williams et al. 2014). In adult zebrafish, Cu NPs suppressed beneficial bacterial strains to non-detectable levels (Merrifield et al. 2013). In addition, Ag NPs depleted the gut microbiome in Nile tilapia (Sarkar et al. 2015). The effects of NPs on the microbiome of invertebrates are not assessed yet. However, it is known that the well being of *Daphnia magna* in respect to their growth, survival and fecundity is strongly dependent on their microbiota (Sison-Mangus et al. 2014). It is not far off to expect that NPs with antimicrobial properties (e.g., Ag NPs) may disrupt the microbial community of filter feeders in particular and subsequently affect its health.

Behavioral responses

Behavioral changes represent an important mechanism of environmental stress response. They appear to be among the most sensitive indicators for visual toxicity and impairments will reveal effects at the community and ecosystem level. Changes can be triggered internally by biochemical processes (neurotoxicity, hormones, energy metabolism) or externally by avoidance. Furthermore, behavior can be assessed in individuals (e.g., locomotion) and in communities (e.g., predator-prey and social interactions). Up to the present, NPs have been mainly assessed for their effects on individual behavior. There are indications that biochemical processes underlie the behavioral response, but more insights are needed.

Swimming responses of larval zebrafish are affected after exposure to Au, Ag, CuO and TiO_2 NPs (Chen et al. 2011, Kim et al. 2013, Powers et al. 2011, Sun et al. 2016). Interestingly, differences in NP coating and size were observed. Polyvinylpryrrolidone (PVP) coated Ag NPs caused hypoactivity in small sizes and hyperactivity in larger dimension. A size dependency in behavioral response was also found in adult zebrafish exposed to SiO_2 NPs (Li et al. 2014). Smaller particles (15 nm) decreased locomotive activity and disrupted advanced learning and memory cognitive behaviors to a greater extent than their bigger (50 nm) counterparts. The feeding (and shoaling) behavior of fish can be affected by polystyrene NPs, increasing the time to consume their food significantly which might be related to the disrupted lipid metabolism, indicating reduced energy reserves in exposed fish (Cedervall et al. 2012, Mattsson et al. 2014). Also, invertebrates show behavioral alterations when exposed to NPs. For example, Cu NPs reduce feeding activity of the shredder *Allogamus ligonifer* (Pradhan et al. 2015).

Trophic transfer

Transfer of NPs through the aquatic food chain requires attention, since ingestion is a major route of NP uptake. Through trophic transfer, organisms can be exposed to higher concentrations than from waterborne exposure. For example, *Daphnia magna* accumulate ZnO NPs in their gut and then fish is served a concentrated form of NPs. In this manner, ZnO NPs reached more than tenfold higher levels in fish than through aqueous exposure (Skjolding et al. 2014). Also, the amphipod *Leptocheirus plumulosus* accumulates quantum dots to a greater extent when exposed through algal food than in water (Jackson et al. 2012). In trophic transfer, NPs adsorbed to the organism to be eaten may play a significant role, whereas absorption is of primary importance for toxicity and biodistribution.

Outlook Towards an AOP Development for NPs

Nanomaterials and nanotechnology are a scientific breakthrough in industry and consumer products. The production of NPs is growing rapidly and therefore environmental concentrations will increase over time. However, impact of NPs on community and population levels in ecosystems is not assessed. In this chapter, the current understanding of NP effects on different biological levels was reviewed in order to evaluate opportunities and challenges to develop an AOP for NPs. In an AOP, a pollutant effect cascades from one biological level to the next. Biochemical interactions are the basic level and related to the functionality of a tissue or an organ. At higher biological levels, it is then evaluated whether such effects change the performance of the organism and whether this altered performance can affect the ecosystem unction. The development of AOPs for NPs can expedite the significance of the various events measured at cellular level. Moreover, AOP development is a regulatory driven plea.

In order to understand where molecular events are initiated, uptake routes need to be determined and fate of tissues and cells assessed. There are a number of techniques available to assess uptake and biodistribution of NPs, each with certain limitations. For NPs that can be made visible with fluorescent laser, fluorescent, confocal and light sheet microscopy are advised methods to track NPs in biota, the latter being the most promising technique. For non-fluorescent NPs, Raman spectroscopy is the technique of choice for bio-imaging. An important site of uptake is the intestinal tract. Thus, as initial step of an AOP development, molecular mechanisms involved in cellular uptake as well as binding and processing of NPs should be identified in the intestinal tract. A lion's share of the particles might be accumulated in the gut and not cross the epithelium membrane. There are indications that NPs disrupt the gut microbiome which can have adverse effects on organism's health. This pathway is yet unexplored for NPs but might evolve into a future AOP with an altered microbiome as initiating event and subsequent health impacts as key events.

In this chapter, it becomes obvious that NPs crossing the membrane can trigger several cellular responses (Fig. 6), depending on the NP's intrinsic and extrinsic properties. Thus, different AOPs may be developed for different NPs. Oxidative stress and inflammation have been identified as major pathways affected. With this knowledge, the foundation is laid to develop AOPs for NPs. However, there is currently a knowledge gap connecting the cellular response with observed adverse outcomes at individual or population level such as decreased growth and survival as well as different behavioral alterations. Due to this missing link, the predictive potential of *in vitro* to *in vivo* is still in its infancy. In view of the limited availability of such data, future research should fill this knowledge gap.

In addition, we identified four research directions which need more attention when developing AOPs for NPs: (1) long term NP exposures are needed as they are likely to be more important for population decline (McKee and Filser 2016), (2) threshold values for the environment are needed for risk assessments, (3) more data on biodegradation of NPs and excretion pathways need to be added, and (4) benthic organisms need to be included in the assessments to understand whether these target organisms are at risk or well adapted, as they are living in a world of natural colloids. Ecotoxicology and environmental fate research communities will have to work together to identify cascading key events. Once established, adverse outcomes should be verified in ecologically relevant scenarios and at environmentally relevant concentrations, as NP behavior and fate in different environments plays a pivotal role for potential toxic effects. A developed AOP allows the bulk of screening analysis

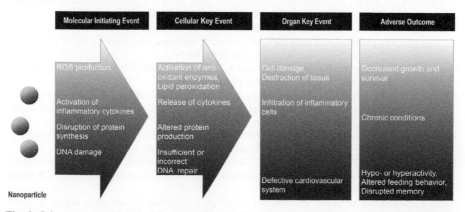

Fig. 6. Scheme summarizing the key event across biological levels and adverse outcomes described for NPs. Molecular initiating events are not defined yet, but may cover a broad spectrum including disruption of protein synthesis. The connections between measured cellular effects and observed adverse outcomes are not established yet. (Figure adapted from the AOP knowledge base; http://www.aopkb.org/.)

to be conducted *in vitro* in a high-throughput manner. Risk reduction for aquatic environments can then be carried out by limiting or avoiding exposures that trigger these toxicological responses.

References

Adam, N., F. Leroux, D. Knapen, S. Bals and R. Blust. 2014. The uptake of ZnO and CuO nanoparticles in the water-flea *Daphnia magna* under acute exposure scenarios. Environ. Pollut. 194: 130–137.

Adam, N., C. Schmitt, L. De Bruyn, D. Knapen and R. Blust. 2015. Aquatic acute species sensitivity distributions of ZnO and CuO nanoparticles. Sci. Total Environ. 526: 233–242.

Arvizo, R.R., O.R. Miranda, M.A. Thompson, C.M. Pabelick, R. Bhattacharya, J. David Robertson et al. 2010. Effect of nanoparticle surface charge at the plasma membrane and beyond. Nano Lett. 10: 2543–2548.

Asharani, P.V., Y. Lianwu, Z. Gong and S. Valiyaveettil. 2011. Comparison of the toxicity of silver, gold and platinum nanoparticles in developing zebrafish embryos. Nanotoxicology. 5: 43–54.

Auffan, M., J. Rose, O. Proux, D. Borschneck, A. Masion, P. Chaurand et al. 2008. Enhanced adsorption of arsenic onto maghemites nanoparticles: As(III) as a probe of the surface structure and heterogeneity. Langmuir. 24: 3215–22.

Auffan, M., J. Rose, J.-Y. Bottero, G.V. Lowry, J.-P. Jolivet and M.R. Wiesner. 2009. Towards a definition of inorganic nanoparticles from an environmental, health and safety perspective. Nat. Nanotechnol. 4: 634–41.

Bar-Ilan, O., R.M. Albrecht, V.E. Fako and D.Y. Furgeson. 2009. Toxicity assessments of multisized gold and silver nanoparticles in zebrafish embryos. Small. 5: 1897–1910.

Barnes, C.A., A. Elsaesser, J. Arkusz, A. Smok, J. Palus, A. Leśniak et al. 2008. Reproducible comet assay of amorphous silica nanoparticles detects no genotoxicity. Nano Lett. 8: 3069–3074.

Bergin, I.L. and F.A. Witzmann. 2013. Nanoparticle toxicity by the gastrointestinal route: evidence and knowlege gaps. Int. J. Biomed. Nanosci. Nanotechnol. 3: 1–2.

Blokhina, O., E. Virolainen and K.V. Fagerstedt. 2003. Antioxidants, oxidative damage and oxygen deprivation stress: A review. Ann. Bot. 91: 179–194.

Brun, N.R., M. Lenz, B. Wehrli and K. Fent. 2014. Comparative effects of zinc oxide nanoparticles and dissolved zinc on zebrafish embryos and eleuthero-embryos: Importance of zinc ions. Sci. Total Environ. 476-477: 657–666.

Canesi, L., C. Ciacci, M. Betti, R. Fabbri, B. Canonico, A. Fantinati et al. 2008. Immunotoxicity of carbon black nanoparticles to blue mussel hemocytes. Environ. Int. 34: 1114–1119.

Carnovale, C., G. Bryant, R. Shukla and V. Bansal. 2016. Size, shape and surface chemistry of nano-gold dictate its cellular interactions, uptake and toxicity. Prog. Mater. Sci. 83: 152–190.

Cedervall, T., I. Lynch, S. Lindman, T. Berggard, E. Thulin, H. Nilsson et al. 2007. Understanding the nanoparticle-protein corona using methods to quantify exchange rates and affinities of proteins for nanoparticles. Proc. Natl. Acad. Sci. USA. 104: 2050–2055.

Cedervall, T., L.A. Hansson, M. Lard, B. Frohm and S. Linse. 2012. Food chain transport of nanoparticles affects behaviour and fat metabolism in fish. PLoS One. 7: 1–6.

Chen, G., M.G. Vijver and W.J.G.M. Peijnenburg. 2015. Summary and analysis of the currently existing literature data on metal-based nanoparticles published for selected aquatic organisms: Applicability for toxicity prediction by (Q)SARs. ATLA Altern. to Lab. Anim. 43: 221–240.

Chen, M., J. Yin, Y. Liang, S. Yuan, F. Wang, M. Song et al. 2016. Oxidative stress and immunotoxicity induced by graphene oxide in zebrafish. Aquat. Toxicol. 174: 54–60.

Chen, R., L. Huo, X. Shi, R. Bai, Z. Zhang, Y. Zhao et al. 2014. Endoplasmic reticulum stress induced by zinc oxide nanoparticles is an earlier biomarker for nanotoxicological evaluation. ACS Nano. 8: 2562–2574.

Chen, T., C. Lin and M. Tseng. 2011. Behavioral effects of titanium dioxide nanoparticles on larval zebrafish (*Danio rerio*). Mar. Pollut. Bull. 63: 303–308.

Chithrani, B.D., A.A. Ghazani and W.C.W. Chan. 2006. Determining the size and shape dependence of gold nanoparticle uptake into mammalian cells. Nano Lett. 6: 662–668.

Chithrani, B.D. and W.C.W. Chan. 2007. Elucidating the mechanism of cellular uptake and removal of protein-coated gold nanoparticles of different sizes and shapes. Nano Lett. 7: 1542–1550.

Choi, H.S., W. Liu, P. Misra, E. Tanaka, J.P. Zimmer, B. Itty Ipe et al. 2007. Renal clearance of nanoparticles. Nat. Biotechnol. 25: 1165–1170.

Choi, J.E., S. Kim, J.H. Ahn, P. Youn, J.S. Kang, K. Park et al. 2010. Induction of oxidative stress and apoptosis by silver nanoparticles in the liver of adult zebrafish. Aquat. Toxicol. 100: 151–9.

Christen, V., M. Capelle and K. Fent. 2013. Silver nanoparticles induce endoplasmatic reticulum stress response in zebrafish. Toxicol. Appl. Pharmacol. 272: 519–528.

Christen, V., M. Camenzind and K. Fent. 2014. Silica nanoparticles induce endoplasmic reticulum stress response, oxidative stress and activate the mitogen-activated protein kinase (MAPK) signaling pathway. Toxicol. Reports. 1: 1143–1151.

Colvin, V.L. 2003. The potential environmental impact of engineered nanomaterials. Nat. Biotechnol. 21: 1166–1170.

Dawson, K.A., A. Salvati and I. Lynch. 2009. Nanotoxicology: nanoparticles reconstruct lipids. Nat. Nanotechnol. 4: 84–85.

Deng, Z.J., M. Liang, M. Monteiro, I. Toth and R.F. Minchin. 2011. Nanoparticle-induced unfolding of fibrinogen promotes Mac-1 receptor activation and inflammation. Nat. Nanotechnol. 6: 39–44.

Dominguez, G.A., S.E. Lohse, M.D. Torelli, C.J. Murphy, R.J. Hamers, G. Orr et al. 2015. Effects of charge and surface ligand properties of nanoparticles on oxidative stress and gene expression within the gut of *Daphnia magna*. Aquat. Toxicol. 162: 1–9.

Esmaeili, F., M.H. Ghahremani, B. Esmaeili, M.R. Khoshayand, F. Atyabi and R. Dinarvand. 2008. PLGA nanoparticles of different surface properties: Preparation and evaluation of their body distribution. Int. J. Pharm. 349: 249–255.

EU. 2011. Commission recommendation of 18 October 2011 on the definition of nanomaterial (2011/696/EU). Off. Journal L. 38–40.

Fang, C.Y., V. Vaijayanthimala, C.A. Cheng, S.H. Yeh, C.F. Chang, C.L. Li et al. 2011. The exocytosis of fluorescent nanodiamond and its use as a long-term cell tracker. Small. 7: 3363–3370.

Federici, G., B.J. Shaw and R.D. Handy. 2007. Toxicity of titanium dioxide nanoparticles to rainbow trout (*Oncorhynchus mykiss*): gill injury, oxidative stress, and other physiological effects. Aquat. Toxicol. 84: 415–30.

Foucaud, L., M.R. Wilson, D.M. Brown and V. Stone. 2007. Measurement of reactive species production by nanoparticles prepared in biologically relevant media. Toxicol. Lett. 174: 1–9.

Fröhlich, E. 2016. Cellular elimination of nanoparticles. Environ. Toxicol. Pharmacol. 46: 90–94.

Gao, J., C.T. Mahapatra, C.D. Mapes, M. Khlebnikova, A. Wei and M.S. Sepúlveda. 2016. Vascular toxicity of silver nanoparticles to developing zebrafish (*Danio rerio*). Nanotoxicology. 5390: 1–10.

George, S., S. Pokhrel, T. Xia, B. Gilbert, Z. Ji, M. Schowalter et al. 2010. Use of a rapid cytotoxicity screening approach to engineer a safer zinc oxide nanoparticle through iron doping. ACS Nano. 4: 15–29.

Gilbert, B., S.C. Fakra, T. Xia, S. Pokhrel, L. Mädler and A.E. Nel. 2012. The fate of ZnO nanoparticles administered to human bronchial epithelial cells. ACS Nano. 6: 4921–4930.

Gomes, T., J.P. Pinheiro, I. Cancio, C.G. Pereira, C. Cardoso and M.J. Bebianno. 2011. Effects of copper nanoparticles exposure in the mussel *Mytilus galloprovincialis*. Environ. Sci. Technology. 45: 9356–9362.

Gottschalk, F., T. Sun and B. Nowack. 2013. Environmental concentrations of engineered nanomaterials: Review of modeling and analytical studies. Environ. Pollut. 181: 287–300.

Gratton, S.E.A., P.A. Ropp, P.D. Pohlhaus, J.C. Luft, V.J. Madden, M.E. Napier et al. 2008. The effect of particle design on cellular internalization pathways. Proc. Natl. Acad. Sci. USA. 105: 11613–11618.

Greulich, C., J. Diendorf, T. Simon, G. Eggeler, M. Epple and M. Köller. 2011. Uptake and intracellular distribution of silver nanoparticles in human mesenchymal stem cells. Acta Biomater. 7: 347–354.

Han, Y., S. Li, X. Cao, L. Yuan, Y. Wang, Y. Yin et al. 2014. Different inhibitory effect and mechanism of hydroxyapatite nanoparticles on normal cells and cancer cells *in vitro* and *in vivo*. Sci. Rep. 4: 7134.

Handy, R.D., F. von der Kammer, J.R. Lead, M. Hassellöv, R. Owen and M. Crane. 2008. The ecotoxicology and chemistry of manufactured nanoparticles. Ecotoxicology. 17: 287–314.

Hao, L., Z. Wang and B. Xing. 2009. Effect of sub-acute exposure to TiO_2 nanoparticles on oxidative stress and histopathological changes in juvenile Carp (*Cyprinus carpio*). J. Environ. Sci. 21: 1459–1466.

He, X., W.G. Aker and H.-M. Hwang. 2014. An *in vivo* study on the photo-enhanced toxicities of S-doped TiO$_2$ nanoparticles to zebrafish embryos (*Danio rerio*) in terms of malformation, mortality, rheotaxis dysfunction, and DNA damage. Nanotoxicology. 8: 185–195.

Hemmerich, P.H. and A.H. von Mikecz. 2013. Defining the subcellular interface of nanoparticles by live-cell imaging. PLoS One. 8.

Hotamisligil, G.S. 2010. Endoplasmic reticulum stress and the inflammatory basis of metabolic disease. Cell. 140: 900–917.

Hu, H., Q. Li, L. Jiang, Y. Zou, J. Duan and Z. Sun. 2016. Genome-wide transcriptional analysis of silica nanoparticle-induced toxicity in zebrafish embryos. Toxicol. Res. 5: 609–620.

Jackson, B.P., D. Bugge, J.F. Ranville and C.Y. Chen. 2012. Bioavailability, toxicity, and bioaccumulation of quantum dot nanoparticles to the amphipod Leptocheirus plumulosus. Environ. Sci. Technol. 46: 5550–6.

Johnston, B.D., T.M. Scown, J. Moger, S.A. Cumberland, M. Baalousha, K. Linge et al. 2010. Bioavailability of nanoscale metal oxides TiO$_2$, CeO$_2$, and ZnO to fish. Environ. Sci. Technol. 44: 1144–51.

Kashiwada, S. 2006. Distribution of nanoparticles in the dee-through Medaka (*Oryzias latipes*). Environ. Health Perspect. 114: 1697–1702.

Keller, A.A., H. Wang, D. Zhou, H.S. Lenihan, G. Cherr, B.J. Cardinale et al. 2010. Stability and aggregation of metal oxide nanoparticles in natural aqueous matrices. Environ. Sci. Technol. 44: 1962–1967.

Kanna, P., C. Ong, B.H. Bay and G.H. Baeg. 2015. Nanotoxicity: An interplay of oxidative stress, inflammation and cell death. Nanomaterials. 5: 1163–1180.

Kim, K.T., S.J. Klaine, J. Cho, S.H. Kim and S.D. Kim. 2010. Oxidative stress responses of *Daphnia magna* exposed to TiO$_2$ nanoparticles according to size fraction. Sci. Total Environ. 408: 2268–2272.

Kim, K.T., T. Zaikova, J.E. Hutchison and R.L. Tanguay. 2013. Gold nanoparticles disrupt zebrafish eye development and pigmentation. Toxicol. Sci. 133: 275–288.

Krug, H.F. and P. Wick. 2011. Nanotoxicology: An interdisciplinary challenge. Angew. Chemie—Int. Ed. 50: 1260–1278.

Kwok, K.W.H., M. Auffan, A.R. Badireddy, C.M. Nelson, M.R. Wiesner, A. Chilkoti et al. 2012. Uptake of silver nanoparticles and toxicity to early life stages of Japanese medaka (*Oryzias latipes*): Effect of coating materials. Aquat. Toxicol. 120-121: 59–66.

Kwon, J.Y., H.L. Kim, J.Y. Lee, Y.H. Ju, J.S. Kim, S.H. Kang et al. 2014. Undetactable levels of genotoxicity of SiO$_2$ nanoparticles in *in vitro* and *in vivo* tests. Int. J. Nanomedicine. 9: 173–181.

Lee, K.J., P.D. Nallathamby, L.M. Browning, C.J. Osgood and X.-H.N. Xu. 2007. *In vivo* imaging of transport and biocompatibility of single silver nanoparticles in early development of zebrafish embryos. ACS Nano. 1: 133–143.

Lesniak, A., A. Salvati, M.J. Santos-Martinez, M.W. Radomski, K.A. Dawson and C. Åberg. 2013. Nanoparticle adhesion to the cell membrane and its effect on nanoparticle uptake efficiency. J. Am. Chem. Soc. 135: 1438–1444.

Lewinski, N.A., H. Zhu, H.-J. Jo, D. Pham, R.R. Kamath, C.R. Ouyang et al. 2010. Quantification of water solubilized CdSe/ZnS quantum dots in *Daphnia magna*. Environ. Sci. Technol. 44: 1841–6.

Li, L.-Z., D.-M. Zhou, W.J.G.M. Peijnenburg, C.A.M. van Gestel, S.-Y. Jin, Y.-J. Wang et al. 2011. Toxicity of zinc oxide nanoparticles in the earthworm, *Eisenia fetida* and subcellular fractionation of Zn. Environ. Int. 37: 1098–104.

Li, X., B. Liu, X.-L. Li, Y.-X. Li, M.-Z. Sun, D.-Y. Chen et al. 2014. SiO$_2$ nanoparticles change colour preference and cause Parkinson's-like behaviour in zebrafish. Sci. Rep. 4: 3810.

Limbach, L.K., P. Wick, P. Manser, R.N. Grass, A. Bruinink and W.J. Stark. 2007. Exposure of engineered nanoparticles to human lung epithelial cells: Influence of chemical composition and catalytic activity on oxidative stress. Environ. Sci. Technol. 41: 4158–4163.

Łojkowski, W., H.-J. Fecht and A. Świderka-Środa. 2015. Quo Vadis Nanotechnology? pp. 79–94. *In*: Van de Voorde, M., M. Werner and H.-J. Fecht. (eds.). The Nano-Micro Interface: Bridging the Micro and Nano Worlds. Wiley-VCH, Weinheim, Germany.

Lowry, G.V., K.B. Gregory, S.C. Apte and J.R. Lead. 2012. Transformations of nanomaterials in the environment. Environ. Sci. Technology. 46: 6893–6899.

Lu, F., S.H. Wu, Y. Hung and C.Y. Mou. 2009. Size effect on cell uptake in well-suspended, uniform mesoporous silica nanoparticles. Small. 5: 1408–1413.

Lundqvist, M., J. Stigler, G. Elia, I. Lynch, T. Cedervall and K.A. Dawson. 2008. Nanoparticle size and surface properties determine the protein corona with possible implications for biological impacts. Proc. Natl. Acad. Sci. USA. 105: 14265–14270.

Ma, L., J. Liu, N. Li, J. Wang, Y. Duan, J. Yan et al. 2010. Oxidative stress in the brain of mice caused by translocated nanoparticulate TiO_2 delivered to the abdominal cavity. Biomaterials. 31: 99–105.

Machlin, L.J. and A. Bendich. 1987. Free radical tissue damage: protecitve role of antioxidant nutrients. FASEB J. 1: 441–445.

Mattsson, K., M.T. Ekvall, L.A. Hansson, S. Linse, A. Malmendal and T. Cedervall. 2014. Altered behavior, physiology, and metabolism in fish exposed to polystyrene nanoparticles. Env. Sci. Technol. 49: 553–561.

Mattsson, K., K. Adolfsson, M.T. Ekvall, M.T. Borgström, S. Linse, L.-A. Hansson et al. 2016. Translocation of 40 nm diameter nanowires through the intestinal epithelium of *Daphnia magna*. Nanotoxicology. 10: 1160–1167.

McKee, M.S. and J. Filser. 2016. Impacts of metal-based engineered nanomaterials on soil communities. Environ. Sci. Nano. 3: 506–533.

Meng, H., S. Yang, Z. Li, T. Xia, J. Chen, Z. Ji et al. 2011. Aspect ratio determines the quantity of mesoporous silica nanoparticle uptake by a small gtpase-dependent macropinocytosis mechanism. ACS Nano. 5: 4434–4447.

Merrifield, D.L., B.J. Shaw, G.M. Harper, I.P. Saoud, S.J. Davies, R.D. Handy et al. 2013. Ingestion of metal-nanoparticle contaminated food disrupts endogenous microbiota in zebrafish (*Danio rerio*). Environ. Pollut. 174: 157–163.

Monopoli, M.P., A. Salvati, C. Åberg, K.A. Dawson, C. Åberg, A. Salvati et al. 2012. Biomolecular coronas provide the biological identity of nanosized materials. Nat. Nanotechnol. 7: 779–786.

Moore, M.N. 2006. Do nanoparticles present ecotoxicological risks for the health of the aquatic environment? Environ. Int. 32: 967–976.

Muller, E.B., S. Lin and R.M. Nisbet. 2015. Quantitative adverse outcome pathway analysis of hatching in zebrafish with CuO nanoparticles. Environ. Sci. Technol. 49: 11817–11824.

Nel, A., T. Xia, L. Mädler and N. Li. 2006. Toxic potential of materials at the nanolevel. Science. 311: 622–627.

Nel, A., L. Mädler, D. Velegol, T. Xia, E.M.V. Hoek, P. Somasundaran et al. 2009. Understanding biophysicochemical interactions at the nano-bio interface. Nat. Mater. 8: 543–557.

Noël, C., J.-C. Simard and D. Girard. 2016. Gold nanoparticles induce apoptosis, endoplasmic reticulum stress events and cleavage of cytoskeletal proteins in human neutrophils. Toxicol. *In Vitro*. 31: 12–22.

Nowack, B. and T.D. Bucheli. 2007. Occurrence, behavior and effects of nanoparticles in the environment. Environ. Pollut. 150: 5–22.

Oh, W.-K., S. Kim, M. Choi, C. Kim, Y.S. Jeong, B.-R. Cho et al. 2010. Cellular uptake, cytotoxicity, and innate immune response of silica-titania hollow nanoparticles based on size and surface functionality. ACS Nano. 4: 5301–5313.

Ortega, V.a., B.a. Katzenback, J.L. Stafford, M. Belosevic and G.G. Goss. 2015. Effects of polymer-coated metal oxide nanoparticles on goldfish (*Carassius auratus* L.) neutrophil viability and function. Nanotoxicology. 9: 23–33.

Ostrowski, A., D. Nordmeyer, A. Borenham, C. Holzhausen, L. Mundhenk, C. Graf et al. 2015. Overview about localization of nanoparticles in tissue and cellular context by different imaging techniques. Beilstein J. Nanotechnol. 6: 263–280.

Park, H.-G. and M.-K. Yeo. 2013. Comparison of gene expression changes induced by exposure to Ag, $Cu-TiO_2$, and TiO_2 nanoparticles in zebrafish embryos. Mol. Cell. Toxicol. 9: 129–139.

Park, J.-H., L. Gu, G. von Maltzahn, E. Ruoslahti, S.N. Bhatia and M.J. Sailor. 2009. Biodegradable luminescent porous silicon nanoparticles for *in vivo* applications. Nat. Mater. 8: 331–6.

Park, K., G. Tuttle, F. Sinche and S.L. Harper. 2013. Stability of citrate-capped silver nanoparticles in exposure media and their effects on the development of embryonic zebrafish (*Danio rerio*). Arch. Pharm. Res. 36: 125–133.

Piccinno, F., F. Gottschalk, S. Seeger and B. Nowack. 2012. Industrial production quantities and uses of ten engineered nanomaterials in Europe and the world. J. Nanopart. Res. 14: 1109.

Powers, C.M., T.A. Slotkin, F.J. Seidler, A.R. Badireddy and S. Padilla. 2011. Silver nanoparticles alter zebrafish development and larval behavior: Distinct roles for particle size, coating and composition. Neurotoxicol. Teratol. 33: 708–714.

Poynton, H.C., J.M. Lazorchak, C.A. Impellitteri, B.J. Blalock, K. Rogers, H.J. Allen et al. 2012. Toxicogenomic responses of nanotoxicity in *Daphnia magna* exposed to silver nitrate and coated silver nanoparticles. Environ. Sci. Technol. 46: 6288–6296.

Pradhan, A., P. Geraldes, S. Seena, C. Pascoal and F. Cássio. 2015. Natural organic matter alters size-dependent effects of nanoCuO on the feeding behaviour of freshwater invertebrate shredders. Sci. Total Environ. 535: 94–101.

Rees, P., M.R. Brown, H.D. Summers, M.D. Holton, R.J. Errington, S.C. Chappell et al. 2011. A transfer function approach to measuring cell inheritance. BMC Syst. Biol. 5: 31.

Salvati, A., C. Aberg, T. dos Santos, J. Varela, P. Pinto, I. Lynch et al. 2011. Experimental and theoretical comparison of intracellular import of polymeric nanoparticles and small molecules: toward models of uptake kinetics. Nanomedicine. 7: 818–826.

Santo, N., U. Fascio, F. Torres, N. Guazzoni, P. Tremolada, R. Bettinetti et al. 2014. Toxic effects and ultrastructural damages to *Daphnia magna* of two differently sized ZnO nanoparticles: Does size matter? Water Res. 53: 339–350.

Sarkar, B., M. Jaisai, A. Mahanty, P. Panda, M. Sadique, B.B. Nayak et al. 2015. Optimization of the sublethal dose of silver nanoparticle through evaluating its effect on intestinal physiology of Nile tilapia (*Oreochromis niloticus* L.). J. Environ. Sci. Heal. Part A. 50: 814–823.

Savolainen, K., U. Backman, D. Brouwer, B. Fadeel, T. Fernandes, T. Kuhlbusch et al. 2013. Nanosafety in Europe 2015–2025: Towards safe and sustainable nanomaterials and nanotechnology innovations. Finnish Institute of Occupational Health.

Scown, T.M., E.M. Santos, B.D. Johnston, B. Gaiser, M. Baalousha, S. Mitov et al. 2010. Effects of aqueous exposure to silver nanoparticles of different sizes in rainbow trout. Toxicol. Sci. 115: 521–534.

Selck, H., R.D. Handy, T.F. Fernandes, S.J. Klaine and E.J. Petersen. 2016. Nanomaterials in the aquatic environment: A European Union-United States perspective on the status of ecotoxicity testing, research priorities, and challenges ahead. Environ. Toxicol. Chem. 35: 1055–1067.

Service, R.F. 2004. Nanotechnology grows up. Science. 304: 1732–1734.

Shang, L., K. Nienhaus and G.U. Nienhaus. 2014. Engineered nanoparticles interacting with cells: Size matters. J. Nanobiotechnology. 12: 5.

Sison-Mangus, M.P., A.A. Mushegian and D. Ebert. 2014. Water fleas require microbiota for survival, growth and reproduction. ISME J. 9: 59–67.

Skjolding, L.M., M. Winther-Nielsen and A. Baun. 2014. Trophic transfer of differently functionalized zinc oxide nanoparticles from crustaceans (*Daphnia magna*) to zebrafish (*Danio rerio*). Aquat. Toxicol. 157: 101–108.

Skjolding, L.M., G. Ašmonaitė, R.I. Jølck, T.L. Andersen, H. Selck, A. Baun et al. 2017. An assessment of the importance of exposure routes to the uptake and internal localisation of fluorescent nanoparticles in zebrafish (*Danio rerio*), using light sheet microscopy. Nanotoxicology. 3: 351–359.

Smith, C.J., B.J. Shaw and R.D. Handy. 2007. Toxicity of single walled carbon nanotubes to rainbow trout (*Oncorhynchus mykiss*): respiratory toxicity, organ pathologies, and other physiological effects. Aquat. Toxicol. 82: 94–109.

Song, L., M.G. Vijver, G. de Snoo and W.J.G.M. Peijnenburg. 2015. Assessing toxicity of copper nanoparticles across five cladoceran species. Environ. Toxicol. Chem. 8: 1863–1869.

Sun, L., Y. Li, X. Liu, M. Jin, L. Zhang, Z. Du et al. 2011. Cytotoxicity and mitochondrial damage caused by silica nanoparticles. Toxicol. Vitr. 25: 1619–1629.

Sun, Y., G. Zhang, Z. He, Y. Wang, J. Cui and Y. Li. 2016. Effects of copper oxide nanoparticles on developing zebrafish embryos and larvae. Int. J. Nanomedicine. 11: 905–918.

Tedesco, S., H. Doyle, J. Blasco, G. Redmond and D. Sheehan. 2010. Oxidative stress and toxicity of gold nanoparticles in *Mytilus edulis*. Aquat. Toxicol. 100: 178–186.

Thurn, K.T., E.M.B. Brown, A. Wu, S. Vogt, B. Lai, J. Maser et al. 2007. Nanoparticles for applications in cellular imaging. Nanoscale Res. Lett. 2: 430–441.

Truong, L., S.C. Tilton, T. Zaikova, E. Richman, K.M. Waters, J.E. Hutchison et al. 2013. Surface functionalities of gold nanoparticles impact embryonic gene expression responses. Nanotoxicology. 7: 192–201.

Tsai, Y.-Y., Y.-H. Huang, Y.-L. Chao, K.-Y. Hu, L.-T. Chin, S.-H. Chou et al. 2011. Identification of the nanogold particle-induced endoplasmic reticulum stress by omic techniques and systems biology analysis. ACS Nano. 5: 9354–9369.

Unfried, K., C. Albrecht, L.-O. Klotz, A. Von Mikecz, S. Grether-Beck and R.P.F. Schins. 2007. Cellular responses to nanoparticles: Target structures and mechanism. Nanotoxicology. 1: 52–71.

Valavanidis, A., T. Vlahogianni, M. Dassenakis and M. Scoullos. 2006. Molecular biomarkers of oxidative stress in aquatic organisms in relation to toxic environmental pollutants. Ecotoxicol. Environ. Saf. 64: 178–89.

Van Pomeren, M., N.R. Brun, W.J.G.M. Peijnenburg and M.G. Vijver. 2017. Exploring uptake and biodistrbution of particles in biota. Accepted. Aquat. Toxicol.

Verma, A., O. Uzun, Y. Hu, Y. Hu, H.-S. Han, N. Watson et al. 2008. Surface-structure-regulated cell-membrane penetration by monolayer-protected nanoparticles. Nat. Mater. 7: 588–595.

Waissi-Leinonen, G.C., E.J. Petersen, K. Pakarinen, J. Akkanen, M.T. Leppänen and J.V.K. Kukkonen. 2012. Toxicity of fullerene (C60) to sediment-dwelling invertebrate *Chironomus riparius* larvae. Environ. Toxicol. Chem. 31: 2108–2116.

Williams, K., J. Milner, M.D. Boudreau, K. Gokulan, C.E. Cerniglia and S. Khare. 2014. Effects of subchronic exposure of silver nanoparticles on intestinal microbiota and gut-associated immune responses in the ileum of Sprague-Dawley rats. Nanotoxicology. 5390: 1–11.

Wu, Y., Q. Zhou, H. Li, W. Liu, T. Wang and G. Jiang. 2010. Effects of silver nanoparticles on the development and histopathology biomarkers of Japanese medaka (*Oryzias latipes*) using the partial-life test. Aquat. Toxicol. 100: 160–167.

Xia, T., M. Kovochich, J. Brant, M. Hotze, J. Sempf, T. Oberley et al. 2006. Comparison of the abilities of ambient and manufactured nanoparticles to induce cellular toxicity according to an oxidative stress paradigm. Nano Lett. 6: 1794–1807.

Xia, T., M. Kovochich, M. Liong, L. Mädler, B. Gilbert, H. Shi et al. 2008. Comparison of the mechanism of toxicity of zinc oxide and cerium oxide nanoparticles based on dissolution and oxidative stress properties. ACS Nano. 2: 2121–2134.

Zhang, H., K.E. Burnum, M.L. Luna, B.O. Petritis, J.S. Kim, W.J. Qian et al. 2011. Quantitative proteomics analysis of adsorbed plasma proteins classifies nanoparticles with different surface properties and size. Proteomics. 11: 4569–4577.

Zhang, W., Y. Ji, X. Wu and H. Xu. 2013. Trafficking of gold nanorods in breast cancer cells: Uptake, lysosome maturation and elimination. ACS Appl. Mater. Interfaces. 5: 9856–9865.

Zhao, X., S. Wang, Y. Wu, H. You and L. Lv. 2013. Acute ZnO nanoparticles exposure induces developmental toxicity, oxidative stress and DNA damage in embryo-larval zebrafish. Aquat. Toxicol. 136-137: 49–59.

Zhu, M., G. Nie, H. Meng, T. Xia, A. Nel and Y. Zhao. 2013. Physicochemical properties determine nanomaterial cellular uptake, transport, and fate. Acc. Chem. Res. 46: 622–631.

Zhu, X., J. Wang, X. Zhang, Y. Chang and Y. Chen. 2009. The impact of ZnO nanoparticle aggregates on the embryonic development of zebrafish (*Danio rerio*). Nanotechnology. 20: 195103.

9

Development of a Management Tool for Environmental Assessment of Organo-nitrogen Pesticides

In Surface Water from Everglades and Biscayne National Parks and Big Cypress National Preserve, South Florida, USA

Natalia Quinete,[1,]* *Joffre Castro,*[2] *Ingrid Zamora-Ley,*[1]
Adolfo Fernadez,[1] *Gary Rand*[3] and *Piero Gardinali*[4]

Introduction

Pesticides are widely used in the agriculture to control weeds, insects, and fungal pests. In South Florida, USA, approximately 21,170 tons of pesticides were used annually in the agriculture from 2007–2009, which includes 169 active ingredients, composed of 46 fungicides, 36 herbicides, 66 insecticides, and 21 other pesticides

[1] Southeast Environmental Research Center (SERC), Florida International University, 6 SE 2nd Ave, Miami, FL 33131, USA.
[2] Everglades National Park, South Florida Ecosystem Office, 950 N Krome Avenue, Homestead, Florida, 33030, USA.
[3] Ecotoxicology & Risk Assessment Laboratory, Department of Earth and Environment, Florida International University Biscayne Bay Campus, 3000 N.E. 151st Street, North Miami, Florida 33181, USA.
[4] Southeast Environmental Research Center (SERC) & Department of Chemistry and Biochemistry, Florida International University, 11200 SW 8th Street, Modesto A. Maidique Campus, Miami, Florida, 33199, USA.
* Corresponding author: nataliaquinete@yahoo.com.br

(FDACS 2010). After the withdrawal and ban of organochlorine pesticides (OCPs), these have been replaced by other classes of pesticides, such as organonitrogen, organophosphorus, and carbamate pesticides, which are very attractive and universally used due to their low cost, wide range of efficacy, and less persistence in the environment than OCPs (Tankiewicz et al. 2010).

Organonitrogen Pesticides (ONP), which include a large number of different types of compounds containing aniline, neonicotinoid, quinoline, triazole, oxazolone and amide in their chemical structures, comprise a group of currently used herbicides for control of annual broadleaf and grass weeds, primarily used in citrus, corn and sugarcane crops, but also in landscape vegetation to some extent. These herbicides often enter the surrounding waters through aerial deposition, field runoff, and groundwater discharge. In fact, the presence of ONP and their metabolites in non-target surface water bodies has been reported worldwide in the range of low ng L^{-1} to several μg L^{-1} in areas of intensive agricultural activity (Byer et al. 2011, Du Preez et al. 2005, Fulton et al. 2004, Gómez-Gutièrrez et al. 2006, Konstantinou et al. 2006, Miles and Pfeuffer 1997, Nogueira et al. 2012, Wilson and Boman 2011).

In South Florida canals, atrazine, simazine, bromacil and norflurazon were frequently detected in surface waters from 1990 to 2006 (Miles and Pfeuffer 1997, Fulton et al. 2004, Carriger and Rand 2008a,b, Schuler and Rand 2008), present in some locations at concentrations exceeding the U.S. Environmental Protection Agency (U.S. EPA) water quality criteria for freshwater plants (10 μg L^{-1}; US EPA 2003). More recently, Wilson and Boman (2011) evaluated the temporal distribution and concentrations of five commonly used herbicides in the South Florida watershed, reporting that spatial trends in pesticide detections followed use patterns, and that atrazine was the most detected herbicide in the canals. The presence of terrestrial-use herbicides in surface water is of great concern due to the potential risks of adverse effects to the aquatic ecosystem. For example, several classes of herbicides (triazine, triazinones, uracils, phenylureas) are photosystem II (PSII) inhibitors (Moreland 1980). Therefore, these compounds block electron transport and energy production by binding to specific target protein (site of toxic action) of the PSII complex in chloroplast thylakoid membranes which stops CO_2 fixation and production of ATP and $NADPH_2$, causing lipid and protein damage which eventually results in plant death (Vencill 2002, Schuler and Rand 2008). Atrazine, one of the most frequently detected herbicides in water, has been shown to be an endocrine disruptor compound in humans and animals, representing high risk during pregnancy, possibly causing birth defects and adverse effects on sexual development (Abarikwu et al. 2013, Agopian et al. 2013, Kucka et al. 2012, Hayes et al. 2006, Hayes et al. 2011).

Currently, there is a major effort to restore the South Florida ecosystem by increasing the freshwater flows to the Everglades and to Florida and Biscayne Bays, which could also result in the increase of contaminant levels, particularly pesticides, being transferred into the southeastern coasts. Therefore, in the present study, a comprehensive survey was conducted between November 2006 to February 2009, elucidating the occurrence and distribution of 17 organonitrogen pesticides (ONPs) in surface waters within the Everglades National Park (ENP), Biscayne National Park (BNP) and Big Cypress National Preserve (BICY). In addition, a contamination index for the studied area based on 85th percentile was developed.

Material and Methods

Study area description

ENP is located at the south end of the Florida peninsula and is characterized by a low, flat, wet plain covered by a wide grassy river with alternating ridges and sloughs, covering an area of 6110 km². The freshwater portion of the park represents about one-third of the original Everglades, which extended from Lake Okeechobee, in the north, to Florida Bay (FB), in the south, for 160 km and from the Coastal Pineland Ridge, in the east, to the Big Cypress Flatwoods, in the west, for 60 km. This extensive freshwater ecosystem comprised wet prairies, sawgrass marshes, cypress and mangrove forests, and coastal lagoons and bays, which continues to provide a mosaic of wildlife habitats. In the late 1940s, the federal government implemented a major water control project to provide water supply and flood protection for south Florida, which substantially changed the hydrology and ecology of the Everglades. Today in the Everglades, an extensive network of canals and structures allow the rapid redistribution of flows throughout the system but also facilitate the movement of pollutants, including agricultural pesticides, into surface waters (Scott et al. 2002, Harman-Fetcho et al. 2005). The Canal 111 (C-111) freshwater basin is a buffer zone that separates the wetlands of ENP from highly productive subtropical agricultural lands and urban development areas. Most of the water discharged into ENP and the southern estuaries, as Florida Bay, are a mixture of rainfall and runoff from urban and agricultural areas of southeast Florida. The issue of environmental impacts and water management has been addressed by the South Florida Water Management District (SFWMD) and the Corps of Engineers in a series of remedial actions since the 1980s and, most recently, with the Comprehensive Everglades Restoration Plan (CERP) that seeks to address both hydrology and water quality issues (SFWMD 2002). The pesticide monitoring network included 60 stations (Fig. 1), where surface water was collected on a regular basis from canals and parks' lands and waters.

Sample collection

Water samples were collected between November 2006 and February 2009 from 30 stations within and around ENP, 9 stations within BICY, 11 stations within BNP, 6 stations within the canal and control structures of the C-111 canal, 3 stations in Loveland Slough (C-111E) and one reference station isolated from the network of canals (Rocket) (Fig. 1). ENP is divided into the following areas: C111 Canal basin (C-111-1/2/3), Highway Creek (C111-4), East Boundary (EB), Florida Bay (FB); Shark River Slough (SRS 1/2/3), Shark River (SRS4), Taylor Slough (TS1/2/3), Taylor Slough/Florida Bay (TS4), Tamiami Trail (TT) and West Boundary (WB). Canals and Control Structures are divided into the areas: L31 Canal (332B), C113 Canal (S176E), C111 Canal (S-176S), Structure 178 (S-178), Structure 178 Buffer (S-178B) and Structure 18C (S18C). Loveland Slough is divided into three areas: C111-212, C111-217 and C111-217B. Some stations were located along areas where anthropogenic inputs were likely, such as the east boundaries of ENP, canals entering BNP and along TT. Areas not likely to be impacted by the implementation of CERP

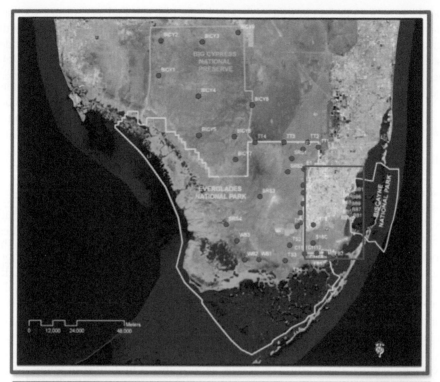

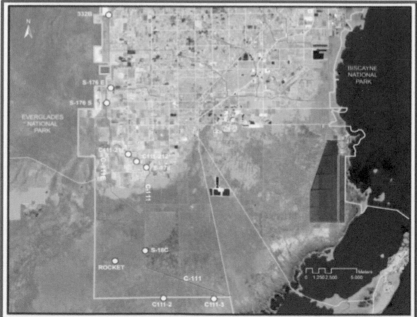

Fig. 1. Surface water sampling locations at Everglades, Biscayne National Parks and Big Cypress National Preserve, in South Florida.

and the resulting changes in water deliveries were also selected as controls, such as sites in western ENP. Sampling was periodically and generally timed to coincide with agricultural production and included sampling during both growing (high pesticide usage) and non-growing (low pesticide usage) seasons. The sampling points at each location are displayed in Fig. 1. Samples were collected in 1-Liter amber glass bottles and maintained under refrigeration ($< 4°C$) until analysis.

Chemicals

All material and glassware used were previously cleaned, combusted in a muffle furnace for 6 hours at 400°C and rinsed with dichloromethane, hexane, methanol and acetone prior to the analysis to avoid contamination. Certified organonitrogen pesticide standards were purchased from Ultra Scientific, Analytical Solutions (N. Kingstown, RI, USA). Stock solutions of individual analytes ($200–1000$ ng μL^{-1}) were prepared in acetone. The working spiking solution was prepared by diluting the stock solution to 2 μg mL^{-1} with hexane. Then, 50 μL of the working spiking solution was added to the spiked sample before the beginning of the extraction. Atrazine d5 (ethylamino d5) at 100 μg mL^{-1} in acetone was obtained from Dr. Ehrenstofer GmbH (EQ Laboratories, Atlanta, GA, USA) and used as surrogate standard in recovery control tests. Working solutions of atrazine d5 were prepared at 1 μg mL^{-1} by dilution in hexane. Tetrachloro-m-xylene (TCMX, Supelco, St. Louis, MO, USA) was used as internal standard. Stock solutions of TCMX at 100 μg mL^{-1} were prepared and working solutions at 1 μg mL^{-1} in hexane were prepared by further dilution. Stock and working solutions were prepared with pesticide quality or equivalent solvent, methanol, n-hexane, pentane, acetone and dichloromethane (Fisher Scientific, Fairlawn, NJ, USA) and stored at $-18°C$. Ultrapure water (18.2 $M\Omega$ cm^{-1}) was obtained by a Nanopure Infinity Ultrapure Water system.

Analysis and instrumentation

Prior to water sample extractions, 20–30 g of sodium chloride was added to the samples to increase ionic strength. 100 μL of working solution of atrazine-d5 was added to every sample prior to the extraction step. 1-Liter water samples were processed by liquid-liquid extraction with 50 mL methylene chloride. The extraction was repeated twice using fresh portions of solvent. All extracts were combined and concentrated to 1 mL using a rotary evaporator and 100 μL of TCMX were added to the samples for the GC/MS analysis. Sample extracts were analyzed by gas chromatography (Trace GC Ultra, Thermo Scientific, West Palm Beach, FL, USA) tandem mass spectrometry (TSQ Quantum XLS, Thermo Scientific, West Palm Beach, FL, USA) in electron impact ionization (EI) mode using selected ion monitoring (SIM) on a 30 meter, 0.25 mm i.d., 0.25 μm phase thickness RiX 5 Sil MS fused silica capillary column with integrated guard column (Restek, Bellefonte, PA, USA). Chromatographic conditions were as follows: 2 μL of sample was injected in the splitless mode; the column oven was programmed for an initial temperature of 100°C for 1 min, and subsequently for a rate of 6°C min^{-1} to 300°C and held for 1 min; helium was used as

Table 1. List of the target herbicides and the selected ions for monitoring (SIM).

Compounds	Monitored Ions (m/z)
Molinate	126.00, 187.00
Atraton	169.00, 196.00, 211.00
Simazine	173.00, 186.00, 201.00
Prometon	168.00, 210.00, 225.00
Atrazine	200.00, 215.00
Propazine	172.00, 214.00, 229.00
Terbuthylazine	173.00, 214.00, 229.00
Secbumeton	169.00, 196.00, 210.00
Metribuzin	198.00, 199.00
Alachlor	146.00, 160.00, 188.00, 237.00
Simetryne	170.00, 198.00, 213.00
Ametryne	170.00, 212.00, 227.00
Prometryne	184.00, 226.00, 241.00
Terbutryne	185.00, 226.00
Bromacil	190.00, 205.00
Metolachlor	162.00, 238.00
Butachlor	160.00, 176.00, 188.00
TCMX (IS)	242.00, 244.00, 246.00
Atrazine D5 (SURR)	205.00, 220.00, 222.00

IS: internal standard; SURR: surrogate

the carrier gas (at a flow rate of 1.5 mL min^{-1}). The injector, transfer line and source temperatures were maintained at 280, 280 and 250°C, respectively. Target herbicides were quantified in SIM mode using the selected ions listed in Table 1.

Quality control

In order to guarantee the quality of the analytical data, target compounds were spiked at a concentration of 100 ng L^{-1} and were analyzed through the same analytical procedures as every sample. Matrix spike recoveries for all target analytes ranged from 56 to 118% (mean ± SD: 97 ± 12%). Surrogate recoveries ranged from 50 to 234 (mean ± SD: 118 ± 36%). External calibration standards were prepared in hexane at concentrations ranging from 2.5 to 1000 ng mL^{-1}. All standard calibration curves exhibited excellent linearity (correlation coefficient > 0.99). These analytical curves were revalidated after every set of twenty samples. Quality control samples included a method/procedural blank, a matrix spike, and a matrix spike duplicate with every sample set. Procedural blanks were run with every 20 samples or with every sample set by passing water and reagents through the entire analytical procedure to routinely

Table 2. Method Detection Limit (MDL) of the studied herbicides in water.

Compounds	MDLs (ng/L)
Molinate	0.95
Atraton	0.92
Simazine	0.99
Prometon	0.77
Atrazine	0.94
Propazine	0.88
Terbuthylazine	0.87
Secbumeton	0.82
Metribuzin	0.86
Alachlor	0.84
Simetryne	0.82
Ametryne	0.41
Prometryne	0.96
Terbutryne	0.54
Bromacil	10.0
Metolachlor	0.50
Butachlor	0.87

monitor contamination in reagents and glassware. Method detection limits (MDLs) for each compound in surface water are shown in Table 2.

Results and Discussion

Concentrations and frequency of pesticide detection in water samples

Atrazine (76%) and metolachlor (38%) were the most frequently detected herbicides in surface water (n = 316 samples) between November 2006 and February 2009 in the studied area. Atrazine concentrations ranged from < 0.94 to 359 ng L^{-1}, while metolachlor ranged from < 0.5 to 18 ng L^{-1}. Some other herbicides such as simazine, atraton, prometron, metribuzin, alachlor and simetryne were also detected but less frequently (< 15%), as displayed in Fig. 2. The spatial and temporal distribution of the studied herbicides are presented in Figs. 3 and 4(a,b), respectively.

The highest level of herbicides was observed in Tamiami Trail, followed by the S178 structure, both areas suffering strong anthropogenic impacts (Fig. 3). February (dry season) norrmaly coincides with the highest pesticide application in the agricultural area and pesticide run-off from the fields is expected to be reduced (Fulton et al. 2004). As presented in Fig. 4a, atrazine and metolachlor levels were the highest in the months following pesticide use (March, May and July 2008),

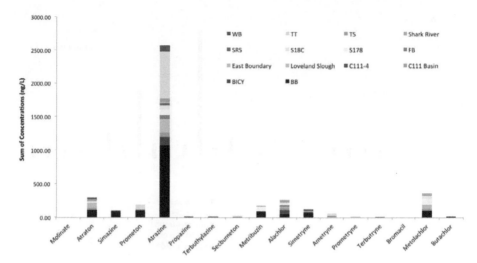

Fig. 2. Pesticide distribution in the studied area.

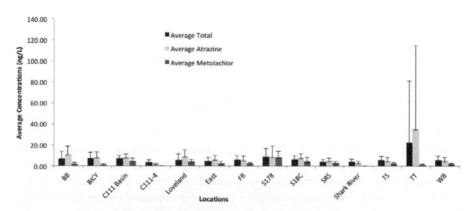

Fig. 3. Spatial distribution of the studied herbicides.

although the same profile is not so evident during the 2007 sampling event. Seasonal distribution of atrazine (Fig. 4b) showed, in general, the highest average concentration in the dry season (November 2007 to March 2008) in comparison to the wet season (April 2008 to October 2008), suggesting that the potential for runoff also exists in the dry season, especially when intensive spray irrigation is applied, which was also observed previously in the Everglades area by Fulton et al. (2004).

Maximum measured atrazine was 359 ng L^{-1} at Site TT3 in March 2008, which was below the levels (10–20 µg L^{-1}) that might be expected to cause ecological impacts in freshwater or saltwater systems (Solomon et al. 1996, Fulton et al. 2004). The highest concentration of metolachlor (18 ng L^{-1}) found at S178 in January 2008 was well below the toxicity threshold for the most sensitive aquatic macrophyte species tested (96 h EC$_{50}$ of 70 µg L^{-1}) (Fairchild et al. 1998).

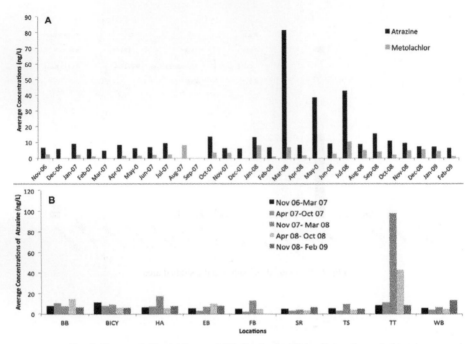

Fig. 4. Temporal (A) and Seasonal (B) distribution of atrazine and metolachlor.

In the United States and Canada, typical atrazine surface water concentrations range from 2 to 50 μ L^{-1}, with peaks of 100 μg L^{-1}, following heavy rain in rivers adjacent to recently sprayed fields (Muir et al. 1978, Hamala and Kollig 1985, Downing et al. 2004). Previous monitoring program conducted in South Florida canals between 1991 and 1995 have reported that triazine herbicides were the most frequently detected compounds with measured values as high as 18 μg L^{-1} for atrazine, 1 μg L^{-1} for ametryn and 2.5 μg L^{-1} for simazine (Miles and Pfeuffer 1997). In general, atrazine concentrations in South Florida surface waters typically ranged from < 2.16 to 337 ng L^{-1}, while metolachlor ranged from < 6.7 to 34 ng L^{-1} (Fulton et al. 2004). These levels are very similar to the ones reported in the present study. However, higher atrazine concentrations in South Florida surface waters have been observed in previous studies (Miles and Pfeuffer 1997, Schuler and Rand 2008, Wilson and Boman 2011). During a sampling event conducted between 2005 and 2008 in South Florida canals, atrazine and norflurazon were the most frequently detected (87–95% of samples) herbicides with maximum concentrations of up to 6.97 μg L^{-1} (Wilson and Boman 2011). Bromacil, metolachlor and simazine were less frequently detected (1.8–36%), reaching up to 4.96 μg L^{-1}, 1.55 μg L^{-1} and 1.35 μg L^{-1}, respectively (Wilson and Boman 2011).

Previous studies have also showed that these herbicides will most likely not accumulate in sediments (Kock-Schulmeyer et al. 2013, Brondi et al. 2011, Villaverde et al. 2008), which was supported by unpublished findings from our group in a first assessment of the studied herbicides in sediments from the Everglades.

Development of a management tool for environmental assessment

The studied group of compounds has been shown to have relatively low bioconcentration factors, indicating that phytoplankton and aquatic macrophytes are the most sensitive species, given that they possess the specific target site for these herbicides (Schuler and Rand 2008). It has been observed that 200 μg L^{-1} atrazine significantly reduced chlorophyll a, phototrophic carbon assimilation and bacterial biomass, but stimulated heterotrophic bacterial productivity, while chlorophyll a was also significantly reduced by 20 μg L^{-1} atrazine (Downing et al. 2004). The only compound for which a national water quality guideline is currently available is atrazine; however, the maximum concentration reported in this study (0.36 μg L^{-1}) does not reach the lowest criterion of 3.00 μg L^{-1}.

In the absence of guidelines and in order to evaluate the areas of potential contamination and to assess which herbicides represent a major anthropogenic stressor to the system, a contamination index was developed based solely on statistical analysis of the whole chemistry dataset. The proposed tool evaluates the cumulative distribution of all chemicals detected in the samples and ranks them on a frequency curve (Fig. 5). An arbitrary but commonly used criterion was used to define an "elevated concentration" as the 85th centile (O'Connor 2004). This approach has been used by NOAA in the past to rank estuarine samples using the national 50th and 85th centiles of the NS&T national database to classify estuaries along the US coast. Through the analysis of the graphs displayed in Figs. 5–7, two important informations are available: the open circles represent the 85th centile of each compound (i.e., 2.1 ng L^{-1} for molinate and 16.5 ng L^{-1} for atrazine) but also the location of the compound in the overall plot describes its rank among all contaminants tested. Figure 5 allows for the visualization of compounds which are at higher concentrations in the study area; however, no information regarding their geographical distribution is provided.

Similarly, a plot was constructed using the site information. Figure 6 shows the same cumulative frequency distribution, where the information on non-detected

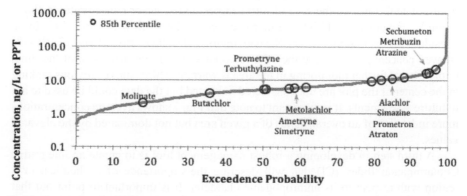

Fig. 5. Cumulative distribution and ranking of ONPs in all water samples analyzed. The 85th centile for each compound is represented as an open circle in the plot.

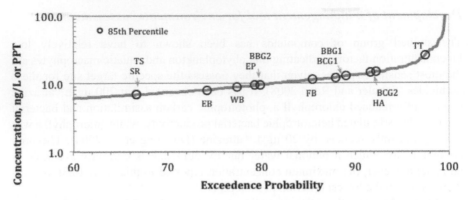

Fig. 6. Cumulative distribution and ranking of studied regions concerned ONPs levels in all water samples analyzed. The 85th centile for each geographical region is represented as open circles in the plot.

compounds was removed for simplicity. In this case, the open circles represent the 85th percentiles of the individual regions for all contaminants. The interpretation of this plot is rather simple, showing the more contaminated areas at the top of the distribution compared to the lower end of the distribution, which is independent from the compounds presented in the site. For example, Tamiami Trail (TT) is located on the top portion of the plot, indicating that the compounds detected in this area showed the highest concentrations of all evaluated sites. This observation is also clearly seen in Fig. 4b, evidencing that this region is dominated by high levels of atrazine (Fig. 3).

Because the 85th centile only represents an "elevated state" and data are heavily dominated by high values, complementary plots could be constructed using the same distributions but showing other relevant benchmarks such as the 25th, 50th or 75th centiles. Figure 7 shows a decision plot where the same data are classified in low, medium and high ranges using the 25th, 50th and 75th centiles. Unlike Figs. 5 and 6, the plot in Fig. 7 represents an average concentration on the region and its rank over the entire study area. Three important parameters could be extracted from this tool. First, in the case of nitrogen pesticides, water concentrations above 10 ng L^{-1} are considered high. Similarly, concentrations below 2.5 ng L^{-1} could be considered as background levels. Second, regions like Big Cypress Group 2 (BCG2) showed concentrations above the 75th regional values more than 50% of the time, implying that further monitoring in the area is warrant. Third, sites or regions ranking in the center of the plot are not considered impacted but the data could be used to aid in future assessments. It is important to note that Fig. 7 shows average concentrations more indicative of an overall status of a given area but not dominated by the elevated values.

A third step in developing a robust management tool is to create an integrative Contamination Index (CI) that will describe the importance of a chemical or a region with respect to its anthropogenic character. It is important to point out that this classification is purely statistical in nature and has no regulatory or ecological implication. Therefore, it simply ranks the compounds of potential concern and

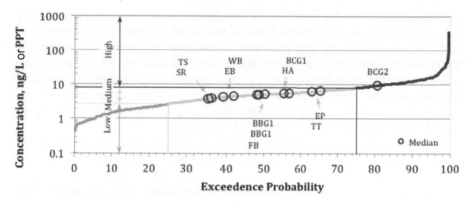

Fig. 7. Cumulative distribution and ranking of studied regions according to their exposure to ONPs in all water samples analyzed. The regions are divided in low (< 25th), medium (between 25th and 50th) and high (> 75th centiles) and regions are plotted as their median concentrations as open circles.

Table 3. Calculated Contamination Index (CI) and ranking for all nitrogen pesticides monitored in surface waters at the 50 collection sites grouped by regions.

	Contamination Index (CI) for Nitrogen Pesticides in Water											Adj. CI
	BBG1	**BBG2**	**BCG1**	**BCG2**	**EB**	**EP**	**FB**	**HA**	**SR**	**TT**	**WB**	**(1-TO-10)**
Alachlor			0.30	0.19				0.12				1
Ametryne										0.83		1
Atraton	0.30				0.21						0.37	1
Atrazine	7.34	0.04	0.06					1.28		31.88		10
Butachlor									0.07			1
Metolachlor	0.65				0.35	1.63		5.45				3
Metribuzin	0.23							0.70				1
Molinate								0.09				1
Prometon	1.22									5.16		2
Prometryne										1.22		1
Secbumeton										0.09		1
Simazine	0.18										0.20	1
Simetryne						0.02					1.32	1
Terbuthylazine				0.04								1
Adj. CI (1-TO-10)	3	1	1	1	1	1	1	3	1	10	1	

the regions more affected by those compounds solely on the contribution of their "elevated concentrations" described by the 85th centiles.

Table 3 shows the Contamination Index (CI) for all analyzed compounds based on their detection in each region. In addition, the far right column and the bottom row provide an overall ranking. Based on the calculations, atrazine is the highest-ranking compound among all analytes and Tamiami trail is the highest ranked region in the study with respect to nitrogen pesticides contamination. Because the calculation aggregates the individual CIs and normalize them to a scale of 1 to 10, both region and contaminants could be classified in terms of their environmental relevance. In this case, atrazine, metolachlor and prometon are the three compounds with the highest CI, yet atrazine clearly dominates. Similarly, the three regions showing the highest anthropogenic signature are TT, HA, and BBG1.

The development of these tools does not require previous knowledge of the chemicals, their effects or an environmental guideline, and they provide a statistical procedure to identify compounds and/or regions where further monitoring is needed. Although a more comprehensive environmental risk assessment is still the best way to proceed in terms of evaluating the impact of nitrogen pesticides in the environment, the presented plots in combination with the CI calculations could be used as an early diagnostic tool before regulatory benchmarks are exceeded.

Acknowledgments

This work was financially supported by the Everglades Fellowship provided by the Department of Interior, Everglades National Park. The CARE Project was funded by the Cooperative Agreement H5297050133 between FIU and Everglades National Park. This is contribution number 855 from the Southeast Environmental Research Center in the Institute of Water & Environment at Florida International University.

References

Abarikwu, S.O., E.O. Farombi and A.B. Pant. 2013. The reproductive toxicity of atrazine, an endocrine disruptor. Toxicology Letters. 221: S215–S215.

Agopian, A.J., Y. Cai, P.H. Langlois, M.A. Canfield and P.J. Lupo. 2013. Maternal residential atrazine exposure and risk for choanal atresia and stenosis in offspring. Journal of Pediatrics. 162(3): 581–586.

Brondi, S.H.G., A.N. de Macedo, G.H.L. Vicente and A.R.A. Nogueira. 2011. Evaluation of the QuEChERS method and gas chromatography-mass spectrometry for the analysis pesticide residues in water and sediment. Bull. Environ. Contam. Toxicol. 86: 18.

Byer, J.D., J. Struger, E. Sverko, P. Klawunn and A. Todd. 2011. Spatial and seasonal variations in atrazine and metolachlor surface water concentrations in Ontario (Canada) EPAing ELISA. Chemosphere. 82: 1155–60.

Carriger, J.F. and G.M. Rand. 2008a. Aquatic risk assessment of pesticides in surface waters in and adjacent to the Everglades and Biscayne National Parks: I. Hazard assessment and problem formulation. Ecotoxicol. 17: 660–679.

Carriger, J.F. and G.M. Rand. 2008b. Aquatic risk assessment of pesticides in surface waters in and adjacent to the Everglades and Biscayne National Parks: II. Probabilistic analyses. Ecotoxicol. 17: 680–696.

Downing, H.F., M.E. Delorenzo, M.H. Fulton, G.I. Scott, C.J. Madden and J.R. Kucklick. 2004. Effects of the agricultural pesticides atrazine, chlorothalonil, and endosulfan on South Florida microbial assemblages. Ecotoxicology. 13(3): 245–260.

Du Preez, L.H, P.J. Jansen van Rensburg, A.M. Jooste, J.A. Carr, J.P. Giesy, T.S. Gross et al. 2005. Seasonal exposures to triazine and other pesticides in surface waters in the western high yield corn production region in South Africa. Environ. Pollut. 135: 131–41.

Fairchild, J.F., D.S. Ruessler and A.R. Carlson. 1998. Comparative sensitivity of five species of macrophytes and six species of algae to atrazine, metribuzin, alachlor, and metolachlor. Environ. Toxicol. Chem. 17: 1830–1834.

Florida Department of Agriculture, Consumer Services (FDACS). 2010. Summary of agricultural pesticide usage in Florida: 2007–2009. FDACS, Division of Agricultural Environmental Services, Bureau of Pesticides, Tallahassee, 2010, 40 p. Available at: http://www.flaes.org/pdf/PUI_narrative_2010.pdf.

Fulton, M.H., G.I. Scott, M.E. DeLorenzo, P.B. Key, D.W. Bearden, E.D. Strozier et al. 2004. Surface water pesticide movement from the Dade County agricultural area to the Everglades and Florida Bay via the C-111 canal. Bull. Environ. Contam. Toxicol. 73: 527– 534.

Gómez-Gutièrrez, A.I., E. Jover, L. Bodineau, J. Albaiges and J.M. Bayona. 2006. Organic contaminant loads into the Western Mediterranean Sea: estimate of Ebro River inputs. Chemosphere. 65: 224–36.

Hamala, J.A. and H.P. Kollig. 1985. The effects of atrazine on periphyton communities in controlled laboratory ecosystems. Chemosphere. 14(9): 1391–408.

Harman-Fetcho, J.A., C.J. Hapeman, L.L. McConnell, T.L. Potter, C.P. Rice, A.M. Sadeghi et al. 2005. Pesticide occurrence in selected south florida canals and biscayne bay during high agricultural activity. J. Agric. Food Chem. 53: 6040–6048.

Hayes, T.B., A.A. Stuart, M. Mendoza, A. Collins, N. Noriega, A. Vonk et al. 2006. Characterization of atrazine-induced gonadal malformations in African clawed frogs (Xenopus laevis) and comparisons with effects of an androgen antagonist (cyproterone acetate) and exogenous estrogen (17b-estradiol): support for the demasculinization/feminization hypothesis. Environ. Health Perspect. 114: 134–41.

Hayes, T.B., L.L. Anderson, V.R. Beasley, S.R. de Solla, T. Iguchi, H. Ingraham et al. 2011. Demasculinization and feminization of male gonads by atrazine: Consistent effects across vertebrate classes. Journal of Steroid Biochemistry and Molecular Biology. 127(1-2): 64–73.

Kock-Schulmeyer, M., M. Olmos, M.L. de Alda and D. Barcelo. 2013. Development of a multiresidue method for analysis of pesticides in sediments based on isotope dilution and liquid chromatography-electrospray-tandem mass spectrometry. Journal of Chromatography A. 1305: 176–187.

Konstantinou, I.K., D.G. Hela and T.A. Albanis. 2006. The status of pesticide pollution in surface waters (rivers and lakes) of Greece: Part I. Review on occurrence and levels. Environ. Pollut. 141: 555–70.

Kucka, M., K. Pogrmic-Majkic, S. Fa, S.S. Stojilkovic and R. Kovacevic. 2012. Atrazine acts as an endocrine disrupter by inhibiting cAMP-specific phosphodiesterase-4. Toxicology and Applied Pharmacology. 265(1): 19–26.

Miles, C. and R. Pfeuffer. 1997. Pesticides in canals of South Florida. Arch. Environ. Contam. Toxicol. 32: 337–345.

Moreland, D.E. 1980. Mechanisms of action of herbicides. Ann. Rev. Plant Physiol. 31: 597–638.

Muir, D.C.G., J.Y. Yoo and B.E. Baker. 1978. Residues of atrazine and N-deethylated atrazine in water from five agricultural watersheds in Quebec. Arch. Environ. Contam. Toxicol. 7: 221–35.

Nogueira, E.N., E.F.G.C. Dores, A.A. Pinto, R.S.S. Amorim, M.L. Ribeiro and C. Lourencettia. 2012. Currently used pesticides in water matrices in central-western Brazil. J. Braz. Chem. Soc. 23(8): 1476–1487.

O′Connor, T.P. 2004. The sediment quality guideline, ERL, is not a chemical concentration at the threshold of sediment toxicity. Mar. Pollut. Bull. 49(5-6): 383–385.

Schuler, L.J. and G.M. Rand. 2008. Aquatic risk assessment of herbicides in freshwater ecosystems of South Florida. Arch. Environ. Contam. Toxicol. 54: 571–583.

Scott, G., M. Fulton, E. Wirth, G. Chandler, P. Key, J. Daugomah et al. 2002. Toxicological studies in tropical ecosystems: An ecotoxicological risk assessment of pesticide runoff in South Florida estuarine ecosystems. J. Agric. Food Chem. 50: 4400–4408.

SFWMD and U.S. Army Corps of Engineers. Central and Southern Florida Project, Comprehensive Everglades Restoration Plan, 2002; 126 pp.

Solomon, K.R., D.B. Baker, P. Richards, K.R. Dixon, S.J. Klaine, T.W. La Point et al. 1996. Ecological risk assessment of atrazine in North American surface waters. Environ. Toxicol. Chem. 15: 31–76.

Tankiewicz, M., M. Fenik and M. Marek. 2010. Determination of organophosphorus and organonitrogen pesticides in water samples. TrAC Trends in Analytical Chemistry. 29(9): 1050–1063.

US EPA (US Environmental Protection Agency). 2003. Ambient aquatic life water quality criteria for atrazine-revised draft. EPA-822-R-03-023. US Environmental Protection Agency, Office of Water, Office of Science and Technology, Health and Ecological Criteria Division, Washington, DC.

Vencill, W.K. 2002. Herbicide Handbook. Lawrence, K.S. Weed Science Society of America.

Villaverde, J., A. Hildebrandt, E. Martinez, S. Lacorte, E. Morillo, C. Maqueda et al. 2008. Priority pesticides and their degradation products in river sediments from Portugal. Sci. Total Environ. 390: 507–13.

Wilson, P.C. and B.J. Boman. 2011. Characterization of selected organo-nitrogen herbicides in south Florida canals: Exposure and risk assessments. Science of the Total Environment. 412-413: 119–126.

10

Conceptual Challenges in the Translation of Toxicological Research into Practice

Low-Dose Hypothesis and Dose-Response Non-monotonicity

Francisco José Roma Paumgartten* and Ana Cecilia Amado Xavier De-Oliveira

"Too much openness and you accept every notion, idea, and hypothesis—which is tantamount to knowing nothing. Too much skepticism—especially rejection of new ideas before they are adequately tested—and you're not only unpleasantly grumpy, but also closed to the advance of science. A judicious mix is what we need."

Carl Sagan- 'Wonder and Skepticism', Skeptical Enquirer (1995), 19(1).

Introduction

The notion that *"the dose makes the poison"* has been a cardinal tenet of toxicology since it emerged as a scientific discipline concerned with the study of nocuous effects of chemicals on living organisms. Enunciated in the 16th century, Paracelsus' famous maxim *"All things are poisonous and nothing is without poison, only the dose makes a thing not poisonous"* already conveyed the idea that virtually all substances might

Laboratory of Environmental Toxicology, Department of Biological Sciences, National School of Public Health, Oswaldo Cruz Foundation, Rio de Janeiro, RJ 21040-361 Brazil.
  E-mail: ana.oliveira@ensp.fiocruz.br
* Corresponding author: paum@ensp.fiocruz.br

eventually cause harm (i.e., be toxic) depending on the doses to which the individual is exposed (Deichmann et al. 1986).[1] The subtle choice of the negative form (*"the dose makes a thing not a poison"*) instead of the affirmative one (the dose makes a thing a poison) to say that to be or not to be harmful depended ultimately on the substance dose, indicates that Paracelsus was well ahead of his time. Modern experimental toxicologists seek for doses and conditions under which a chemical is safe, or the doses and exposure conditions that *"make a thing not a poison"*. To discover the safe dose range of a chemical, experimental toxicologists generally take a top-down view of the dose-response curve, i.e., after identifying an overtly toxic (high) dose level, they look for the highest dose below that level causing no harm. In other words, toxicologists assume that there is a monotonic relationship between doses and toxic responses (i.e., the higher the exposure or dose, the more severe and likely the harmful effect) and that, for each chemical and adverse effect, there would be a "threshold" dose, below which the chemical does not cause the effect.

The assumptions that dose-responses are monotonic, and that there are dose-thresholds for adversity, are major elements underlying the existing testing protocols that cover essentially all regulated nongenotoxic chemicals (Briggs 1996). The repeated-dose toxicity, carcinogenicity and reproductive toxicity studies are designed to evaluate a control and three or more groups treated with the substance. Within the tested dose range, dose levels are spaced by using a multiplication factor (2x, 10x, and so on) so that, at the highest dose, the substance is expected to cause overt toxicity whereas at the lowest dose level, it should produce no discernible effect. The highest tested dose causing no discernible adverse effect is the study-derived NOAEL ("no-observed-adverse effect level") while the lowest tested dose inducing a discernible toxic effect is the LOAEL ("lowest observed adverse effect level") (Duffus et al. 2007). If there is no dose-threshold for the effect (i.e., the dose-threshold assumption is false), one cannot determine a NOAEL, or at least a true NOAEL.[2]

If adverse effects result ultimately from an immediate probabilistic (stochastic) event, and it is fair to assume that there is no dose-threshold (and so no NOAEL) for the chemical or physical agent-caused harmfulness, then risk assessors seek a virtually safe dose range. Virtually safe doses are the doses at which the estimated probability of the initiating event and the ensuing harmful effects are so low that one could assume that they would produce no discernible negative impact on the health of exposed people (Paumgartten 1993).

---

[1] Paracelsus means surpassing Celsus, a Roman encyclopaedist known for his extant medical work. The name was adopted by Phillipus Aureoleus Theophrastus Bombastus von Hohenheim (1493–1541), a Swiss-German physician who wrote *Der Dritte Defense* (*The Third Defense*), an authoritative piece of writing containing his most quoted statement (in German): *"Alle Ding sind Gift und nichts ist ohne Gift; allein die Dosis macht das dies TDing kein Gift ist"* (Deichmann et al. 1986).

[2] Even if there is no threshold for an effect, experiment-derived NOAELs can be determined. The ability to detect a difference between a control and a treated group is dependent on the statistical power of the study, i.e., on the number of animals per group (group size). Larger group sizes are likely to result in lower NOAELs because the study power to detect (smaller) differences increases (and vice versa). Therefore, if group sizes are small, effects at the lowest tested dose may remain undetected, thereby erroneously suggesting that they are NOAELs. Moreover, a study-derived NOAEL is always one of the tested doses and so it depends on the tested dose range and on the interval between the tested doses.

Low-dose Effects and Non-monotonic Dose-response Curves

In 2001, an expert panel established by the *National Toxicological Program* (NTP) from the US *National Institute of Environmental Health Sciences* defined operationally low-dose effects as *"biological changes that occur in the range of human exposures or at doses that are lower than those typically used in the EPA's standard testing paradigm for evaluating reproductive and developmental toxicity"* (NTP 2001). If one replaces human dose (external exposure) with body burden (internal exposure), "low-doses" could be defined as doses that, in experimental animals, give rise to blood concentrations within the range that is measured in the general population (i.e., people not occupationally exposed). In other words, "low doses" in the context of experimental research would be "environmentally relevant" doses of a chemical (Vandenberg et al. 2012). Along this line, "low-dose" hypothesis is the conjecture that some chemicals, particularly the substances that act on the endocrine system (or endocrine active chemicals), can cause low-dose effects or, in other words, the speculation that low doses of some chemicals can bring about biological responses and adverse health effects.

Dose-response non-monotonicity (NMDR), on the other hand, means that the slope of a curve relating doses (or concentrations) to the magnitude of the response (in *in vivo* or *in vitro* test systems) changes its sign from positive to negative or *vice versa* at one (or more than one) point along the tested range of doses (or concentrations). In principle, low-dose effects might occur in both monotonic (the slope does not change sign) and non-monotonic dose-response curves. Most putative low-dose effects reported so far, however, refer to chemicals and biological responses showing non-monotonic dose-effect relationships such as U- (or J-) or inverted U- (or J-) shaped curves (Fig. 1).

The low-dose effects, and *ipso facto* the low-dose hypothesis, took center stage in the 1990s when Frederick vom Saal and coworkers (1997) published their study on the effects of prenatal exposure to 17-β-estradiol (EST) and diethylstilbestrol (DES) on the size (hyperplasia) and the number of androgen receptors (increased) in the prostate gland of adult CF-1 mice. The authors reported a 50% increase in free–serum EST (from 0.21 to 0.32 pg.mL^{-1}) in male mouse fetuses (released through a Silastic capsule implanted under the mother skin from gestation day 13 to 19, GD 13–19) caused a prostate gland enlargement (due to hyperplasia) and an increase in the number of androgen receptors per prostatic cell in adult animals. Nonetheless, as fetal blood serum EST concentrations rose by 2- to 8-fold (0.56, 0.78 and 1.7 pg.mL^{-1}) the background hormone levels (0.21 pg.mL^{-1}), the prostate gland weight declined relative to the weight of the gland of adult males exposed to a 50% increase in free-serum EST levels (to 0.32 pg.mL^{-1}) during fetal life. In the same study, vom Saal et al. (1997) obtained a similar inverted U-shaped dose-response curve for adult mouse prostate weight when groups of pregnant mice were treated orally with doses of DES (a rather potent synthetic estrogen) ranging from 0.002 to 200 ng.g^{-1} bw from GD 11 to 17 (Fig. 2). A subsequent study by the same research group found that prenatal exposure to bisphenol A (BPA), a man-made chemical widely used in plastics, resins, dental sealants, lining in canned food and beverage products, and a myriad of consumer products, caused a non-monotonically dose-dependent effect

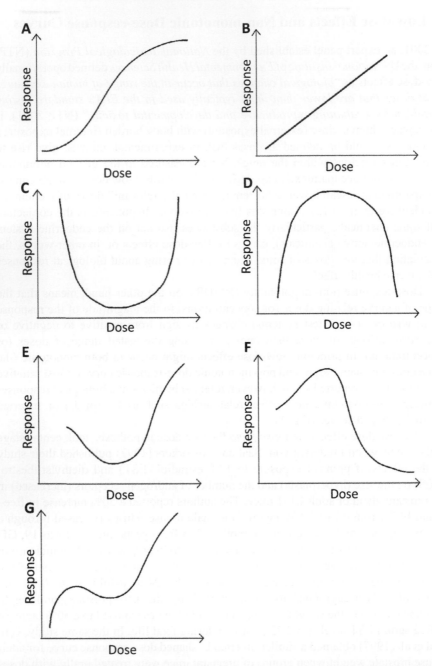

Fig. 1. Examples of monotonic and non-monotonic dose-response curves. Examples of monotonic dose-response curves: **A**–"S" or sigmoid ("logistic") curve (response plotted along the ordinates or y axis against the log of the dose or concentration plotted along the abscissa or x axis) and **B**–linear curve ($y = ax + b$). In both dose-response curves, the slope of the curve never changes sign. Examples of non-monotonic dose-response curves: **C**–U-shaped curve, **D**–inverted U-shaped curve, **E**–J-shaped, **F**–inverted J-shaped and **G**–multiphasic curve. In non-monotonic dose-response curves, the slope of the curve changes sign one or more times.

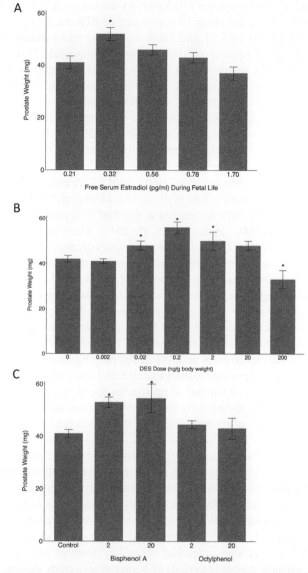

Fig. 2. Inverted U-shaped curves describing the effects of prenatal exposure to supra-physiological levels of 17-β-estradiol (EST) and xenoestrogens on adult prostate weight in CF-1 mice. A. Weights (mg) of prostate gland from adult (8-month old) CF-1 male mice exposed prenatally to supra-physiological levels of free serum EST from gestation day 13 to 19. EST was administered through Silastic capsules implanted under skin, and control (untreated) free serum EST levels were 0.21 pg.mL^{-1}. **B.** Prostate gland weight (mg) in adult male mice born to pregnant females treated orally (gavage) with diethylstilbestrol (DES, 0.002 to 200 ng.g bw^{-1}.day^{-1}) from gestation day 11 to 17. Data are shown as means ± SEM. **C.** Weight of prostate glands (mg) from six-month CF-1 old male mice born to pregnant females treated orally (*via* diet) with bisphenol A (BPA: 2 or 20 pg.kg bw^{-1}.d^{-1}) or octyphenol (OTP: 2 or 20 pg.kg bw^{-1}.d^{-1}) from gestation days 11 to 17. Histogram bar heights are means ± SEM. Differences (p < 0.05) from the group mean prostate weight are indicated by an asterisk (*). Graphs 2A and 2B were modified from vom Saal et al. (1997) and graph 2C was redrawn from Nagel et al. (1997).

(i.e., an inverted U dose-response relationship) on the weight of prostate gland (Nagel et al. 1997). Since the effect of low doses of BPA on prostate development was similar to the effects of EST and DES, vom Saal and colleagues ascribed it to a putative estrogenic activity of this phenolic compound. This interpretation is amazing because BPA has proved to be a very weak estrogenic compound in a variety of screening tests for estrogenic activity. It was shown that BPA, in orders of magnitude, is less potent than EST and DES in *in vitro* assays for screening estrogenic chemicals such as YES (yeast-based estrogen assay) (Gaido et al. 1997, Harris et al. 1997, Andersen et al. 1999, Dhooge et al. 2006), MCF-7 (human breast cancer) cell proliferation assay (Andersen et al. 1999), relative binding displacement of ligand binding to human estrogen α-receptor (Krishnan et al. 1993, Olea et al. 1996, Nagel et al. 1997, Andersen et al. 1999), and STTA assay (stably transfected transcriptional activation assay) (Lee et al. 2012). Moreover, after absorption from the gastrointestinal tract, BPA undergoes a marked first-pass metabolism in the liver (Pottenger et al. 2000, Vandenberg et al. 2010) where uridine 5'-diphospho-glucuronosyltransferases (UGTs) and sulfotransferases promptly convert it into BPA-conjugates (BPA glucuronides and BPA-sulfate conjugates) that are virtually devoid of any agonistic activity on estrogen receptors (Matthews et al. 2001, Shimizu et al. 2002). In the following years, studies by two independent research groups (Ashby et al. 1999, Cagen et al. 1999) failed to replicate the findings reported by Nagel et al. (1997) with low doses of BPA and DES (positive control). Along the same line, a large second-generation toxicity study by Tyl et al. (2008) found no effect of BPA administered *via* diet (control and five doses ranging from 0.003 to 600 mg.kg bw^{-1}.d^{-1}) on the weight of prostate gland of adult CD-1 mice from either the F_1 or the F_2 generation. Furthermore, a number of rat studies found no effect of exposure to a broad range of BPA doses during early development on the weight of prostate gland of adult animals. The lack of reproducibility of the effects (and the inverted U dose-response relationship) of developmental exposures to low doses of BPA and DES on the mouse prostate gland is intriguing. As commented by Paumgartten and De-Oliveira (2014), the failure of studies in rats to replicate the initial findings in mice might eventually arise from inter-species differences in the responsiveness to DES and BPA. There is no scientifically plausible explanation, however, for discrepancies between results from some studies in mice. The studies performed by Ashby et al. (1999) and Cagen et al. (1999), for instance, not only were conducted with the same mouse strain (CF-1), but also mimicked other key features (doses, oral route of administration, prenatal exposure period) of Nagel et al.'s study design.

During the last 25 years, the putative developmental toxicity of low doses of BPA has become a hallmark of the Endocrine Disruption (ED) hypothesis, possibly the most controversial topic of modern toxicology. Unsurprisingly, the reproducibility of data on the effects of low doses of BPA during early development on the adult prostate size and mammary gland architecture (commented elsewhere in this chapter) has been a central issue of this unrelenting debate (Paumgartten and De-Oliveira 2014). Notwithstanding the 5,000 or more safety-related studies on BPA, it is still in dispute whether at current levels of exposure of the general population, BPA causes adverse health effects, and, if so, whether such effects are in some way mediated by an estrogenic activity of this compound (Hengstler et al. 2011, Paumgartten and De-

Oliveira 2014). In an effort to put an end to the BPA controversy, the *US National Toxicology Program* (NTP), *National Institute of Environmental Health Sciences* (NIEHS), and *US Food and Drug Administration* (FDA) launched a consortium-based research program known by the acronym CLARITY-BPA, or "Consortium Linking Academic and Regulatory Insights on BPA Toxicity" (Schug et al. 2013). The objective of CLARITY-BPA is to link a variety of hypothesis-related academic laboratory investigations and Good Laboratory Practice (GLP) and guideline-compliant studies. A recent report informs that the in-life phase of the university-based research studies was completed in January 2014, while the in-life phase of the core chronic studies was completed in January 2015. According to CLARITY-BPA, data from the core chronic study are expected to be publicly available by 2018 (Heindel et al. 2015).

The definition of "low-dose effects", however, is far from being a consensus among toxicologists. "Low-dose effects" and NMDRs of endocrine disrupting chemicals have been debated over-and-over again in a number of conferences. In 2012, a meeting held by the European Food Safety Authority (EFSA) got together approximately 100 researchers and risk assessors who concluded that an adequate and generally accepted definition of low-dose effects and NMDR is necessary to facilitate further discussions on these topics. Shortly thereafter, a poll conducted among attendees of a workshop on ED held in Berlin brought to light a lack of consensus about what should be the definition of low doses (Beausoleil et al. 2013). The results of the survey were as follows: for 41% of respondents, "low-doses" are doses within "*human exposure range and/or environmental levels*", for 18%, low-doses are "*any dose at or below the NOAEL of the most sensitive species tested*", for 7%, low-dose is the "*NOAEL divided by an uncertainty factor which could be flexible or fixed*", for 22%, "*no formal definition was needed*", while for the remaining 12%, the response was "other" (Beausoleil et al. 2013). Four years later, a consensus reached by an international workshop hosted by the German Federal Institute for Risk Assessment (BfR) stated that: "*Non-monotonic dose-response relationships and low-dose effects of endocrine disruptors have been described in the literature*", yet "*... a consensus about these issues is unlikely to emerge in the near future*" (Solecki et al. 2016).

Hormesis: A Specific Type of Dose-response Non-monotonicity

"*Hormesis*", or "*hormetic* behavior", is the phenomenon behind a biphasic dose-response curve characterized by stimulatory responses or beneficial effects in the low dose range and inhibition or damaging effects at higher doses (Calabrese 2008, Mattson 2008). A J-shaped or U-shaped curve (or inverted J- or U-shaped curves, depending on the endpoint evaluated), therefore, illustrates, graphically, a typical *hormetic* phenomenon. Many researchers believe that the beneficial effects of low doses on the cell or on the intact organism arise from adaptive compensatory processes triggered by an initial disruption of homeostasis that, in the higher dose range of a toxicant, becomes overtly detrimental (Mattson 2008).

In the nineteenth century, Hugo Schulz, a German pharmacologist, and Rudolf Arndt, a physician, described what was later called "*hormetic*" phenomenon.

According to these researchers, life processes (e.g., the growth of yeast) are enhanced or stimulated by low doses (or concentrations) of substances that at higher doses (or concentrations) are overtly toxic and lethal. In 1888, based on his own experimental findings and Schulz's studies, Arndt formulated a rule (the Arndt-Schulz law) stating that for every substance, small doses stimulate, moderate doses inhibit, and large doses eventually terminate life processes (Stumpf 2006). It was only in 1943, however, that the American researchers Chester Southam and John Ehrlich introduced the term *hormesis* (adj. *hormetic*) to designate such a stimulatory effect of subinhibitory concentrations of any toxic substance on any organism. The *hormesis* concept did not receive much attention until the 1990s when a series of remarkable articles by Edward Calabrese rescued it (Calabrese et al. 1987, Calabrese and Baldwin 1998, Calabrese 2004). It is noteworthy that revival of *hormesis* theory by Calabrese's articles was more-or-less coincident with the emergence of hypotheses on endocrine disruption and low-dose effects. Nonetheless, despite some obvious resemblances, the low-dose effect concept and the *hormesis* notion do not easily fit in to each other. The "low-dose" phase of a *hormetic* biphasic dose-response curve is generally interpreted as corresponding to an adaptive (beneficial) response to a chemical (or physical) stimulus that at higher doses (strengths) would be harmful, whereas the low-dose hypothesis tacitly assumes that "low-dose effects" (particularly those of endocrine disruptors) would be potentially detrimental to health.

There is little doubt that *hormesis* does in fact occur in a number of cases. Calabrese and coworkers identified in the published literature, for instance, hundreds of studies reporting *hormetic* dose-responses (Calabrese and Baldwin 2001, Calabrese and Blain 2011). Notwithstanding this fact, whether *hormesis* is a broadly generalizable phenomenon or, on the contrary, the exception rather than the rule, remains controversial (Elliott 2000, Mushak 2009, 2013).

The Linear Non-Threshold (LNT) Dose-response Concept

The assumption that there is a dose-threshold for toxic effects implies that there is a range of doses at which a chemical causes no harm, or a dose range at which it is safe. If this assumption proves to be untrue and there is no threshold for adverse effects, then any dose of a chemical might eventually cause harm. Along this line, one generally assumes that nongenotoxic chemicals show a dose-threshold for harmfulness whereas genotoxic agents do not (Briggs 1996).

The notion that there is no dose-threshold for agents causing genetic damage has its origins in 1928, when the American geneticist Hermann Joseph Muller noted that X-rays could produce mutations in the progeny of irradiated fruit flies (*Drosophila melanogaster*) (Muller 1928a,b). Muller also described that the mutation rate increased linearly with the radiation dose, a discovery of great significance that was further confirmed by others (Kathren 2002). Actually, the injurious effects of ionizing radiation have been known for almost as long as X-ray radiation itself. As early as 1897, one year after Wilhelm Röntgen discovered X-rays, Thomas Casper Gilchrist reported skin burns and dermatitis caused by X-rays (Gilchrist 1897), while, a few years later, in 1902, a German physician (Albert Frieben) described a case of occupational skin cancer (on the dorsum of the hand) in a male worker (aged 33 years) of a factory producing X-rays tubes (Frieben 1902).

The harmful effects of ionizing radiation are generally divided into two categories: deterministic effects (e.g., skin burns, erythema, cataracts, sterility, dermatitis, cytotoxicity, tissue necrosis, immune and bone-marrow function depression and reduction in blood counts) and stochastic effects (of random or probabilistic nature) derived from radiation-produced mutations in germ (e.g., genetic effects in the progeny) and somatic cells (e.g., cancer initiation) (Little 2003). The deterministic effects are non-stochastic events that typically occur after a high acute dose exposure (mostly > 0.1 Gy) with a dose-threshold below which no effect occurs. In other words, for deterministic effects (relevant for radiotherapy), it is assumed that there is a dose-threshold and, therefore, a LNT model approach would not be applicable to extrapolate effects from high to low doses. For stochastic effects (mutations), on the other side, one assumes that the probability of their occurrence (but not their severity) is directly proportional or linearly related to the radiation dose, and therefore, there is no dose-threshold for the effect. In other words, theoretically, interaction of a single photon with the biological matter would be sufficient to induce a mutation that could in turn cause a heritable genetic disease (germ cell mutation) or trigger the initiation of a tumor (somatic cell mutation). However, the probability associated to adverse health effects triggered by interactions of a single photon with the genetic material is extremely low (Little 2003).

In 1956, based on the findings reported by Muller and on the idea that mutations (and cancer initiation) are stochastic events, a Genetics Panel held by the Committee on Biological Effects of Radiation of the US National Academy of Sciences recommended that the assessment of genomic risks associated with ionizing radiation should switch from the threshold dose-response model to a linear non-threshold dose-response (LNT) model approach. In the 1970s, the US Environment Protection Agency (US EPA) and the US Food and Drug Administration (US FDA) adopted the LNT concept approach for chemical carcinogens as well (Calabrese 2013).

The universal use of the LNT model approach in cancer risk assessment and in radiation health protection has been questioned by several researchers (Kathren 2002, Luckey 2006, Calabrese 2015, 2016, Feinendegen 2016, Seong et al. 2016). As far as biological effects of radiation are concerned, the LNT model approach to extrapolate effects from high to low doses clashes with the radiation *hormesis* hypothesis. According to the radiation *hormesis* notion, low doses of ionizing radiation—within or just above the natural background levels—stimulate cell DNA repair mechanisms that are not activated in the absence of radiation, thereby being beneficial and protecting the organism against diseases (Luckey 1982, 2006, Feinendegen 2005, 2016). It is of note that acceptance of radiation *hormesis* notion does not imply that immediate DNA damage is not a stochastic phenomenon. Even if the (low) probability of immediate DNA damage per energy deposition event rises linearly with the number of events (i.e., absorbed dose), the (adverse) response of the biological system as a whole would not be linear (and monotonic) because of the (marked) stimulation of DNA repair mechanisms by low doses of radiation (Feinendegen 2016). Analogously, Tuomisto et al. (2006) speculated that dioxin cancer risk could also be a *hormetic* phenomenon involving J-shaped dose-response curves.[3] This provocative hypothesis stands on the results from a single case-control study suggesting that there was an inverse correlation between measured body burden of dioxins and furans (PCDD/Fs) and the risk of soft tissue sarcoma in the normal population exposed to dioxins *via* food. Nonetheless, case-control epidemiology studies are particularly prone to uncontrolled bias and confounding and thus one cannot rule out non-causal explanations for weak associations (Doll 2002). Owing to the lack of robust experimental and epidemiological data to support it, Tuomisto et al.'s (2005) hypothesis is too speculative to be considered. At any rate, in spite of being supported by many scientists, the radiation *hormesis* hypothesis has not been endorsed by health agencies, and LNT approach is generally used for assessing radiation and chemical carcinogenic risks (Luckey 2006).

Experimental Evidence for NMDRs and Low-dose Effects

As previously stated, hundreds of studies describing *hormetic* non-monotonic dose response curves were identified in the literature by Calabrese and Blain (2011), thereby indicating that, at least as far as this specific type of biphasic dose-response is concerned, NMDR is a relatively common phenomenon (see Mushak 2013 for a balanced view). Furthermore, Vandenberg et al. (2012), in one of the most comprehensive narrative reviews[4] of the literature on endocrine-disrupting chemicals published so far, also analyzed a number of cases and concluded that non-monotonic dose responses and low-dose effects are common in studies of hormones and EDs. More recently, Beausoleil et al. (2016) conducted a systematic review of the scientific peer-reviewed literature in the last decade (from 2002 onwards) in the area of food safety and evaluated the evidence for NMDR hypothesis. In this review, dose-response results were evaluated for possible evidence of NMDR by applying six checkpoints and the plausibility of a NMDR was assessed based on the number of fulfilled checkpoints. Overall, the researchers identified 202 *in vivo* data sets (from 49 studies), 311 *in vitro* datasets (from 91 studies) and nine human datasets (from two epidemiological studies). After exclusion of datasets considered unsuitable for analysis (due to dataset limitations and other inadequacies), 179 *in vivo*, 23 *in vitro*

---

[3] Data on the genotoxicity of *2,3,7,8*-TCDD are conflicting and positive (generally weak) as well as clearly negative results have been reported. In the *in vitro* assays, the effects of TCDD were largely negative for a range of genotoxic endpoints (Giri 1986, Paustenbach et al. 1986, ASTDR 1989, IARC-WHO 1997). The *in vivo* animal studies on the genotoxic potential of TCDD yielded predominantly negative results as well (Giri 1986, IARC-WHO 1997). Since putative TCDD-mediated carcinogenicity does not arise from a stochastic initiation event (mutation), LNT approach would not be applicable for extrapolating dioxin cancer risks. However, as pointed out by Slob (1999, 2007), carcinogenesis process as a whole has a stochastic nature because a small sequence of specific individual mutations are required for originating a malignant tumor development and each of these mutations has a certain probability to occur or not. Since it is plausible to think that both genotoxic and nongenotoxic carcinogens may increase these probabilities, the LNT approach has been used for assessing the risk of nongenotoxic carcinogens as well.

[4] Contrasting with systematic reviews of the literature, narrative reviews have the disadvantage that they are prone to bias thereby conveying an unbalanced view on the debated issue. A brief comment on this problem can be found in Paumgartten (2015).

and none human datasets were analyzed and evaluated using the six checkpoints.[5] Results showed that only 6% (10 of 179) *in vivo* datasets (related to four studies) fulfilled all six checkpoints for NMDRs while none of the *in vitro* datasets fulfilled the six checkpoints. The highest number of fulfilled checkpoints in *in vitro* datasets was five (fulfilled by one *in vitro* dataset only). The *in vivo* datasets fulfilling all six criteria for NMDR were studies of substances such as quercetin, resveratrol, alpha-benzene hexachloride and methylmercury. Beausoleil et al.'s systematic review of datasets in the area of food safety therefore indicated that NMDRs occurred in only 6% of cases for which enough data on dose/concentration response relationships were available for analysis (Beausoleil et al. 2016).

At least three large *in vivo* studies of putative EDs were specifically designed to reveal low dose effects and NMDRs if they do in fact occur.

Fussell et al. (2015) examined whether very low doses of the anti-androgenic substance flutamide disrupted endocrine homeostasis and caused endocrine-mediated developmental effects in the rat. The study design was compliant with regulatory testing protocols for pre-postnatal *in vivo* studies and included some additional endpoints such as hormone levels, morphology and histopathological examinations. The tested dose-range was wide and included a "clear effect" dose level (2.5 mg.kg bw^{-1}.d^{-1}), a low-endocrine effect level or LOAEL (0.25 mg.kg bw^{-1}.d^{-1}), a NOAEL for endocrine effects (0.025 mg.kg bw^{-1}.d^{-1}), a further lower dose at 0.0025 mg.kg bw^{-1}.d^{-1} and a dose consistent with an acceptable daily intake or "ADI" (0.00025 mg.kg bw^{-1}.d^{-1} or 100-fold below the NOAEL), so that a possible dose-response non-monotocity would be disclosed, if it did occur. As expected, typical anti-androgenic effects such as nipple retention (the most sensitive measure of anti-androgenic effects), changes in the age at sexual maturation, alterations of anogenital distance/anogenital index and weight of male reproductive organs, as well as gross pathology and histopathological findings, were noted at the LOAEL and the "clear effect" doses. No effect, however, was detected at lower exposures and very low dose levels. Therefore, no evidence was found of non-monotonic dose–response relationships. Flick et al. (2016) conducted a similarly designed rat study with another potent antiandrogenic compound, the fungicide vinclozolin. The doses of vinclozolin were chosen to represent an effect level (20 mg.kg bw^{-1}d^{-1}), the NOAEL (4 mg.kg bw^{-1}d^{-1}) and a dose close to the "ADI" (0.005 mg.kg bw^{-1}.d^{-1}). The anti-androgenic effects were observed at the effect level but not at lower exposures and a non-monotonic dose-response curve was not evident either.

Andrade, Chahoud and coworkers investigated the developmental effects of a range of doses of di-(2-ethylhexyl) phthalate (DEHP), the most commonly used phthalate plasticized and putative ED. Like flutamide and vinclozolin, DEHP is a

---

[5] The six checkpoints for non-monotonicity defined by Beausoleil et al. (2016) were questions as follows: Can apparent NMDR be explained by (1) random fluctuations around a horizontal dose-response (= no effect at all)?, (2) random fluctuations around a monotone dose response (MDR)?, (3) a single potential outlying dose group?, (4) Is the effect size in one of the directions smaller than 5%?, (5) Is the steepness of the dose-response curve outside the range of biologically plausible/realistic dose-response shapes?, (6) Does the apparent NMDR consist of more (or less) than two directions? When the answer to the indicated checkpoint was "no", it was considered fulfilled.

potent antiandrogenic compound that was demonstrated to affect male rat sexual differentiation (Wolf et al. 1999, Parks et al. 2000). The authors conducted a large and extensive dose-response study of the effects of developmental exposure to DEHP (from GD 6 to postnatal day 22) on the reproductive development of male and female rats. The tested dose range included oral dose levels of DEHP that were doses considered relevant for human exposure or "low doses" (0.015, 0.045, 0.135, 0.405 and 1.215 mg.kg bw^{-1}.d^{-1}) as well as high doses typically used in toxicity assays of the plasticizer (5, 15, 45, 135 and 405 mg.kg bw^{-1}.d^{-1}). The effects of this broad range of DEHP doses on distinct male and female development endpoints were reported separately in a series of five articles as follows: the reproductive effects on adult female offspring (Grande et al. 2007), the reproductive effects on adult male offspring (Andrade et al. 2006b), the effects on rat brain (hypothalamic preoptic area) aromatase (Andrade et al. 2006a), the effects on developmental landmarks and testicular histology in male offspring (Andrade et al. 2006c), and the effects on female reproductive development (Grande et al. 2006). The authors described that brain aromatase activity in male rats on PND1 was inhibited at low doses (0.135 and 0.405 mg.kg bw^{-1}.d^{-1}) and increased at high doses (15, 45 and 405 mg.kg bw^{-1}.d^{-1}). This is what gave rise to a NMDR resembling a J-shaped curve (Andrade et al. 2006a). Except for this low-dose effect on brain aromatase, in all other evaluated male and female reproductive development endpoints, effects were observed only at the high dose range (generally 405 mg/kg bw/d). Overall, this rather extensive dose-response evaluation of an antiandrogenic ED consistently failed to demonstrate low dose effects and NMDRs (Andrade et al. 2006b,c, Grande et al. 2006, 2007) except for one of the endpoints (brain aromatase activity) examined on PND1.

Evidence from in vitro test systems and the role of cytotoxicity

Low-concentration effects and non-monotonic (inverted-U) concentration response curves are often observed in *in vitro* test systems. Effects of very low concentrations of TCDD, for instance, were found in *in vitro* assays. Baldridge et al. (2015) described that nanomolar (3.1 × 10^{-9} M), picomolar (3.1 × 10^{-12} M) as well as femtomolar (3.1 × 10^{-15} M) concentrations of TCDD decreased the production of 17-β-estradiol (EST) by human luteinizing granulosa cells (hLGC). The authors also noted that declines in the secretion of EST by hLGC cells correlated with a reduction of mRNA expression levels of *CYP11A1* and *CYP19A1,* two key enzymes (monooxygenases) of steroid-hormone biosynthesis pathways. Although effects in the femtomolar (10^{-15} M) concentration range are to be considered responses to extremely low concentrations even for a potent toxicant and aryl hydrocarbon receptor (*AhR*) ligand as TCDD, Baldridge et al.'s results not only failed to demonstrate a non-monotonic concentration-response, but also found no clear concentration-dependent effect over a very broad range of tested concentrations (i.e., the size of the response of hLGC cells to added TCDD did not change over a six-orders of magnitude concentration-range) (Baldridge et al. 2015).

In *in vitro* tests, changes in the concentration-response curve slope sign often reflect the superimposition of a cytotoxic effect over another (stimulatory) response as substance concentrations rise and attain a toxic concentration range. One example of this is the response of MCF-7 human breast cancer cells to increasing concentrations of natural estrogen 17-β-estradiol (EST) or xenoestrogens (DES) reported by Welshons et al. (2003). MCF-7 is a permanent cell line derived from a human breast malignant tumor that contains estrogen receptors. Upon sustained estrogenic stimulation, MCF-7 cells undergo a marked increase in proliferation and thus a MCF-7 cell based assay has been widely used to screen xenobiotic compounds for estrogenic activity. Welshons et al. (2003) found that proliferation or cell growth (indicated by an augment of cultivated cell DNA per plate well) of MCF-7 cells, kept in an estrogen-free cell culture medium, underwent a 3.5-fold increase as EST levels rose from 0.1 pM to 100 pM (low concentration range), cell growth response attained a *plateau* at EST concentrations between 100 pM and 1.0 μM (intermediate concentration range), and showed a concentration-dependent decline in cell growth response at EST concentrations above 1.0 μM (high concentration range) (Fig. 3A). These findings indicated that stimulation of MCF-7 cell proliferation by low and intermediate concentrations is followed by high-concentration cytotoxicity, giving a curve that relates EST concentration to cell growth response an inverted U shape. In a subsequent experiment, Welshons et al. (2003) derived a clonal cell line (C4-12-5) from MCF-7 that, contrasting to the parental cell line, did not express estrogen receptors, and so it was completely nonresponsive to estrogenic stimulation. As expected, the C4-12-5 estrogen insensitive cells treated with increasing concentrations of EST did not show any growth stimulation response, yet it retained the cytotoxic response noted in MCF-7 cells in the same high concentration range (Fig. 3B). Results, therefore, suggested that cytotoxic responses of both MCF-7 and C4-121-5 cells to high concentrations of 17β-estradiol (EST) were independent of its actions on estrogen receptors. Another experiment (Fig. 3C) with estrogen-responsive MCF-7 cells showed that the presence of a background low concentration (10 pM) of DES (a potent xenoestrogen) in the culture medium averted the growth stimulation effect of low concentrations of EST, but did not change the cytotoxic response to high concentrations of this sex hormone. Overall, this elegant set of experiments by Welshons et al. (2003) unveiled that, in *in vitro* cell based test systems, high concentration cytotoxicity may give concentration-response curves inverted-U-shapes.

It is of note that there are plausible explanations other than cytotoxicity at high concentrations for inverted U-shaped concentration-response curves. A possible mechanistic explanation is given by a mathematical model created by Kohn and Melnick (2002) to examine how xenobiotic ligands that bind to nuclear hormone receptor proteins may affect transcriptional activation of hormone-regulated genes. The model predicts that inverted-U-shaped concentration-response curves are possible outcomes for xenobiotics that activate nuclear receptors in the same manner as the natural ligands, if natural ligand basal levels did not saturate receptor binding sites, and if affinity for co-activator when the xenobiotic is bound to the receptor is weaker than affinity for co-activator when the natural ligand is bound. A further article by Conolly and Lutz (2004) also provided four examples from analyses of pharmacological and toxicological data sets to demonstrate that there may be biologically founded mechanistic explanations for non-monotonic concentration (or dose)-response curves describing the interaction of toxicants with complex biological systems over a broad range of concentrations (doses).

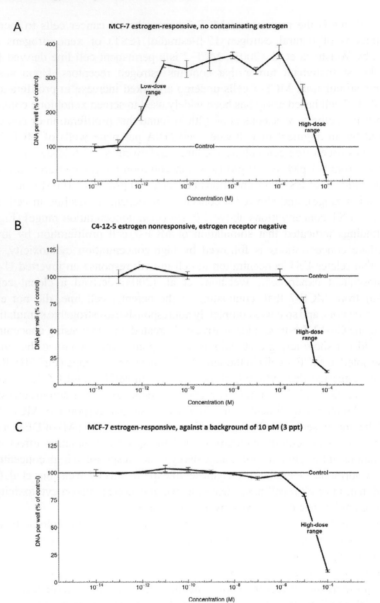

Fig. 3. Non-monotonic concentration-response curves in *in vitro* test systems. Effects of estrogenic stimulation on the proliferation of MCF-7 human breast cancer cells grown in cell culture microplates. Cell proliferation is indicated by increases in amounts of DNA per well (% of untreated control wells). **A.** Stimulation of MCF-7 cells proliferation in estrogen-free culture medium by increasing EST concentration in the medium up to a frankly cytotoxic level. **B.** Lack of a stimulatory response (but not of a cytotoxic response) when EST is added to a culture of C4-12-5 estrogen-receptor negative (and estrogen unresponsive) cell line derived from MCF-7 cells. **C.** Absence of a stimulatory response to EST (but not of a cytotoxic response) of estrogen-responsive MCF-7 cells grown in the presence of a background concentration of a xenoestrogen (10 pM DES) added to an estrogen-free culture medium. Control (100%) values were 1.0, 3.7, and 5.5 μg of DNA per well for *A*, *B*, and *C*, respectively. Values are the mean and SD of determinations in replicate wells (*n* = 3). Graphs were modified version of a figure published in Welshons et al. (2003).

Additionally, cytotoxicity does not explain all types of biphasic concentration-response curves observed in *in vitro* test systems. The superimposition of cytotoxicity, for instance, does not provide an explanation for U-shaped concentration response curves with inhibitory effects noted at low concentrations and stimulatory effects at higher concentrations. An example along this line is the effect of TCDD on the secretion of steroid hormones by antral follicles. Karman et al. (2012) exposed antral follicles (mechanically isolated from the mouse ovary and kept in culture for 96 h) to TCDD (0.1, 1, 10 and 100 nM) or its vehicle (DMSO) alone and measured sex steroid hormone secretion *in vitro*. Results showed that the lowest TCDD concentrations (0.1 and 1 nM) depressed the secretion of progesterone, androstenedione, testosterone and estradiol, inhibitory effects the magnitude of which clearly declined at the highest concentrations tested (10 and 100 nM), i.e., the effect of TCDD on sex steroid secretion displayed a clear non-monotonic (U-shaped) concentration-response relationship (Fig. 4).

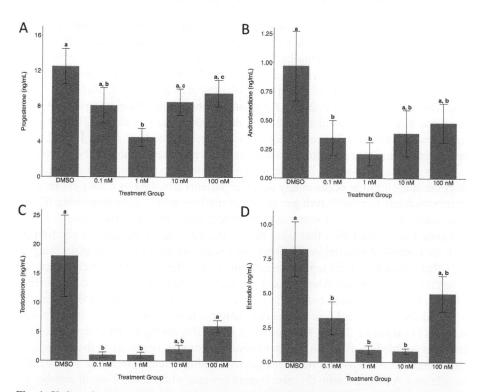

Fig. 4. U-shaped concentration-response curve in *in vitro* test system. Effects of TCDD on mouse antral follicle sex steroid secretion. Antral follicles isolated from young cycling CD1 mice were kept in culture medium and exposed to TCDD (0.1–100 nM) or its vehicle (DMSO) alone for 96 h. Graphs show effects of treatment with TCDD on the release of progesterone (A), androstenedione (B), testosterone (C) and estradiol (D) to the culture medium. Histogram bar heights are means ± SEM (from 8 to 23 cell-culture microplate wells). Means corresponding to the height of histogram bars not sharing the same letters differ from each other (p < 0.05). Graphs were a modified version of a graph shown in Karman et al. (2012).

Evidence from in vivo studies

As aforementioned, low dose-effects and/or non-monotonic dose-response relationships were reported for several substances and *in vivo* and *in vitro* test endpoints. Although low dose effects have been mostly described for endocrine active chemicals and hormone-sensitive endpoints, some typical low dose effects and non-monotonic dose-responses were reported for hormone unrelated outcomes as well. The effect of supra-physiological levels of natural estrogens and low doses of xenoestrogens (DES and BPA) during a critical period of fetal development on the adult prostate size was commented elsewhere in this chapter. In the following lines, three additional examples of low dose effects and/or non-monotonic dose-responses (one of which for an endocrine unrelated outcome) are described and critically appraised.

BPA exposure in the womb and mammary gland development

Studies by Soto, Vandenberg, Markey and others yielded data consistent with the notion that exposure to low doses of BPA during early development (pre- and perinatal exposures) induce long-lasting changes in the histogenesis and architecture of mammary gland tissue such as increased duct branching, ductal hyperplasia and enhanced epithelial cell proliferation rates (Markey et al. 2001, 2005, Muñoz-de-Toro et al. 2005, Vandenberg et al. 2007). All these studies evaluated the offspring of CD-1 mice and Wistar rats treated continuously during pregnancy with BPA (0.25 to 250 $\mu g.kg\ bw^{-1}d^{-1}$) released from an osmotic pump implanted under the skin. If these data on rodents are used for quantitative risk assessment purposes, a hurdle to be overcome is that a human exposure to BPA through a parenteral route is the exception rather than the rule (it might occasionally occur if patients admitted to a hospital receive intravenous infusions with syringes and other medical plastic ware containing BPA). The subcutaneous route of entry used in rodent experiments circumvents the pre-systemic clearance of BPA that takes place after oral ingestions and, in addition to that, the controlled drug delivery system ensures a sustained blood level of unchanged BPA that otherwise would rapidly decline due to an efficient metabolic clearance. In a further study, pregnant Rhesus monkeys were treated orally with a dose of BPA (400 $\mu g.kgbw^{-1}.d^{-1}$) which resulted in 0.68 ± 0.312 ng of unconjugated BPA per mL of blood serum collected four hours after dosing, a level comparable to that found in humans (Tharp et al. 2012). The treatment with BPA during prenatal development, however, yielded no effect on the expression of estrogen receptors in the mammary tissue and equivocal overall results (most reported differences were not statistically significant). A problem with this non-human primate study was the small number of BPA-treated animals (four treated and five control monkeys) and the evaluation of mammary gland histological architecture only at birth.

Although the effects of BPA on the mammary gland development are consistent with a "low-dose effect", so far, the dose-response relationship has remained poorly characterized and, thus, it is unclear whether the dose-response curves along a broader range of BPA doses are monotonic or non-monotonic.

Developmental toxicity of chronic exposures to TCDD

Low dose effects have also been described for a variety of *in vivo* responses to 2,3,7,8-tetrachlorodibenzo-*p*-dioxin (TCDD). It is of note that TCDD is an extremely potent aryl hydrocarbon receptor (*AhR*) ligand and CYP1A inducer, and one of the, if not the most toxic, ubiquitous and persistent environmental contaminant on earth. The kinetics and acute toxicity of TCDD also exhibit marked inter-species variations. Among rodents, for instance, TCDD-LD$_{50}$ varies from 1 μg/kg.bw for guinea pigs to nearly 1000 μg.kg bw^{-1} for hamsters (IPCS 1989, IARC 1997). The half-life of TCDD in rodents is about 2–4 weeks, while it is approximately 10 years in humans (IPCS 1989, IARC 1997, Pollitt 1999, Schecter et al. 2006, Sany et al. 2015). Compared to rabbits and rodents, humans are relatively resistant to TCDD-caused lethality. Taking into account that TCDD body burden (lipid adjusted) in the general population was estimated to be around 2 parts per trillion (ppt) in 2000, with a trend of steady decline in the following years (Aylward and Hays 2002), effects of "environmentally relevant doses", or "low doses", should indeed be effects of extremely low doses (concentrations) on test systems.

It is of note that the *AhR* not only mediates the induction of genes coding for metabolizing enzymes (e.g., CYP1A) by xenobiotic compounds (e.g., TCDD), but it also plays an important role in cell development, differentiation and function. Along this line, recent studies indicate that, in the absence of xenobiotic interference, the *AhR* takes part in a variety of endogenous processes such as control of perinatal growth, fertility, hepatic and vascular development, immunity, hematopoiesis, stem cell expansion and cancer (Stockinger et al. 2014, Esser and Rannug 2015). As suggested by Esser and Rannug (2015), the toxic effects induced by TCDDs and some PCB congeners (potent *AhR* ligands) could arise from a perturbation of normally tightly controlled and transient *AhR*-regulated cell functions caused by an uncontrolled or persistent activation of the *AhR*. High levels of *AhR* expression were detected in hematopoietic stem cells, cells of the innate immune system, T-cells subsets and B-cells, and ligands of this transcription factor were shown to change the function and fate of these cells of the immune system. Unsurprisingly, the immune system has proved to be a physiological system particularly sensitive to TCDD-mediated toxicity.

TCDD at doses of ≥ 1 μg.kg bw^{-1} in mice and ≥ 3 μg.kg bw^{-1} in rats causes a pronounced thymus involution, while single doses of 10–30 ng.kg bw^{-1} induced a decrease in the percentage and absolute numbers of CD4$^+$ CD29$^{(bright)}$ T-cells and CD20$^+$ B-cells in the marmoset *Callithrix jacchus* (Neubert et al. 1993,1994). Along the same line, Ishimura et al. (2009) described that "low doses" of TCDD (0.1, 1, 10 ng per mouse) given to NFS/*sld* mutant mice on days 0, 1 and 2 after birth, induced auto-immunity-type lesions in the salivary glands of 6-month-old animals. The NFS/*sld* mutant mice thymectomized three days after birth is a model for human Sjögren syndrome, a T cell-mediated autoimmune disorder characterized by lymphocytic infiltrates and destruction of exocrine glands, particularly the salivary glands. Ishimura et al.'s results, therefore, suggested that low doses of TCDD given to neonatal NFS/*sld* mice (without thymectomy) might disrupt early thymus differentiation and the development of T-cell immune tolerance thereby predisposing the animals to the development of autoimmunity later in life.

Chahoud et al. (1992) investigated the effects of a range of single doses of TCDD (0, 0.5, 1, 3 and 5 µg.kg bw⁻¹, sc) on the rat testis. The authors found that doses as high as 3 and 5 µg.kg⁻¹ decreased (60% of the controls) the number of spermatids per testis due to a dissolution of the germinal epithelium, whereas no effect was noted at the two lowest doses (0.5 and 1 µg.kg bw⁻¹). Therefore, under the conditions of Chahoud et al.'s study, the NOAEL for TCDD-caused testicular toxicity in rats was set at 1 µg.kg bw⁻¹ (as a single dose). Based on Chahoud et al.'s data, Vandenberg et al. (2012) selected a NOAEL of 1 µg/kg bw/day for effects on the testes as a cut-off dose for what should be considered as "low-dose" in studies of TCDD[6] and, by doing so, identified 18 studies that had examined effects of low-doses of TCCD on male fertility endpoints such as epididymal sperm counts, ejaculated sperm counts, daily sperm production, sperm transit time and proportion of abnormal sperm. According to Vandenberg et al. (2012), 12 out of 16 rodent studies examining low-dose TCDD on epididymal sperm count found significant detrimental effects on this parameter whereas the other four studies did not. A predominance of positive over negative study results for low dose effects of TCDD was also obtained for the other male fertility endpoints.

Modulation of cytochrome P450 2A5 activity by bacterial Lypopolysaccaride (LPS)

De-Oliveira et al. (2015) evaluated the activity of CYP2A5 in the liver of female DBA-2 mice challenged with a broad range of LPS doses (0, 0.025, 0.05, 0.1, 0.2, 0.5, 1, 2, 5, 10 and 20 mg.kg bw⁻¹ ip). The results showed that immunostimulation with LPS depressed CYP2A5 activity at low doses (0.025–2.0 mg.kg bw⁻¹) but not at higher doses (> 2 mg.kg bw⁻¹) (Fig. 5). Increases in the blood serum levels of pro-inflammatory cytokines and NO, and depressions of the activities of liver CYP1A and CYP2B, however, occurred only at the high dose range (Fig. 5). A U-shaped dose-response curve, therefore, describes how liver CYP2A5 activity changes across a range of doses of LPS extending into the low dose region (low doses of LPS are those that caused no clinically visible signs of immunostimulation). De-Oliveira et al.'s findings also demonstrated that CYP2A5 was down-regulated by low doses of LPS that did not alter activities of other liver monooxygenases (CYP1A and CYP2B) and were insufficient to elicit any increase in pro-inflammatory cytokines and NO blood levels. The depression of CYP2A5 activity, however, was attenuated and

---

[6]   The NOAEL (1 µg.kg bw⁻¹) reported by Chahoud et al. (1992) was obtained for treatment with a single dose of TCDD administered to rats by sc injections, whereas Vandenberg et al. (2012) defined the same cut-off dose (1 µg.kg bw⁻¹.d⁻¹) for repeated-dose treatments. Since TCDD plasma half-life in rats is 2–4 weeks, depending on the duration of treatment and time-interval between two sequential administrations, with repeated-dose experiments, much higher body burdens of TCDD may be attained before a steady-state body burden is achieved. Thus, the cut-off dose set by Vandenberg et al. for identifying "low-dose effect" in studies gives rise to an internal dose higher than that achieved by the NOAEL established by Chahoud et al. for adverse effects of TCDD on the rat testis.

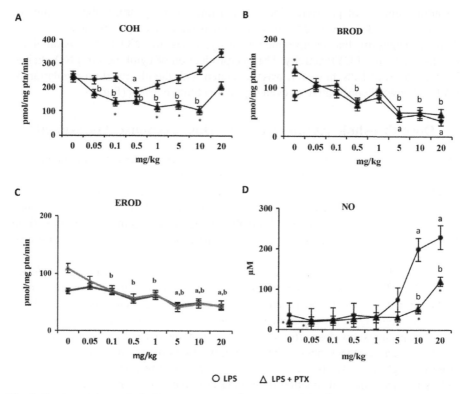

O LPS   △ LPS + PTX

Fig. 5. *In vivo* non-monotonic dose-response unrelated to an endocrine mode of action. Changes of liver cumarin-7-hydroxylase (COH) activity (a marker for CYP2A5) in the liver of female DBA-2 mice treated with increasing doses of LPS (0, 0.05, 0.1, 0.5, 1, 5, 10 or 20 mg.kg bw⁻¹, i.p., N = 10 per dose group) alone (full circles: ●) are described by a U-shaped dose-response curve. In mice co-treated with LPS and the anti-inflammatory drug pentoxifylline (▲; PTX 2 × 100 mg.kg bw⁻¹, i.p.), the U dose-response that had been noted for LPS alone changed into a monotonic inhibitory effect (up to the second highest dose of LPS tested, 10 mg.kg bw⁻¹ i.p.). Activities of BROD (CYP2B9/10) and EROD (CYP1A), on the other side, were consistently inhibited over the whole range of LPS doses tested in the experiment, and the slope of the dose-response curve did not change sign. The reversal of the low-dose LPS-induced depression of CYP2A5 was coincident with the overproduction of nitric oxide (NO) and pro-inflammatory cytokines (not shown in Fig. 5). Data are means ± SEM. Letter "a" indicates that the value differs from control value in the LPS-treated group; "b" indicates that the value differs from control value in the PTX+LPS treated group. An asterisk (*) indicates that the mean value in the PTX+LPS-treated group differs from the mean value in the LPS-treated group for the same dose (ANOVA and Dunnett's multiple comparison test or Student's t-test, P < 0.05).

eventually reversed at higher doses of LPS that down-regulated activities of CYP1A and CYP2B and raised blood pro-inflammatory cytokines and NO levels (Fig. 5). The link between inflammatory signaling pathways and *CYP* genes transcriptional regulation is still poorly understood and so is how CYP2A5 activity shifts from down to up regulation as the strength of the inflammatory stimulus (LPS doses) increases. Nonetheless, De-Oliveira et al. (2015) also noted that when overproduction of pro-inflammatory cytokines (e.g., TNF, IL-6, IL-17A, IFN-γ) and NO was blocked by administration of pentoxifylline (an anti-inflammatory drug), the activities of CYP1A, CYP2B and CYP2A5 were all down-regulated by high doses of LPS, thereby suggesting that overproduction of cytokines and NO is not required for down-regulation of CYP activity. The overproduction of cytokines and NO elicited by high doses of LPS, however, was associated with the observed up-regulation of CYP2A5 toward constitutive or even supra-constitutive levels (Fig. 5).

Dose-threshold Assumption and Dose-response Assessment

Dose response assessment (DRA) is one of the four steps of the current paradigmatic approach to health risk assessment set forth by the US National Academy of Sciences (National Research Council, NRC) in 1983.[7] The DRA step consists of the evaluation of effects in the tested dose range, and the extrapolation from the observable range to low doses/risks. The tested or observable range is the "point of departure" from where extrapolation begins by either a linear non-threshold (LNT) or a non-linear (threshold-based) approach.

Since adequate amounts of data are seldom available for a full range of doses, establishing dose-response functions usually requires extrapolating a limited amount of data from high dose (concentration) experimental studies in animals to low doses (concentrations) typically experimented by humans. If it is assumed that a particular chemical presents low dose effects and non-monotonic dose-response relationships, DRA in risk assessment faces a challenge. Low dose effects cannot be extrapolated from the high dose effects occurring in non-linear dose-response curves (NMDRs) unless the mathematical function describing how the effect changes as function of dose across the full range of tested and environmentally relevant doses had been established. Using the law of mass action and assuming a number of factors and mechanistic events, Kohn and Melnick (2002) predicted differential equations that would describe a theoretical inverted U-shaped curve. In practice, however, mechanistic events underlying a NMDR and the mathematical function that describe it are unknown. At any rate, if a NOAEL for the "low-dose effect" could be determined in experimental studies, it would still be possible to establish a safe dose-range for humans. Nonetheless, supporters of low-dose hypothesis maintain that *"experimental data provide evidence for the lack of a threshold for EDCs"* and that even if there existed in fact a *"mechanistic threshold"* for EDs, *"such a threshold cannot be demonstrated experimentally"* (Sheehan 2006, Vandenberg et al.

---

[7] According to the NRC risk assessment/risk management paradigm, risk assessment analysis involves four key steps, i.e., (1) hazard identification; (2) dose response assessment; (3) exposure assessment and (4) risk characterization. Hazard identification and dose-response assessment are sequential steps of toxicity evaluation; the former identifies substances that may pose health hazards and describes the effects that may occur in humans, while the latter step characterizes the relationship between the exposure and the resultant health effects. Toxicity evaluation and (human) exposure assessment leads to risk characterization, the final step of the risk assessment analysis that precedes the risk management analysis (National Research Council 1983).

2012, Bergman et al. 2013, Gore et al. 2013, for a balanced view see: Rhomberg and Goodman 2012, Dietrich et al. 2013, Lamb et al. 2014).[8]

The existence, or not, of a dose-threshold for "low dose effects" of EDs is a key challenging issue whenever the translation of toxicological research data into actions to protect public health is on the table.[9] As highlighted by Wout Slob (1999, 2007) a dose-threshold for toxicity may have a biological (i.e., "*dose of a compound below which the organism does not suffer from any adverse effect*"), an experimental (i.e., "*dose below which no effects are observed*") and a mathematical definition (i.e., "*dose below which the response is zero, and above which it is non-zero*"). Notwithstanding the current dispute on the existence, or not, of a dose-threshold for cancer and some non-cancer toxicity endpoints, according to Slob (1999), clearly, in the sense conveyed by the experimental definition, thresholds do exist because "*any experiment has a nonzero detection limit*". Nonetheless, Slob noted that, in the strict sense conveyed by the mathematical definition, thresholds cannot be measured because any method of measurement has a limited capacity to detect effects (i.e., a limit of detection) and a finite precision. Therefore, in this strict sense, the existence of thresholds cannot be proven, nor can it be disproven by empirical data. In the case of a LNT model, the assumption that a dose-threshold does not exist was based on the reasoning that, theoretically, only one single molecule (or photon) could provoke a mutation related to cancer, or to a genetic disease in the progeny, thereby making a difference between a zero and nonzero response. Those who are skeptical about the nonexistence of thresholds for genotoxic carcinogens, on the other side, argue that, owing to homeostatic responses and repair mechanisms, organisms should be able to handle small amounts of toxicants, and thus a "practical dose-threshold" should exist.

Slob (2007) pointed out that the concept of dose-threshold is "totally impractical" because even if the existence of a dose-threshold (i.e., a dose below which the effect is assumed to be zero) was highly plausible based on mechanistic or toxicological arguments, or could be "proven", one would not be able to estimate it from any dose-response data. This reasoning seems to hold particularly true regarding the existence, or not, of a dose-threshold for putative "low-dose" effects of EDs. From a practical standpoint, Slob (2007) suggested to appoint a particular non-zero effect size (small but within the range of observation) or Benchmark response (BMR), and

---

[8] In support of the notion that there is no threshold for EDs at a population level, Gore et al. (2013) argued that "*because of the range of susceptibility to environmental chemicals across the population, such as that from age, pre-existing conditions, and genetic variation*", and "*because there are documented exposure to multiple chemicals, including EDCs, in the population*", it would be "*more appropriate to consider a lack of threshold at a population level.*" The limitations of epidemiological observational studies to find out a dose-threshold are notorious due to a number of inherent methodological limitations including a flawed (generally retrospective) quantitative estimation of the exposure.

[9] If one assumes that there are "low-dose effects" and a NMDR, and that there is no dose-threshold, then there is no risk management alternative but to impose a ban on the chemical.

the associated Benchmark Dose (BMD).[10] It is of note that estimation of BMD for health effects such as cancer or developmental damage may be problematic if we are dealing with quantal variables and very low risk levels or response rates (below one in one thousand, or 10^{-3}). Toxicological research rarely gives rise to observed quantal rates of response below 1/50 or 1/100. As noted by Piegorsch (2008), however, this is of less concern when data are obtained in a continuous scale and BMR is based on a percent change in response, e.g., a 5% change in organ or body weight. At any rate, the reported ED low-dose effects were generally taken in continuous scales and thus appointment of BMRs for estimating BMD does not seem to be a problem in this context.

Concluding Remarks

The concepts of low-dose effects and dose-response non-monotonicity and the existence, or not, of dose-thresholds for adverse effects are challenging issues whenever a risk assessment is undertaken and toxicological data are translated into risk management actions. Evidence is accumulating that NMDRs, including *hormetic* responses, do in fact occur with a number of chemical and physical agents and biological responses. Nonetheless, a recent systematic review of the literature (Beausoleil et al. 2016) and the outcome of a few large studies designed to disclose NMDRs if they do occur, suggested that dose-response non-monotonicity is the exception rather than rule.

Low-dose (concentration) effects have also been reported for a number of chemicals and biological responses (Vandenberg et al. 2012), yet a consensus has not been reached among toxicologists on what should be considered a "low-dose effect". Some of the reported "low-dose effects" of BPA, for example, represent responses to doses as high as eight to twelve times the doses humans are typically exposed to in the environment (Teeguarden and Hanson-Drury 2013). Moreover, the statistical power required to detect small effects is a practical hurdle to disclose a real low dose effect. Although vom Saal and coworkers called them "large effects from small exposures" (Welshons et al. 2003), low dose effects are, as a rule, small effects from small exposures. If sample sizes are small, random fluctuations of the response cannot be ruled out, and thus the detection of low-dose effects is unreliable, and the experiments insensitive, to distinguish monotonic from nonmonotonic dose responses. In other words, a reliable detection of "small effects" from low doses requires large sample sizes and an appropriate and robust (sensitive) statistical analysis. Moreover, a consistent replication of low dose effect results within and between laboratories is necessary (scientific reproducibility) as well.

The existence or not of a dose-threshold (or a zero response) for toxicity can never be proven nor can it ever be disproven, and thus to debate whether should exist

---

[10] The benchmark dose (BMD) is the dose that corresponds to a specific adverse response (BMR) compared to the response in unexposed subjects (background). The lower 95% confidence limit is termed the benchmark dose level (BMDL) (Filipsson et al. 2003).

a dose-threshold for ED-mediated "low dose effects" is to take part in a Byzantine discussion (Bergman et al. 2013, Dietrich et al. 2013, Gore et al. 2013). In any case, taking a pragmatic view on the problem, a BMR that is small yet large enough to be observed, and its associated BMD could be set forth and used for risk assessment and management purposes.

Recently, Chahoud and Grote (2016) proposed a new *in vivo* testing strategy for chemicals taking the estimated or measured human exposure levels as the starting point for dose selection (i.e., a bottom-up approach), that is, tested doses would be 100- (i.e., the background exposure level times the classical safety factor of 100), 500- and 1000-fold the estimated human body burden. According to the authors, this pragmatic approach would make extrapolation from high to low dose levels unnecessary (because low doses are automatically tested), and would put aside the assumption of linearity of dose-response. Apparently, Chahoud and Grote (2016) assumed that current levels of environmental exposure (human body burden) to chemicals should *a priori* be considered "safe" exposure levels. Moreover, it remains unclear how this "pragmatic" bottom-up testing approach would lead to the establishment of safe dose ranges, and how experimental data thus obtained would be translated into feasible risk management recommendations.

In conclusion, even if we assume that low dose effects and NMDRs occur in a number of cases, Paracelsus' famous statement remains essentially valid, since chemical-caused harmfulness still depends on the dose or level of exposure. It is up to toxicologists to establish, through well-designed experiments, meticulous observation and rigorous data analysis, the dose range and exposure conditions under which "*a thing is not poison*".

Acknowledgments

The authors are grateful to their students and coworkers for making the Laboratory of Environmental Toxicology a scientifically inspiring environment. Thanks to a good dose of enthusiasm, and students' and coworkers' tenacious work, it was possible to overcome obstacles otherwise insurmountable, such as a chronic underfunding and lack of institutional support. FJRP was the recipient of a fellowship for scientific productivity granted by the National Council for Scientific and Technological Development (CNPq). ACAXO research projects were partially supported by grants from CNPq (PAPES-FIOCRUZ) and Rio de Janeiro State Agency for Supporting Research (FAPERJ). The authors declare no conflicts of interest.

References

Andersen, H.R., A.M. Andersson, S.F. Arnold, H. Autrup, M. Barfoed, N.A. Beresford et al. 1999. Comparison of short-term estrogenicity tests for identification of hormone-disrupting chemicals. Environ. Health Perspect. 107 Suppl 1: 89–108.

Andrade, A.J., S.W. Grande, C.E. Talsness, C. Gericke, K. Grote, A. Golombiewski et al. 2006a. A dose response study following *in utero* and lactational exposure to di-(2-ethylhexyl) phthalate (DEHP): Reproductive effects on adult male offspring rats. Toxicology. 228(1): 85–97.

Andrade, A.J., S.W. Grande, C.E. Talsness, K. Grote and I. Chahoud. 2006b. A dose-response study following *in utero* and lactational exposure to di-(2-ethylhexyl)-phthalate (DEHP): non-monotonic dose-response and low dose effects on rat brain aromatase activity. Toxicology. 29; 227(3): 185–92.

Andrade, A.J., S.W. Grande, C.E. Talsness, K. Grote, A. Golombiewski, A. Sterner-Kock et al. 2006c. A dose-response study following *in utero* and lactational exposure to di-(2-ethylhexyl) phthalate (DEHP): effects on androgenic status, developmental landmarks and testicular histology in male offspring rats. Toxicology. 225(1): 64–74.

Ashby, J., H. Tinwell and J. Haseman. 1999. Lack of effects for low dose levels of bisphenol A and diethylstilbestrol on the prostate gland of CF1 mice exposed *in utero*. Regul. Toxicol. Pharmacol. 30(2 Pt 1): 156–66.

ASTDR—Agency for Toxic Substances and Disease Registry US Public Health Service, and US Environment Protection Agency (US EPA). 1989. Toxicological profile for *2,3,7,8*-tetrachlorodibenzo-p-dioxin (ATSDR/TP-88/23). 129 p.

Aylward, L.L. and S.M. Hays. 2002. Temporal trends in human TCDD body burden: decreases over three decades and implications for exposure levels. J. Expo. Anal. Environ. Epidemiol. 12(5): 319–28.

Baldridge, M.G., G.T. Marks, R.G. Rawlins and R.J. Hutz. 2015. Very low-dose (femtomolar) *2,3,7,8*-tetrachlorodibenzo-p-dioxin (TCDD) disrupts steroidogenic enzyme mRNAs and steroid secretion by human luteinizing granulosa cells. Reprod. Toxicol. 52: 57–61.

Beausoleil, C., J.N. Ormsby, A. Gies, U. Hass, J.J. Heindel, M.L. Holmer et al. 2013. Low dose effects and non-monotonic dose responses for endocrine active chemicals: science to practice workshop: workshop summary. Chemosphere. 93(6): 847–56.

Beausoleil, C., A. Beronius, L. Bodin, G.G.H. Bokkers, P.E. Boon, M. Burger et al. 2016. Review of non-monotonic dose-responses of substances for human risk assessment. EFSA (European Food Safety Authority) supporting publication 2016: EN-2027. 290 pp.

Bergman, Å., A.M. Andersson, G. Becher, M. van den Berg, B. Blumberg, P. Bjerregaard et al. 2013. Science and policy on endocrine disrupters must not be mixed: a reply to a "common sense" intervention by toxicology journal editors. Environ. Health. 27; 12: 69.

Briggs, G.B. 1996. Risk assessment policy for evaluating reproductive system toxicants and the impact of responses on sensitive populations. Toxicology. 111(1-3): 305–13.

Cagen, S.Z., J.M. Waechter Jr, S.S. Dimond, W.J. Breslin, J.H. Butala, F.W. Jekat et al. 1999. Normal reproductive organ development in CF-1 mice following prenatal exposure to bisphenol A. Toxicol. Sci. 50(1): 36–44.

Calabrese, E.J., M.E. McCarthy and E. Kenyon. 1987. The occurrence of chemically induced hormesis. Health Phys. 52(5): 531–41.

Calabrese, E.J. and L.A. Baldwin. 1998. Hormesis as a biological hypothesis. Environ. Health Perspect. 106 Suppl 1: 357–62.

Calabrese, E.J. and L.A. Baldwin. 2001. The frequency of U-shaped dose responses in the toxicological literature. Toxicol. Sci. 62(2): 330–8.

Calabrese, E.J. 2004. Hormesis: from marginalization to mainstream: a case for hormesis as the default dose-response model in risk assessment. Toxicol. Appl. Pharmacol. 197(2): 125–36.

Calabrese, E.J. 2008. Converging concepts: adaptive response, preconditioning, and the Yerkes-Dodson Law are manifestations of hormesis. Ageing Res. Rev. 7(1): 8–20.

Calabrese, E.J. and R.B. Blain. 2011. The hormesis database: the occurrence of hormetic dose responses in the toxicological literature. Regul. Toxicol. Pharmacol. 61(1): 73–81.

Calabrese, E.J. 2013. Origin of the linearity no threshold (LNT) dose-response concept. Arch. Toxicol. 87: 1621–1633.

Calabrese, E.J. 2015. On the origins of the linear no-threshold (LNT) dogma by means of untruths, artful dodges and blind faith. Environ. Res. 142: 432–42.

Calabrese, E.J. 2016. LNTgate: How scientific misconduct by the U.S. NAS led to governments adopting LNT for cancer risk assessment. Environ. Res. 148: 535–46.

Chahoud, I., J. Hartmann, G.M. Rune and D. Neubert. 1992. Reproductive toxicity and toxicokinetics of *2,3,7,8*-tetrachlorodibenzo-p-dioxin. 3. Effects of single doses on the testis of male rats. Arch. Toxicol. 66(8): 567–72.

Chahoud, I. and K. Grote. 2016. Is there a need in regulatory toxicity testing for evaluating chemicals at doses eliciting general toxicity? Toxicology. 363-364: 46–7.

Conolly, R.B. and W.K. Lutz. 2004. Nonmonotonic dose-response relationships: mechanistic basis, kinetic modeling, and implications for risk assessment. Toxicol. Sci. 77(1): 151–7.

Deichmann, W.B., D. Henschler, B. Holmstedt and G. Keil.1986. What is there that is not poison? A study of the Third Defense by Paracelsus. Arch. Toxicol. 58(4): 207–13.

De-Oliveira, A.C., K.S. Poça, P.R. Totino and F.J. Paumgartten. 2015. Modulation of cytochrome P450 2A5 activity by lipopolysaccharide: low-dose effects and non-monotonic dose-response relationship. PLoS One. 10(1): e0117842.

Dhooge, W., K. Arijs, I. D'Haese, S. Stuyvaert, B. Versonnen, C. Janssen et al. 2006. Experimental parameters affecting sensitivity and specificity of a yeast assay for estrogenic compounds: results of an interlaboratory validation exercise. Anal. Bioanal. Chem. 386(5): 1419–28.

Dietrich, D., S. von Aulock, H.W. Marquardt, B.J. Blaauboer, W. Dekant, J. Kehrer et al. 2013. Open letter to the European Commission: scientifically unfounded precaution drives European Commission's recommendations on EDC regulation, while defying common sense, well-established science, and risk assessment principles. Arch. Toxicol. 87(9): 1739–41.

Doll, R. 2002. Proof of causality: deduction from epidemiological observation. Perspect. Biol. Med. 45(4): 499–515.

Duffus, J.H., M. Nordberg and D.M. Templeton. 2007. Glossary of terms used in toxicology, 2nd edition (IUPAC Recommendations 2007). Pure Appl. Chem. 79(7): 1153–1344.

Elliott, K.C. 2000. A case for caution: an evaluation of Calabrese and Baldwin's studies of chemical hormesis. Risk: Health, Safety and Environment. 11(2): 177–196.

Esser, C. and A. Rannug. 2015. The aryl hydrocarbon receptor in barrier organ physiology, immunology, and toxicology. Pharmacol. Rev. 67(2): 259–79.

Feinendegen, L.E. 2005. Evidence for beneficial low level radiation effects and radiation hormesis. Br. J. Radiol. 78(925): 3–7.

Feinendegen, L.E. 2016. Quantification of adaptive protection following low-dose irradiation. Health Phys. 110(3): 276–80.

Filipsson, A.F., S. Sand, J. Nilsson and K. Victorin. 2003. The benchmark dose method—review of available models, and recommendations for application in health risk assessment. Crit. Rev. Toxicol. 33(5): 505–42.

Flick, B., S. Schneider, S. Melching-Kollmuss, K.C. Fussell, S. Gröters, R. Buesen et al. 2016. Investigations of putative reproductive toxicity of low-dose exposures to vinclozolin in Wistar rats. Arch. Toxicol. 2016 [ahead of print].

Frieben, A. 1902. Demonstration eines Cancroids des rechten Handrückens, das sich nach langdauernder Einwirkung von Röntgenstrahlen bei einem 33 jährigen Mann entwickelt hatte Fortsch. Röntgenstrahlen. 6: 106.

Fussell, K.C., S. Schneider, R. Buesen, S. Groeters, V. Strauss, S. Melching-Kollmuss et al. 2015. Investigations of putative reproductive toxicity of low-dose exposures to flutamide in Wistar rats. Arch. Toxicol. 89(12): 2385–402.

Gaido, K.W., L.S. Leonard, S. Lovell, J.C. Gould, D. Babaï, C.J. Portier et al. 1997. Evaluation of chemicals with endocrine modulating activity in a yeast-based steroid hormone receptor gene transcription assay. Toxicol. Appl. Pharmacol. 143(1): 205–12.

Gilchrist, T.C. 1897. A case of dermatitis due to the x-rays. Bull. Johns Hopkins Hospital. 8(71): 17–22.

Giri, A.K. 1986. Mutagenic and genotoxic effects of 2,3,7,8-tetrachlorodibenzo-p-dioxin, a review. Mutat. Res. 168(3): 241–8.

Gore, A.C., J. Balthazart, D. Bikle, D.O. Carpenter, D. Crews, P. Czernichow et al. 2013. Policy decisions on endocrine disruptors should be based on science across disciplines: a response to Dietrich et al. Andrology. 1(6): 802–5.

Grande, S.W., A.J. Andrade, C.E. Talsness, K. Grote and I. Chahoud. 2006. A dose-response study following *in utero* and lactational exposure to di(2-ethylhexyl)phthalate: effects on female rat reproductive development. Toxicol. Sci. 91(1): 247–54.

Grande, S.W., A.J. Andrade, C.E. Talsness, K. Grote, A. Golombiewski, A. Sterner-Kock et al. 2007. A dose-response study following *in utero* and lactational exposure to di-(2-ethylhexyl) phthalate (DEHP): reproductive effects on adult female offspring rats. Toxicology. 229(1-2): 114–22.

Harris, C.A., P. Henttu, M.G. Parker and J.P. Sumpter. 1997. The estrogenic activity of phthalate esters *in vitro*. Environ. Health Perspect. 105(8): 802–11.

Haseman, J.K., A.J. Bailer, R.L. Kodell, R. Morris and K. Portier. 2001. Statistical issues in the analysis of low-dose endocrine disruptor data. Toxicol. Sci. 61(2): 201–10.

Hassoun, E.A., S.C. Wilt, M.J. Devito, A. Van Birgelen, N.Z. Alsharif, L.S. Birnbaum et al. 1998. Induction of oxidative stress in brain tissues of mice after subchronic exposure to *2,3,7,8*-tetrachlorodibenzo-p-dioxin. Toxicol. Sci. 42(1): 23–7.

Heindel, J.J., R.R. Newbold, J.R. Bucher, L. Camacho, K.B. Delclos, S.M. Lewis et al. 2015. NIEHS/FDA CLARITY-BPA research program update. Reprod. Toxicol. 58: 33–44.

Hengstler, J.G., H. Foth, T. Gebel, P.J. Kramer, W. Lilienblum, H. Schweinfurth et al. 2011. Critical evaluation of key evidence on the human health hazards of exposure to bisphenol A. Crit. Rev. Toxicol. 41(4): 263–91.

IARC-WHO. International Agency for Research on Cancer–World Health Organization. 1997. Polychlorinated dibenzo-*para*-dioxins and dibenzofurans. IARC Monographs on the evaluation of carcinogenic risks to humans. Vol. 69. IARC-WHO. Lyon, France, 687 p.

IPCS-WHO. International Programme on Chemical Safety–World Health Organization. 1989. Polychlorinated Dibenzo-para-Dioxins and Dibenzofurans. Environmental Health Criteria no. 88. ICPS-WHO. Geneva, Switzerland, 192 p.

Ishimaru, N., A. Takagi, M. Kohashi, A. Yamada, R. Arakaki, J. Kanno et al. 2009. Neonatal exposure to low-dose *2,3,7,8*-tetrachlorodibenzo-p-dioxin causes autoimmunity due to the disruption of T cell tolerance. J. Immunol. 182(10): 6576–86.

Karman, B.N., M.S. Basavarajappa, Z.R. Craig and J.A. Flaws. 2012. *2,3,7,8*-Tetrachlorodibenzo-p-dioxin activates the aryl hydrocarbon receptor and alters sex steroid hormone secretion without affecting growth of mouse antral follicles *in vitro*. Toxicol. Appl. Pharmacol. 261(1): 88–96.

Kathren, R.L. 2002. Historical development of the linear non-threshold dose-response model as applied to radiation. Pierce Law Review. 1(1-2): 5–30.

Kohn, M.C. and R.L. Melnick. 2002. Biochemical origins of the non-monotonic receptor-mediated dose-response. J. Mol. Endocrinol. 29(1): 113–23.

Krishnan, A.V., P. Stathis, S.F. Permuth, L. Tokes and D. Feldman. 1993. Bisphenol-A: na estrogenic substance is released from polycarbonate flasks during autoclaving. Endocrinology. 132(6): 2279–86.

Lamb, J.C. 4th, P. Boffetta, W.G. Foster, J.E. Goodman, K.L. Hentz, L.R. Rhomberg et al. 2014. Critical comments on the WHO-UNEP State of the Science of Endocrine Disrupting Chemicals 2012. Regul. Toxicol. Pharmacol. 69(1): 22–40.

Lee, H.K., T.S. Kim, C.Y. Kim, I.H. Kang, M.G. Kim, K.K. Jung et al. 2012. Evaluation of *in vitro* screening system for estrogenicity: comparison of stably transfected human estrogen receptor-α transcriptional activation (OECD TG455) assay and estrogen receptor (ER) binding assay. J. Toxicol. Sci. 37(2): 431–7.

Little, M.P. 2003. Risks associated with ionizing radiation. Br. Med. Bull. 68: 259–75.

Luckey, T.D. 1982. Physiological benefits from low levels of ionizing radiation. Health Phys. 43(6): 771–89.

Luckey, T.D. 2006. Radiation hormesis: the good, the bad, and the ugly. Dose Response. 4(3): 169–90.

Markey, C.M., E.H. Luque, M. Munoz De Toro, C. Sonnenschein and A.M. Soto. 2001. *In utero* exposure to bisphenol A alters the development and tissue organization of the mouse mammary gland. Biol. Reprod. 65(4): 1215–23.

Markey, C.M., P.R. Wadia, B.S. Rubin, C. Sonnenschein and A.M. Soto. 2005. Long-term effects of fetal exposure to low doses of the xenoestrogen bisphenol-A in the female mouse genital tract. Biol. Reprod. 72(6): 1344–51.

Matthews, J.B., K. Twomey and T.R. Zacharewski. 2001. *In vitro* and *in vivo* interactions of bisphenol A and its metabolite, bisphenol A glucuronide, with estrogen receptors alpha and beta. Chem. Res. Toxicol. 14(2): 149–57.

Mattson, M.P. 2008. Hormesis defined. Ageing Res. Rev. 7(1): 1–7.

Melnick, R., G. Lucier, M. Wolfe, R. Hall, G. Stancel, G. Prins et al. 2002. Summary of the National Toxicology Program's report of the endocrine disruptors low-dose peer review. Environ. Health Perspect. 110(4): 427–3.

Muller, H.J. 1928a. The measurement of gene mutation rate in drosophila, its high variability, and its dependence upon temperature. Genetics. 13(4): 279–357.

Muller, H.J. 1928b. The production of mutations by X-Rays. Proc. Natl. Acad. Sci. USA. 14(9): 714–26.

Muñoz-de-Toro, M., C.M. Markey, P.R. Wadia, E.H. Luque, B.S. Rubin, C. Sonnenschein et al. 2005. Perinatal exposure to bisphenol-A alters peripubertal mammary gland development in mice. Endocrinology. 146(9): 4138–47.

Mushak, P. 2009. Ad hoc and fast forward: the science of hormesis growth and development. Environ. Health Perspect. 117(9): 1333–8.

Mushak, P. 2013. How prevalent is chemical hormesis in the natural and experimental worlds? Sci. Total Environ. 443: 573–81.

Nagel, S.C., F.S. vom Saal, K.A. Thayer, M.G. Dhar, M. Boechler and W.V. Welshons. 1997. Relative binding affinity-serum modified access (RBA-SMA) assay predicts the relative *in vivo* bioactivity of the xenoestrogens bisphenol A and octylphenol. Environ. Health Perspect. 105(1): 70–6.

National Research Council. 1983. Risk assessment in the federal government. Managing the process. National Academy Press, Washington, DC.

Neubert, R., R. Stahlmann, M. Korte, H. van Loveren, J.G. Vos, G. Golor et al. 1993. Effects of small doses of dioxins on the immune system of marmosets and rats. Ann. N. Y. Acad. Sci. 685: 662–86.

Neubert, R., G. Golor, L. Maskow, H. Helge and D. Neubert. 1994. Evaluation of possible effects of *2,3,7,8*-tetrachlorodibenzo-p-dioxin and other congeners on lymphocyte receptors in *Callithrix jacchus* and man. Exp. Clin. Immunogenet. 11(2-3): 119–27.

Olea, N., R. Pulgar, P. Pérez, F. Olea-Serrano, A. Rivas, A. Novillo-Fertrell et al. 1996. Estrogenicity of resin-based composites and sealants used in dentistry. Environ. Health Perspect. 104(3): 298–305.

Parks, L.G., J.S. Ostby, C.R. Lambright, B.D. Abbott, G.R. Klinefelter, N.J. Barlow et al. 2000. The plasticizer diethylhexyl phthalate induces malformations by decreasing fetal testosterone synthesis during sexual differentiation in the male rat. Toxicol. Sci. 58(2): 339–49.

Paumgartten, F.J.R. 1993. Risk assessment for chemical substances: The link between toxicology and public health. Cad Saude Publica. 9(4): 439–447.

Paumgartten, F.J.R. 2013. The Brazilian hazard-based cut-off criteria for pesticide registration: a critical appraisal. Vigil. Sanit. Debate. 1(1): 3–10.

Paumgartten, F.J.R. and A.C.A.X. De-Oliveira. 2014. The bisphenol A toxicological paradox: The more we learn the less we know for sure. Environmental Skeptics and Critics. 3(4): 65–82.

Paumgartten, F.J. 2015. Commentary: Estrogenic and anti-androgenic endocrine disrupting chemicals and their impact on the male reproductive system. Front. Public Health. 3: 165.

Paustenbach, D.J., H.P. Shu and F.J. Murray. 1986. A critical examination of assumptions used in risk assessments of dioxin contaminated soil. Regul. Toxicol. Pharmacol. 6(3): 284–307.

Piegorsch, W. 2008. Low-dose extrapolation. Encyclopedia of Quantitative Risk Analysis and Assessment. John Wiley & Sons, Ltd.

Pollitt, F. 1999. Polychlorinated dibenzodioxins and polychlorinated dibenzofurans. Regul. Toxicol. Pharmacol. 30(2 Pt 2): S63–8.

Pottenger, L.H., J.Y. Domoradzki, D.A. Markham, S.C. Hansen, S.Z. Cagen and J.M. Waechter Jr. 2000. The relative bioavailability and metabolism of bisphenol A in rats is dependent upon the route of administration. Toxicol. Sci. 54(1): 3–18.

Rhomberg, L.R. and J.E. Goodman. 2012. Low-dose effects and nonmonotonic dose-responses of endocrine disrupting chemicals: has the case been made? Regul. Toxicol. Pharmacol. 64(1): 130–3.

Sany, S.B.T., R. Hashim, A. Salleh, M. Rezayi, D.J. Karlen, B. Marzieh et al. 2015. Dioxin risk assessment: mechanisms of action and possible toxicity in human health. Environ. Sci. Pollut. Res. 22: 19434–19450.

Schecter, A., L. Birnbaum, J.J. Ryan and J.D. Constable. 2006. Dioxins: an overview. Environ. Res. 101(3): 419–28.

Schug, T.T., J.J. Heindel, L. Camacho, K.B. Delclos, P. Howard, A.F. Johnson et al. 2013. A new approach to synergize academic and guideline-compliant research: the CLARITY-BPA research program. Reprod. Toxicol. 40: 35–40.

Seong, K.M., S. Seo, D. Lee, M.J. Kim, S.S. Lee, S. Park et al. 2016. Is the linear no-threshold dose-response paradigm still necessary for the assessment of health effects of low dose radiation? J. Korean Med. Sci. 31 Suppl 1: S10–23.

Sheehan, D.M. 2006. No-threshold dose-response curves for nongenotoxic chemicals: findings and applications for risk assessment. Environ. Res. 100(1): 93–9.

Shimizu, M., K. Ohta, Y. Matsumoto, M. Fukuoka, Y. Ohno and S. Ozawa. 2002. Sulfation of bisphenol A abolished its estrogenicity based on proliferation and gene expression in human breast cancer MCF-7 cells. Toxicol. *In Vitro.* 16(5): 549–56.

Slezak, B.P., G.E. Hatch, M.J. DeVito, J.J. Diliberto, R. Slade, K. Crissman et al. 2000. Oxidative stress in female B6C3F1 mice following acute and subchronic exposure to *2,3,7,8*-tetrachlorodibenzo-p-dioxin (TCDD). Toxicol. Sci. 54(2): 390–8.

Slob, W. 1999. Thresholds in toxicology and risk assessment. Int. J. Toxicol. 18: 259–268.

Slob, W. 2007. What is a practical threshold? Toxicol. Pathol. 35(6): 848–9.

Solecki, R., A. Kortenkamp, Å. Bergman, I. Chahoud, G.H. Degen, D. Dietrich et al. 2016. Scientific principles for the identification of endocrine-disrupting chemicals: a consensus statement. Arch. Toxicol. [ahead of print]

Southam, C.M. and J. Ehrlich. 1943. Effects of extract of western red-cedar heartwood on certain wood-decaying fungi in culture. Phytopathology. 33: 517–524.

Stockinger, B., P. Di Meglio, M. Gialitakis and J.H. Duarte. 2014. The aryl hydrocarbon receptor: multitasking in the immune system. Annu. Rev. Immunol. 32: 403–32.

Stumpf, W.E. 2006. The dose makes the medicine. Drug Discov. Today. 11(11-12): 550–5.

Teeguarden, J.G. and S. Hanson-Drury. 2013. A systematic review of Bisphenol A "low dose" studies in the context of human exposure: a case for establishing standards for reporting "low-dose" effects of chemicals. Food Chem. Toxicol. 62: 935–48.

Tharp, A.P., M.V. Maffini, P.A. Hunt, C.A. VandeVoort, C. Sonnenschein and A.M. Soto. 2012. Bisphenol A alters the development of the rhesus monkey mammary gland. Proc. Natl. Acad. Sci. USA. 109(21): 8190–5.

Tuomisto, J., J. Pekkanen, H. Kiviranta, E. Tukiainen, T. Vartiainen, M. Viluksela et al. 2006. Dioxin cancer risk—example of hormesis? Dose Response. 3(3): 332–41.

Tyl, R.W., C.B. Myers, M.C. Marr, C.S. Sloan, N.P. Castillo, M.M. Veselica et al. 2008. Two-generation reproductive toxicity study of dietary bisphenol A in CD-1 (Swiss) mice. Toxicol. Sci. 104(2): 362–84.

Vandenberg, L.N., M.V. Maffini, P.R. Wadia, C. Sonnenschein, B.S. Rubin and A.M. Soto. 2007. Exposure to environmentally relevant doses of the xenoestrogen bisphenol-A alters development of the fetal mouse mammary gland. Endocrinology. 148(1): 116–27.

Vandenberg, L.N., I. Chahoud, J.J. Heindel, V. Padmanabhan, F.J. Paumgartten and G. Schoenfelder. 2010. Urinary, circulating, and tissue biomonitoring studies indicate widespread exposure to bisphenol A. Environ. Health Perspect. 118(8): 1055–70.

Vandenberg, L.N., T. Colborn, T.B. Hayes, J.J. Heindel, D.R. Jacobs Jr, D.H. Lee et al. 2012. Hormones and endocrine-disrupting chemicals: low-dose effects and nonmonotonic dose responses. Endocr. Rev. 33(3): 378–455.

vom Saal, F.S., B.G. Timms, M.M. Montano, P. Palanza, K.A. Thayer, S.C. Nagel et al. 1997. Prostate enlargement in mice due to fetal exposure to low doses of estradiol or diethylstilbestrol and opposite effects at high doses. Proc. Natl. Acad. Sci. USA. 94(5): 2056–6.

Welshons, W.V., K.A. Thayer, B.M. Judy, J.A. Taylor, E.M. Curran and F.S. vom Saal. 2003. Large effects from small exposures. I. Mechanisms for endocrine-disrupting chemicals with estrogenic activity. Environ. Health Perspect. 111(8): 994–1006.

Wolf, Jr, C., C. Lambright, P. Mann, M. Price, R.L. Cooper, J. Ostby et al. 1999. Administration of potentially antiandrogenic pesticides (procymidone, linuron, iprodione, chlozolinate, p,p'-DDE, and ketoconazole) and toxic substances (dibutyl- and diethylhexyl phthalate, PCB 169, and ethane dimethane sulphonate) during sexual differentiation produces diverse profiles of reproductive malformations in the male rat. Toxicol. Ind. Health. 15(1-2): 94–118.

11

Conventional Wastewater Treatment Plants as a Discharge and Source Point for Biota Exposure to Micro-pollutants

IIIIIIIIIIIIIIIIIIIIIIIIIIIIIIIIIIIIIIIIIIIIIIIIIIIIIIIIIIIIIIIIIIIIIIIIIIIIIIIIIIIIIIIIIIIIIIIIIIIIIIIIIIIIIIIIIIIIIIIIIIIIIIIIIIIIIIIIIIIIIIIIIIIII

Francis Orata Omoto

Introduction

Most conventional wastewater treatment plants (WWTPs) are not designed to effectively remove micro-pollutants (MPs) and other chemicals of emerging concerns (CECs), including metabolites that are generated through biotransformation and other processes. As a result, the MPs may escape from the WWTPs treatment process *via* effluent and discharged into aquatic environment. The focus for advanced wastewater treatment processes is on drinking water, and often not on WWTPs effluents. Hence the risks posed by direct transfer of MPs from WWTPs to receiving water, and subsequently to drinking water.

Over the past decade, the rapid increase and advancement in chemical analytical instrument sensitivity has led to detection of a wide range of biologically active contaminants that are also referred to as organic MPs, in lower than pg L^{-1} concentration levels (Wille et al. 2012). Herein, MPs are defined as chemicals that are both organic and inorganic in nature, and which are generally found in low concentrations in the environment. These MPs may include CECs and trace elements. CECs are chemicals which have been recently identified in the environment and are believed to cause adverse effects on ecosystems and humans and are also still

Department of Pure and Applied Chemistry, Masinde Muliro University of Science and Technology, Kakamega, 190-50100, Kenya.
E-mail: fraora@yahoo.com

insufficiently regulated (Murray et al. 2010). In contrast to micro-pollutants, macro-pollutants are compounds which are common in various environmental matrices and include acids, salts, nutrients, and organic matter (Schwarzenbach et al. 2006). MPs therefore include several hydrophobic pollutants such as heavy metals, dioxins, polycyclic aromatic hydrocarbons (PAHs), polychlorinated biphenyls (PCBs), flame retardants, but also more polar (hydrophilic) compounds that are designed to be biologically active such as pesticides, pharmaceuticals and other naturally produced bioactive compounds.

The presence of MPs in WWTP effluent may enter receiving water like rivers which, in turn, are the source of drinking water. Although there is dilution effect of the MPs in receiving waters, the MPs may enter the food chain through aquatic microorganisms; benthos and subsequent processes such as bioconcentration, bioaccumulation and biomagnification can significantly increase the concentration to several orders of magnitude higher in the receiving biota. WWTP effluents are thus considered as the vector or/and the source of these compounds into the environment (Kasprzyk-Hordern et al. 2009) since they are not efficient in the removal of MPs from effluents.

The absence of involving advanced wastewater treatment technologies in conventional WWTPs is a major concern and, therefore, this chapter presents data evidence that drinking water alone is not the only exposure route or media for MPs to human, but also WWTPs effluent, received into surface water and directly to the food chain through aquatic biota, among other exposure routes. The underlying statement of this chapter is that advanced WWTPs can function as the main remedial step in the MPs' removal from wastewater, and in addition, it can be supplemented by advanced treatment for drinking water. A review of the current status, challenges and perspectives of WWTPs with regard to MPs can help in designing their preventive and removal measures and also lay a framework for future studies on wastewater treatment. The implementation of these recommendations will significantly reduce the exposure risk of biota to MPs. The objectives of this chapter are: (i) to evaluate the efficiency of conventional WWTPs in removal of MPs from wastewater, (ii) to evaluate processes such as biodegradation, adsorption and other oxidative processes and their effectiveness in the removal of MPs from WWTPs, (iii) to link the MPs in WWTPs effluent and their transfer to biota, and (iv) to recommend various options to improve MPs' removal from municipal wastewaters, with a special focus on combined treatment technologies that can enhance efficient removal of MPs.

Review of Micro-pollutants, Wastewater Treatment Plants and Biota

WWTPs are the most important discharge and source point for MPs' continuous release into the environmental matrices which include biota. This section reviews MPs, WWTPs process as related to, and effect on biota. Micro-pollutants cause unwanted effects in the aquatic environment. The best treatment methods to remove MPs from wastewater are based on their physical and chemical properties.

Micro-pollutants and their sources

Micro-pollutants are substances or residue from substances that are used in modern society and have been known to be persistent and bioactive (Benner et al. 2013). The major sources of MPs are industrial, agricultural, domestic and hospital. The MPs include pharmaceuticals, personal care products, agricultural chemicals, pesticides, trace and radioelements, industrial chemicals, combustion products, chlorinated solvents, biocides, flame retardants among others. All these sources' percentage (%) contribution to wastewater varies significantly. In the case of pharmaceuticals as an example, Kumar et al. (2010) reported that the emission of pharmaceuticals per person measured in wastewater in residential areas is about 10% of the emission measured in hospital wastewater. However, hospitals and health care facilities' contribution to the total pharmaceutical emission is relatively small (20%) compared to residential areas (80%) (RIVM 2012). The reason for this is that much more people live in residential areas than in hospitals and health care centers. Agricultural sector, and thus livestock farming, contributes to 20% of pharmaceuticals found in wastewater. Some MPs, such as perfluoroalkyl substances (PFASs), can originate from any of the mentioned sources (Chirikona et al. 2015). In modern urban centres, liquid waste from various sources such as hospital, domestic, agricultural and industrial that contain MPs are often channeled to WWTPs before being released to other aquatic ecosystems as effluent and also often as sludge. WWTPs also receive rainwater run-off from urban areas, which can also be a significant source of MPs, especially from cottage industries. For example, Orata et al. (2008) reported the observed small cottage industries' contribution to the presence of perfluorooctanoic acid (PFOA) and perfluorooctane sulfonate (PFOS) in drainage systems within Lake Victoria catchment area. Figure 1 shows the cycle of MPs in wastewater and various environmental compartments.

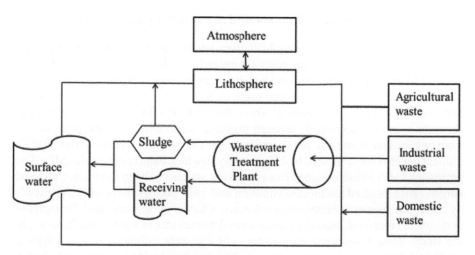

Fig. 1. Sources and the cycle of micro-pollutants in water and pathways for their introduction into aquatic environment.

Atmospheric dust deposition is part of the geochemical cycles of several elements and organic compounds, and its chemical composition could provide valuable information about sources of air pollution in specific areas (Santos et al. 2013). The atmosphere receives MPs in substantial amounts and in a complex mixture of different chemical species. In the atmosphere, chemicals can undergo reactions to produce new compounds or they can be produced through the transformation of their respective precursor chemicals. It has been established that these pollutants can be transported over very long distances (Hunga et al. 2013) to even remote areas without local sources containing MPs. Once in the atmosphere, deposition to the lithosphere is apparent. This can occur in terms of storm water runoff, i.e., urban surface runoff which is recognized as one of the major sources of pollution to receiving waters (Gromaire et al. 2001).

Many classes of MPs originate from manmade sources, i.e., nanomaterials that are used in clothing and many other human activities, hormones such as synthetic and natural estrogens and androgens, metabolites and transformation products of man-made chemicals that are produced from biological, chemical and physical breakdown reactions in WWTPs. Other example is Bisphenol A (2, 2-bis-4-hydroxyphenylpro-pane), a synthetic xenoestrogen which is used in the production of polycarbonate, epoxy resins, flame retardants, among other uses. Bisphenol A is involved in the production of adhesives, powder paints, automotive lenses, protective window glazing, building materials, compact disks and optical lenses (Staples et al. 1998). Synthetic chelating agents such as Ethylenediamino tetraacetae (EDTA) and diethylenetriamino pentaacetate (DTPA) are manmade MPs that find many uses and applications in industries, e.g., in the textile, photo, and pulp and paper industries as well as in galvanic enterprises and households. These chelating agents have recently been detected in WWTPs (Reemstma et al. 2006), and have been proven to be widely distributed in aquatic systems (Bernhard et al. 2006).

Biota exposure to micro-pollutants and the resulting toxic effects

Technological measures to remove MPs from wastewater at the WWTPs stage are often not considered because the costs are judged to be high. As a result, preference and emphasis are put at the drinking water treatment stage with the assumption that drinking water is the major exposure route of MPs into human beings. In contrast, MPs enter the food chain directly from the WWTP effluent release to aquatic ecosystem, and not necessarily through drinking water. Direct consumption of fish from wastewater treatment ponds or from surface waters receiving the WWTP effluent which is contaminated by MPs is a way in which biota is exposed to MPs. The presence of MPs in fish obtained from receiving waters has been reported. Orata and Birgen (2016) studied the bioconcentration and interspecies uptake of heavy metals by three fish species (*Oreochromis niloticus*, *Clarius gariespinus* and *Protopterus aethiopicus*) receiving naturally contaminated wastewater in wastewater lagoons. In the study, tissue bioconcentration factors (BCFs) were estimated within a typical municipal wastewater lagoon in Kenya. The results obtained suggest that heavy metals uptake by the fish species and their transfer to various tissue organs do not exclusively depend on concentration levels by aqueous exposure alone but largely depends on their feeding mode, diet and biochemical needs of individual fish species. Zn, Pb, Zn, Cu, and Zn concentrations of up to 11.72, 11.27, 5.29, 4.12 and 4.74 µg g^{-1} for muscle, skin, liver, scales and gills, respectively, were determined (Orata and Birgen 2016). Levels of Perfluorooctane Sulfonate (PFOS) and Perfluorooctanoic Acid (PFOA) in Nile tilapia (*Oreochromis niloticus*) obtained from Winam gulf of Lake Victoria, Kisumu, Kenya was reported by Orata et al. (2008). Winam gulf receives effluent from Kisumu WWTPs. MPs enter the organism body by all pathways of exposure, which are ingestion, inhalation, and dermal absorption. MPs are believed to cause long-term hazards to aquatic organisms, human and other terrestrial organisms through bioaccumulation and biomagnification processes which increase the concentration levels within the food chain. The presence of MPs in the environment has been linked to toxic biological effects, including estrogenicity, mutagenicity and genotoxicity. Synthetic and natural estrogens and androgens, DDT and other pesticides, bisphenol A (BPA) and phthalates used in children's products, personal care products and flame retardants are categorized as endocrine disrupting compounds (EDCs) (Wille et al. 2012). EDCs are an exogenous or manmade chemical, or mixture of chemicals, that interferes with any aspect of hormone action. These effects include changes in sex hormones associated with exposure to bisphenol A in men (Tetreault et al. 2012). Some MPs such as PFASs are known to be non-biodegradable, persistent and bioaccumulative (Ahrens 2011). Neuroendrocinal alterations and oxidative stress in freshwater mussels (Gillis et al. 2014), and probable impact to the whole aquatic food web downstream of WWTPs has been reported. The biocide triclosan affects river biofilms and algae community structure at concentrations potentially lower than 0.5 µg L^{-1} (Ricart et al. 2010). Halden (2005) identified WWTPs as a major pathway and/or one of the secondary routes of human indirect exposure to biocides *via* the environment. Figure 2 shows the role of effluent and sludge from WWTPs in MPs, i.e., biocides and their metabolites cycles in the environment and how it is linked to air, food, wastewater and sediments which are exposure media or agents for pollution.

Direct or primary pathway of exposure for human to MPs is through inhalation, ingestion or dermal absorption. The indirect or secondary routes involve the passage of MPs through a chain of other environmental media, and processes which may concentrate the MPs. Such processes which concentrate the MPs within the environmental cycles are bioconcentration, bioaccumulation and biomagnification. PFASs have been associated with adverse effects for humans, for example, complications in birth weight, fertility disorders, phenomena of early menopause in women, carcinogenesis and thyroid malfunction (Rahman et al. 2014). Of particular concern in this respect are pharmaceutically active compounds (PhACs) which are designed to be active at very low concentrations (Plósz et al. 2013). For example, the antiepileptic carbamazepine may alter freshwater community structure and ecosystem dynamics at a concentration of 0.2–2 µg L^{-1} (Jarvis et al. 2014). Several antibiotics were also reported to significantly inhibit algae and cyanobacteria growth in concentrations as low as 1–5 µg L^{-1}, which is close to the concentrations found in WWTP effluents (Ebert et al. 2011). Moreover, MPs such as PhACs may exist in the

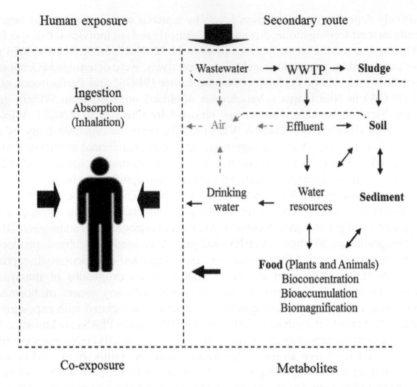

Human exposure   Secondary route

Co-exposure   Metabolites

Fig. 2. Routes of exposure of human to MPs, i.e., biocides. Modified from Halden (2005).

environment as mixtures and raise concerns because the combined environmental effects are largely unknown (Stackelberg et al. 2004, Tixier et al. 2003). Therefore, the resulting new mixtures and metabolites arising from degradation processes can also cause adverse health effects that are yet to be understood. The different combined effects may be simple addition of a toxic effect (non-interactive or additive action), an effect which is less than the sum of the separate constituents and toxic effects caused by MPs synergism (Hernando et al. 2006, Kim et al. 2007) and antagonism (Boxall et al. 2003), especially by PhACs. PhACs are another serious concern because of the rise of antibiotic-resistant organisms in the environment, posing additional hazard to the microbial ecosystems.

Transfer of MPs to biota through sludge

Sludge from WWTPs is applied as fertilizer to farmland (Wu et al. 2010). Concerns have been raised about the exposure to MPs through crops. A study by Klenow et al. (2013) observed that foods of plant origin (e.g., fruit and vegetables) were found to be important for the dietary exposure to PFASs. There have been cases of soil contamination, where application of sewage sludge that is contaminated with PFOS/PFOA and other PFASs was used as soil fertilizers (Washington et al.

2010). Moreover, further runoff from this sludge contaminated soils also resulted in contaminated surface water and drinking water reservoirs (Kröfges et al. 2007). In another study, Verstegren et al. (2013) identified the consumption of silage by red Swedish cow to be the dominant intake pathway for all PFAAs, which then bioaccumulate and biomagnify (Conder et al. 2008) in cow tissues. Therefore, MPs that are adhered to biosolids can be transferred through filtration process to sludge. Use of contaminated sludge from WWTPs as fertilizer is also an exposure media to biota. A study by Ventatesan and Halden (2014) linked about 70% of chemicals detected in biosolids to those also detected in humans.

Conventional wastewater treatment plants processes

WWTPs are designed to efficiently and consistently control a wide range of substances, such as particulates, carbonaceous substances, nutrients and pathogens. However, little or no effort is put particularly in removal of MPs from WWTPs (Luo et al. 2014). Hence, the evaluation of the fate and removal of MPs during wastewater treatment is imperative for the optimization of treatment processes in order to prevent the release of these potentially harmful MPs (van Beelen 2007). Many effluents still show the presence of MPs even after the treatment processes, which is a course of concern for the effectiveness of WWTP. For example, one class of persistent organic pollutants (POPs) measured in sewage sludge are the polychlorinated dibenzo-p-dioxins and furans (PCDD/Fs), despite the strict regulations for their use and disposal in some countries. PCDD/Fs are listed among the 12 initial POPs, under annex C, for continuing minimization and where feasible, to be ultimately eliminated under the Stockholm Convention (2001).

The fate of MPs in WWTPs is under the control or influence of 'internal factors' and 'external factors'. Internal factors are MPs-related, and are the characteristics of MPs (e.g., hydrophobicity, biodegradability, and volatility). Some of the important external factors that influence the efficiency of conventional WWTPs are: (i) the Sludge Retention Time (SRT), which is the contact time of the wastewater with the activated sludge and is an important design parameter for the efficiency of removal of compounds. Researchers have demonstrated that existing biological wastewater treatment processes can remove a broad array of MPs to a certain extent (Joss et al. 2006). Approaches to further improve the biological processes to remove MPs, such as pharmaceuticals, by using long solids retention time (SRT) in activated sludge systems is recommended to increase efficiency (Clare et al. 2005, Suarez et al. 2010). However, techniques such as SRT cannot effectively enhance biotransformation rate of some MPs such as carbamazepine; (ii) Dissolved Oxygen, which is required by microorganisms in the purification process, for degradation of organic content of the influent as well as for the reduction of the nutrient load; (iii) Bioreactor processes, which involves mixing bacteria flocs with water; (iv) Oxygen depletion (BOD and COD status) of WWTPs often coursed by nutrients load and; (v) the turbidity and general visibility which prevents light penetration in WWTPs. However, it should be noted that external factors alone cannot effectively remove MPs that are known to be persistent in wastewater. Therefore, a review at the internal factors that influence the efficiency of removal of MPs is important. These internal factors are: (i) The

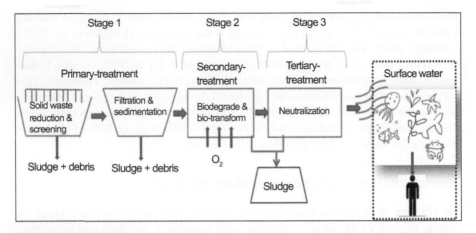

Fig. 3. Stages and processes involved in a conventional wastewater treatment plant.

physical, chemical and structural properties such as molecular weight and structure, functional group of MPs that determines their lipophilicity and hydrophilicity in water, sorption properties and volatility in aqueous media; (ii) Toxicity of MPs towards the microorganisms that are involved in the MPs biodegradation process; (iii) The design and engineering aspects of the WWTPs, and (iv) the transformation of MPs that results in other chemical species and metabolites. Figure 3 shows the processes involved in influent treatment within conventional WWTPs, and the potential transfer of micro-pollutants into receiving surface water.

The sequence of the processes can be divided into three stages, which are the primary, secondary and tertiary stages, which are described in brief below. After treatment, residues from WWTPs are then discharged to receiving water bodies where further transformation or natural transport takes place.

First stage: primary treatment

Primary treatment is basically mechanical where solid waste is removed from the influent by means of adsorption, filtration and sedimentation. In the primary stage, solid particles which act as adsorbents for various pollutants including MPs are removed through sedimentation that is aided by gravity as sludge, and then separated by filtration. Most MPs that are highly lipophilic significantly sorb onto sludge and sediments. One of the factors that affect sorption is the octanol-water partition coefficient (Kow), and can be frequently used to predict absorption of MPs on solids. Rogers (1996) provided a general rule of thumb for applying K_{ow} to the estimation of sorption: log Kow < 2.5 indicates low sorption potential, 2.5 < log Kow < 4 indicates medium sorption potential, and log Kow > 4 indicates high sorption potential. Yamamoto et al. (2007) found that pharmaceuticals of high molecular weight and high octanol/water partition coefficients (Kow), such as analgesics (e.g., acetoaminophen, ibuprofen, mefenamic acid) and estrogens can be removed by rates from 76% to 96% by sorption to activated sludge. Thus, biosolids are known to represent a 'sink' for hydrophobic organic compounds of limited biodegradability.

Second stage: secondary treatment

Micro-pollutants in the aqueous output of the primary stage go to the next treatment stage. In the secondary process, microorganisms are used to biodegrade and bio-transform both organic contaminants as well as reduce the nutrient load (van Beelen 2007). Often, in this purification step, dissolved organic matter is progressively converted into a solid mass by using indigenous, waterborne bacteria. A parent compound is lost in the process by mechanisms of chemical and physical transformation, biodegradation, sorption to solids (Jelic et al. 2011) and also volatilization which occurs to a minor degree (Verlicchi et al. 2012). The fate of MPs in WWTPs strongly depends on their sorption behavior, especially those that are hydrophobic. Sorption behavior also influences their availability for biotransformation due to increased exposure to transforming and degrading microorganism. However, recent advances in WWTPs technologies use activated sludge and trickling filter with long solids retention time (SRT) in activated sludge systems (Clara et al. 2005, Suarez et al. 2010) to enhance the degradation process. Simulations have shown that the fate of the pollutants is influenced by the sludge retention time of the system, i.e., a higher removal is observed in long retention time systems and the physicochemical properties of the pollutants, i.e., their persistence in the WWTP conditions (Cloutier et al. 2012). Suárez et al. (2010) identified 10% higher removal efficiency for fluoxetine, citalopram and ethinylestradiol pharmaceuticals when prolonged sludge retention time was applied. Activated sludge plant uses a process that use dissolved oxygen to promote the growth of a biological floc that substantially removes organic material (van Beelen 2007). The process is a multi-chamber reactor unit that makes use of microorganisms to degrade organic substances and remove nutrients from wastewater. To maintain aerobic conditions, a well-timed supply of oxygen in an aerated tank is required. The bacteria use the waste to grow and transform it to energy, water, CO_2 and new cell material. In the trickling filter, wastewater is aerated as it flows through a media bed with large surface area. Wastewater should flow in a thin film over the media to allow time for treatment. The media serves as a substrate where a biological film grows and is fed by the nutrients contained in the wastewater. The process of bio-transformation in the secondary process involves the conversion of ammonia to nitrite and nitrate and finally to nitrogen gas. Joss et al. (2006) demonstrated that the existing biological wastewater treatment processes can remove a broad array of MPs only to a certain extent. Non-degradable MPs, metabolites and new chemicals resulting from chemicals' biotransformation are passed on to the tertiary treatment stage. Therefore, non-degradable MPs, metabolites from biodegradable MPs, and new chemicals from biotransformation process are passed on to the tertiary stage.

Third stage: tertiary treatment

In the final (tertiary) treatment step, the organic solids which are mainly sludge, are neutralized and then disposed or re-used. Tertiary treatment processes are "user specific" and the treatment is focused on water use for certain purposes. Thus, the requirement for tertiary treatment processes is generally based on public and environmental health objectives. The final effluent can be discharged onto a natural surface water body (receiving water) as shown in Fig. 2.

Efficiency and effectiveness of WWTPs in removal of MPs

The efficiency of WWTPs to remove MPs from effluent varies with the nature of the chemical compound in question. Comparing removal of non-conventional organic MPs such as dioxane and conventional ones such as elemental metals, it can be observed that the removal rate of metals can reach 70% (Lee et al. 2015) while removal rate of non-conventional MPs are lower. For example, the removal rates of selenium was 18% and was found to be lower than the removal rate of 1, 4-dioxane, which was 30%. Relatively hydrophobic MPs which are biodegradable, such as some pharmaceuticals, several personal care products (PCPs) and other household chemicals, are usually well removed (> 70%) in WWTPs, either by sorption onto sewage sludge or by biodegradation (Lee et al. 2015). Other chemicals that have shown a higher efficiency removal by sorption also include heavy metals, persistent organic pollutants (POPs), brominated flame retardants, surfactants, plastic additives, hormones, and several PCPs (Lee et al. 2015). In some cases, effluent concentrations of MPs have been found to be higher than those detected in the influent (Lee et al. 2015). This observation can be due to combined result of accumulation of persistent MPs in WWTP, and inflow of MPs through other alternative transport means such as surface run off to the WWTP. For example, Köck-Schulmeye et al. (2013) found concentration of pesticides in the effluent higher than in the corresponding influent. These authors hypothesized that atmospheric deposition, deconjugation of metabolites and/or transformation products of the pesticides, hydrolysis, and desorption from particulate matter during wastewater treatment were responsible for the higher concentrations in the effluent (Köck-Schulmeye et al. 2013). Pesticide molecules have different physical and functional groups, which affect their elimination from WWTPs. For example, diuron, which is a carbamate, can be removed up to 60% at the primary treatment stage (Stasinakis et al. 2009). However, higher concentrations of diedrine, which is an organochlorine, were observed (Katsoyiannis and Samara 2004) due to the potential transformation of aldrine to diedrine. The primary removal of organochlorine pesticides exhibited lower correlation with the log of octanol-water partition coefficient (Kow) showing that their removal from conventional WWTP processes cannot be attributed only to sorption, but to other mechanisms as well (Katsoyiannis and Samara 2004). In another study, the removal of thiazine herbicide (atrazine and simazine) and their degradation products, desethylatrazine and desisopropylatrazine, from the primary wastewater treatment and biological treatment processes were found to be ineffective (as low as 40%) (Meakins et al. 1994). Bernhard et al. (2006) studied the biodegradation of persistent polar pollutants in wastewater and found no removal for EDTA from WWTPs. In other studies, both influent and effluent showed an almost steady concentration level EDTA ranging from 107 to 134 µg L^{-1} (Bernhard et al. 2006, Reemtsma et al. 2006). The low EDTA removal was confirmed by a study by Knepper et al. (2004) in which influent and effluent samples were taken from different conventional activated sludge treatment plants in Spain, Germany, Austria, the Netherlands, and Belgium. A range of studies have monitored PFASs in WWTPs and sewage treatment plants (STPs) in various countries (Sinduka et al. 2013, Sepulvado et al. 2011, Guo et al. 2010). One of the reasons why PFASs are so ubiquitous in the environment is their persistence in WWTPs and the environment. Previous studies regarding PFASs in WWTP show that these compounds cannot be effectively removed by conventional treatment processes (Yu et al. 2013, Guo et al. 2010, Schultz et al. 2006). Sources of PFASs to the environment include STP effluents, landfill effluents, and fire training facilities (Ahrens 2011). Chirikona et al. (2015) calculated the discharge loads of PFAAs homologues into the drainage systems of Lake Victoria, Kenya catchment from five WWTPs. The total daily discharge load for the five WWTPs was 1013 mg day^{-1}, and Kisumu WWTP had the highest daily discharge load (656 mg day^{-1}). Kisumu is the largest city on the Lake Victoria shore, in Kenya. Previous study on the efficiency of flame retardants removal from WWTPs gave results that ranged between 0% and 35% (Bernhard et al. 2006). However, a study by Kim et al. (2014) on the occurrence and fate of four novel brominated flame retardants (NBFRs) in WWTPs, observed a median removal efficiency, i.e., decabromodiphenylethane (DBDPE), 1,2-bis(2,4,6-tribromophenoxy) ethane (BTBPE), hexabromobenzene (HBB), and pentabromoethylbenzene (PBEB) to be 81 to 93, 76 to 98, 61 to 97, and 54 to 97% respectively. In another study, Wu et al. (2013) reported on the efficiency of six PAHs (fluoranthene, benzo[b]fluoranthene, benzo[k]fluoranthene, benzo[a] pyrene, benzo[ghi]perylene and indeno[1,2,3-cd]pyrene) in different WWTPs. The removal efficiencies of six PAHs were 73–83% at biological treatment units, and 24–56% at the aerated grit stage, respectively. The efficiency of MPs removal from WWTPs and the main factors or processes that influence their effective removal are displayed in Table 1.

WWTPs as a source of metabolites and new chemicals

Biotransformation may not completely mineralize MPs but instead transform the parent compound to a metabolite or cause formation of new chemicals by means of chemical reactions. Many researchers have demonstrated or reported transformational products (Melcer et al. 2007, Soares et al. 2008, Katsoyiannis and Samara 2004) resulting from MPs' presence in WWTPs. In addition, there are observed cases where the concentration of MPs in effluent exceeds that in the influent for some chemical analytes. The observation suggests that conjugated forms of micropollutants enter WWTPs and retransform, or deconjugate, back to their parent form (Plósz et al. 2010). Khunjar et al. (2011) found evidence of biologically mediated conjugation of chemicals by ammonia oxidizing and heterotrophic bacteria in WWTPs that resulted in compounds that have the potential to retransform back to their parent form in the environment. These observations can also be explained by the presence of some substances (e.g., metabolites and/or transformation products) in the influent, which can subsequently be transformed back to parent compounds during biological treatment (Kasprzyk-Hordern et al. 2009), or desorbed from solid particles (Köck-

Table 1. Important micro-pollutants, subgroups, examples and efficiency and effectiveness of removal from WWTPs.

Classes of MPs	Categories	Examples	Efficiency & Effectiveness in WWTP	Factors/Process influencing removal efficiency
Agricultural Pesticides and chemical fertilizers	Pesticides (Fungicides, insecticides, rodenticides, herbicides, etc.)	Organophosphates, Carbamates, Organochlorines, Phenylpyrazole, pyrethroids	Not Effective/ Not Efficient	Adsorption, Persistence, Toxicity
	Fertilizers	Ammonium	Effective	Biodegradation
		Phosphate	Effective	
		Nitrogen	Effective	
Pharmaceuticals & Personal care Products	Personal care products	Additives, Fragrances, Surfactants, Cosmetics, Toiletries	Not Effective	Biodegradation, Sorption
	Antibiotics	B-lactams, Tetracyclines, Macrolides, Quinolones, Sulphonamides	Not Efficient	Toxicity, Adsorption
	Antiepileptic	Carbamazepine	Not Effective	Persistence
	Non-steroidal anti-inflammatory drugs	Aspirin, Fluoxetine, diazepam	Not Effective	Biodegradation, Adsorption
	Painkillers	Naproxen, Ibuprofen, Diclofenac	Not Efficient	Persistence, Biodegradation, Adsorption
	Psycostimulants	Caffeine	Not Efficient	Biodegradation, Adsorption
	Antidepressants	Monoamine oxidase inhibitors (MAOIs), serotonin reuptake inhibitors (SSRIs), Serotonin-noradrenalin reuptake inhibitors (SNRIs)	Not Efficient	Biodegradation
	Cardiovascular drugs	Calcium-channel blockers, e.g., nefedine, Beta-Blockers	Not Efficient	Biodegradation, Adsorption
	Phthalates	Dibutyl, diethyl, dimethyl phthaletes,	Not Efficient	Biodegradation, Adsorption
	Synthetic xenoestrogens	Bisphenol A	Not Efficient	Biodegradation, Adsorption
	Synthetic Hormones	17α ethinylestradial (EE2)	Not Efficient	Biodegradation, Adsorption
Naturally occurring Airborne Estrogens	Steroid oestrogens	17β-oestradiol	Not Efficient	Biodegradation, Adsorption
	Phyto-oestrogens	Isoflavones	Non known	Biodegradation, Adsorption

Table 1 contd. ...

...Table 1 contd.

Classes of MPs	Categories	Examples	Efficiency & Effectiveness in WWTP	Factors/Process influencing removal efficiency
Particles	Crystalline silica	Quartz, christobalite, tridymite	Effective with sedimentation and flocculation processes	Adsorption, Toxicity
	Asbestos	Crocidolite, Chrysotile		
	Toxic trace elements	–		
	Diesel fuel	–		
	Biomass from wildfires	–	–	Biodegradation, Adsorption
Engineered nanomaterials	Zinc oxide (ZnO) NPs	–	Not Effective	Adsorption, Toxicity
	Silver (Ag) NPs			
	Carbon nanotubes	–	–	Adsorption
Trace and radioelements	Heavy metals	Zn, Pb, Se, Hg, Cu, Cr, Cd,	Not Efficient	Adsorption, Toxocity
	Other Micro-elements	F	Not Efficient	Adsorption, Toxicity
	Radioelements	U, Th, Pa, Ra, Rn, Po, Rb, Bi, Po	Not Efficient	Adsorption, Toxicity
Industrial Chemicals	Brominated flame retardants (BFRs)	Polybrominated diphenyl ethers (Deca-BDE, Octa-BDE, Penta-BDE)	Not Effective	Persistence, Adsorption
	Per- and Polyfluorinated Substances	PFOS, PFOA, PFBA	Not Effective	Persistence, Adsorption
	Trichloroethylene (TCE)	–	Not Effective	Persistence, Adsorption
	Benzene	Degraded to phenols	Not Effective	
	Polyaromatic hydrocarbons (PAHs)	Naphthalene, Acenaphthene, Phenanthrene, Anthracene, pyrene, Benzo[a]anthracene, Benzo[a]pyrene, etc.	Not Efficient	Persistence, Adsorption, Toxicity
	Polychlorinated dibenzodioxins	Dibenzo-þ-dioxin (DD)	Not Effective	Toxicity, Adsorption
	Polyclorinated biphenyls (PCBs)	–	Not Effective	Adsorption
	Coordination complexes	Ethylenediamino tetraacetate (EDTA) Diethylenetriamino pentaacetate (DTPA)	–	Adsorption
	Methyl isocyanate	-	Not Effective	Adsorption
	Anti-oxidants (Food additives)	Butylated hydroxyanisole	–	Adsorption, biodegradation

References: Powell et al. 2008, Swartz et al. 2006, Jurgens et al. 2002, Nakada et al. 2006, Treadgold et al. 2012, Togola and Budzinski 2008, WHO 2008, EUREAU 2001
–Not indicated.

Schulmeyer et al. 2013). Example of new chemicals that can potentially be formed in WWTP is halonitromethanes, which constitutes one class of emerging disinfection by-products (Song et al. 2010). Song et al. (2010) observed that municipal WWTP effluents contained some reactive halonitromethanes precursors, possibly the by-products of biological treatment processes and/or some moiety of industry or household origin, which form halonitromethanes by ozonation/chrorination or ozonation/chloramination processes (Song et al. 2010).

Factors/Processes influencing removal efficiency

Removal of MPs from wastewater is influenced by water partition coefficient (Kow), ready biodegradability, toxicity, persistence, among other factors. These factors are outlined below:

Adsorption and the octanol/water partition coefficient (Kow)

To predict if a compound is likely to adsorb on biosolids and subsequently partition into sludge in WWTPs, the Kow value can be used. In general, pollutants with low Kow values may be considered relatively hydrophilic (especially if Henry's Law constant is also low); they tend to have high water solubility, small soil/sediment adsorption coefficients, and small bioconcentration factors for aquatic life. Conversely, chemicals with high Kow values (e.g., greater than 10^4 (log Kow > 4)) are very hydrophobic and adsorb to soil/sediments and tend to bioaccumulate. Polycyclic aromatic hydrocarbons such as Acenaphththylene (log Kow = 4) and Anthracene (Log Kow = 4.68) can therefore be classified as hydrophobic substances, and their sorption on soils and sediments and, thus, sludge in WWTPs is significant. Adsorption, which is the main mechanism by which the primary treatment functions, and partially also in secondary treatment, is compound specific. Study by Carballa et al. (2004) reported 40% removal efficiency for fragrances from the primary treatment stage of WWTP, while more than 75% of steroid hormones are removed from the secondary treatment process (Suarez et al. 2010). Cardiovascular drugs such as β-blockers have a removal efficiency of about 38% to 73%, while phthalates have removal efficiency of between 15%–62% by the sorption processes (Luo et al. 2014). High removal of Bisphenol A > 90% shown by low effluent concentrations has been reported from WWTPs, and has been attributed to biodegradation and biotransformation processes as the main removal pathway for Bisphenol A (Nakada et al. 2006).

Biodegradation

Structural features of organic compounds have been studied to determine compounds that enhance or inhibit their biodegradability (Tunkel et al. 2000). The Japanese Ministry of International Trade and Industry (MITI) test protocol data set examined the ability of microorganisms in aqueous suspension to degrade about 900 organic chemicals inhibiting a diverse range of functional groups (Takatsuki et al. 1995). From MITI test protocol data set examination, a readily degradable substance was defined as the experimentally showed consumption of dissolved O_2 exceeding more than 60% of the theoretical oxygen demand needed to complete mineralization of the organic chemical within 28 days. Application of this theory was used to test the ready degradability of PFASs that were commercially available in the market where it was observed that PFOS and PFOA were not readily biodegradable (Quinete et al. 2009). According to Tunkel et al. (2000), a given structural moiety influences the aerobic degradation of compounds. For example, it is widely seen that compounds including hydrolysable groups, like carboxylic acid esters (C(O)OR), anides (C(O) NR_2) and anhydrides or phosphorous acid esters are readily degradable (Loonen et al. 1999). In contrast, some structural features consistently diminish the ease of biodegradability; for example, chloro and nitro groups, particularly on aromatic ring (Loonen et al. 1999, Tunkel et al. 2000). Such structural activity relationships of aerobic biodegradation prove capable of predicting qualitatively compounds lability in 80 to 90% of the cases.

Toxicity to microorganisms in WWTP

Toxicity of the MPs on microorganisms in WWTPs can also adversely affect their removal efficiency by biodegradation process. Biodegradation is a significant removal pathway for some pharmaceuticals and steroid hormones but of minor importance for antibiotics and pesticides, which in return stops the bioactivities of the microorganisms. PhACs are designed to be bioactive at very low concentration levels and their inefficient removal from WWTPs may potentially be of environmental concern (Grung et al. 2008). This inefficiency of WWTPs in the removal of PhACs has resulted to the development of antibiotic resistant bacteria strains and mutations (Christen et al. 2010, Santos et al. 2010), and also PhACs synergistic and antagonistic adverse health effects on biota (Boxall et al. 2010, Pomati et al. 2006). The removal of pharmaceuticals from WWTPs shows great variability from < 25% to > 75% (Verlicchi et al. 2012), and it is compound specific (Luo et al. 2014). Study by Stasinakis et al. (2013) reported that EDC removal from WWTPs during primary treatment was from 13% to 43%. The impact of eight household MPs (erythromycin, ofloxacin, ibuprofen, 4-nonylphenol, triclosan, sucralose, PFOA and PFOS (PFAAs)) on the laboratory bacterial strain *Escherichia coli* MG1655 and on activated sludge from a WWTP was studied by Pasquini et al. (2013). In the same study, growth-based toxicity tests on *E. coli* were performed for each MPs and MP removal was also assessed. Ibuprofen, erythromycin, ofloxacin, 4-nonylphenol and triclosan were removed from wastewater, mainly by biodegradation. Sucralose and PFOA were not removed from wastewater at all, and PFOS was slightly eliminated by adsorption on sludge (Pasquini et al. 2013). In a similar study, Li and Zhang (2010) studied the biodegradation and adsorption of antibiotics in the activated sludge process. In the study, it was observed that cefalexin and two sulfonamide antibiotics were predominantly removed by biodegradation in both freshwater and saline sewage systems, while ampicillin, norfloxacin, ciprofloxacin, ofloxacin, tetracycline, roxithromycin, and trimethoprim were mainly removed by adsorption. Although conventional biological wastewater treatment processes are effective for the removal of some antibiotics (β-lactams, sulfonamides, trimethoprim, macrolides, fluoroquinolones, and tetracyclines), many have been reported to occur even after the secondary treatment process of effluents (Le-Minha et al. 2010) in WWTPs in concentrations of 10 ng L^{-1} to 1,000 ng L^{-1}.

Persistence

Several MPs can persist for long periods of time in the environment and can accumulate and pass from one species to the next through the food chain. Persistent compounds included surfactants, fire-retardant chemicals, pesticides, fragrance compounds, hormones, and pharmaceutical (Levine et al. 2006). Examples of these persistent MPs are the one listed under the Stockholm Convention on Persistent Organic Pollutants so that they can be addressed globally, including the organ-chlorine pesticides, polychlorinated biphenyls (PCBs), polychlorinated dibenzo-p-dioxins (dioxins), polychlorinated dibenzofurans (furans) and recently PFOS, PFOSF and related precursor substances which were added in May 2009 as the first fluorinated POPs in the Stockholm Convention POPs list (Stockholm Convention 2010, Stockholm Convention 2009; http://www.pops.int) due to their Persistent Organic Pollutants (POPs) properties.

Receiving waters and drinking water contamination

Contamination of surface waters by MPs released from municipal WWTPs may lead to drinking water contamination. This is because surface waters are one of the main sources of drinking water all around the world. Several MPs such as pharmaceuticals, biocides, personal care products, plastic additives or sweeteners have been detected at low concentrations (< 1–100 ng L^{-1}) in finished drinking waters in many countries and their origin traced back to wastewater as the source (Benner et al. 2013). The decrease in levels of MPs in drinking water as compared to effluent is due to the varying degrees of natural attenuation (Pal et al. 2010) such as dilution in surface water, sorption onto suspended solids and sediments, direct and indirect photolysis and aerobic biodegradation, within the effluent receiving waters. Specifically, for PCPs, Gómez et al. (2012) found that the natural attenuation is more likely to resuls from river water dilution or sorption to solids, than from degradation. In drinking water production, conventional refining processes remove numerous MPs (Stackelberg et al. 2004, Westerhoff et al. 2005).

Proposed improvement of wastewater treatment plants and effluent treatment

In order to protect aquatic ecosystems and to preserve drinking water resources, reduction of the inputs of MPs in surface waters is necessary (Eggen et al. 2014). Various studies have highlighted the need to remove MPs from the treated wastewater before discharge into aquatic ecosystem due to their negative effect on human and animal health and ecotoxicological effects (Escher et al. 2011). Le-Minha et al. (2010)

recommended that tertiary treatment should have advanced treatment processes, which includes tertiary media filtration, ozonation, chlorination, UV irradiation, activated carbon adsorption, nano-filtration and reverse osmosis, and should be used to fully manage environmental and human exposure to these contaminants in water recycling schemes.

MP removal technologies from aqueous media are already available and because of the unknown environmental risk posed by the numerous MPs, the preventive action ought to be taken based on the precautionary principle (Plósz et al. 2013). Figure 4 demonstrates in form of a flow diagram, the situation of MPs removal from effluent for conventional WWTs treatment compared to the proposed treatment which is recommended in this chapter.

In the current conventional treatment, practice largely relies on biodegradation process, and advanced treatment processes are often applied for drinking water only, while for the proposed/recommended case, the advanced treatment processes are applied for both effluent as well as for drinking water. In the latter scenario, MPs are removed effectively from the effluent, and thus reduce the risk posed by MPs to aquatic biota residing in receiving water. It is expected that regarding advanced effluent treatments at WWTP, interferences due to variety of matrices in effluent can affect the process. Moreover, "secondary" pollution from atmospheric depositions or from surface run-offs may contaminate receiving water. This justifies the advanced treatment of drinking water. The recommended advanced wastewater treatment

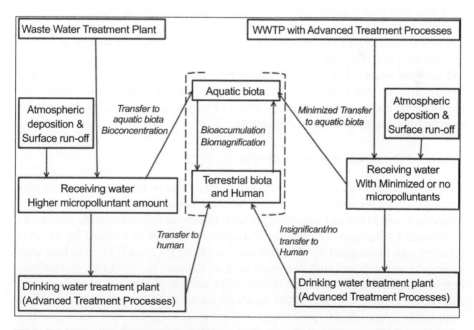

Fig. 4. The proposed and the conventional wastewater flow diagram. For the conventional treatment, the advanced wastewater treatment is shown only for drinking water while for the proposed treatment, the advanced wastewater treatment is shown for effluent and drinking water.

involves the following processes: enhanced biological treatment, advanced oxidation processes (AOPs), use of specialized sorbents and ultrafiltration and membrane technology outlined (in Section 2.8.1 to 2.8.4) as follows:

Enhanced biological treatment

Some bacteria mineralize the MPs by using them as a source of carbon and energy at the secondary treatment. The secondary treatment uses a wide variety of micro-organisms. They convert biodegradable materials through the absorption of soluble and suspended particles contained in wastewater into simple products such as carbon dioxide and additional biomass, or nitrate and nitrogen gas. Enhancing biological wastewater treatment has received much attention in the recent past. The technology's advancement over microorganisms use in waste water treatment are those that: (i) exploit microbial diversity; complex microbial consortia composed by bacteria-bacteria, bacteria-archea and bacteria-fungi are developed to enhance biological degradation of MPs. Oxidase enzymes have great potential as biocatalysts for MP and organic waste breakdown; (ii) exploit metabolic diversity; new bioprocesses to treat wastewater can be developed by exploiting the diverse metabolic capabilities of microbes, and (iii) exploit biocatalyst diversity where many enzymes are "promiscuous" biocatalysts capable of transforming a variety of substrates that share structural similarity with their primary substrate (Singhal and Perez-Garcia 2016). Identification and isolation of bacteria that can specifically biodegrade particular MPs was demonstrated in a study by Onunga et al. (2015). In this study, the capacity of native bacteria to degrade carbofuran in soils obtained from Nzoia River basin in Kenya was investigated. A gram positive, rod-shaped bacterium capable of degrading carbofuran was isolated through liquid cultures with carbofuran as the only carbon and nitrogen source. The isolate degraded 98% of 100 μg mL^{-1} carbofuran within 10 days with the formation of carbofuran phenol as the only detectable metabolite. Identification and isolation of the most effective microorganisms such as bacteria for specific MPs degradation is recommended.

Advanced Oxidation Processes (AOPs)

Advanced oxidation processes have been applied in wastewater treatment to varying degrees of success depending on the chemical compounds, to degrade organic compounds and to convert non-biodegradable pollutants into substances that can be assimilated by bacteria. The choice of oxidant to be used is dictated by its good selectivity for the targeted MP. Oxidants such as Ozone (O_3) and H_2O_2 have been used separately or combined with processes such as Fenton ($Fe^{2+} + H_2O_2$), electrolysis, sonolysis (Ultrasounds) and light driven AOPs such as photolysis, photo-catalysis, and Photo-Fenton (Stasinakis 2008). AOPs are successful to transform toxic organic compounds (e.g., drugs, pesticides, endocrine disruptors) into biodegradable substances. AOPs, in general, are cheap to install but involve high operating costs due to the input of chemicals and energy required (Cominelis et al. 2008). To limit the costs, AOPs are often used as pre-treatment combined with biologic treatment (Pulgarin et al. 1999). The combination of several AOPs is an efficient way to increase pollutant removal and reduce costs. Quinete et al. (2009) showed that PFOA and PFOS increased degradation with time of exposure to UV radiation and even more accentuated degradation when it was applied alongside H_2O_2. For perfluorobutane sulfonate (PFBS), degradation due to UV and oxidation exposure method was not significant within 120 min. Other methods of carbofuran detoxification, such as oxidation with ozone, photodegradation, fenton degradation, ozonation, membrane filtration and adsorption (Yang et al. 2011) have been used. In another example, oxidation by physico-chemical techniques is also used for water treatment to decolor and degrade the organic compounds and to convert non-biodegradable pollutants into substances that can be assimilated by the bacteria in a downstream biological treatment process. One specific example of AOPs that has received much attention is electro-oxidative degradation.

Electro-oxidative degradation

The electrochemical oxidation or electrooxidation processes could be a reasonable option to treat organic compounds due to the implementation ease and high oxidation rates attained. The pharmaceutical active compounds' suitability for electrochemical oxidation was tested by cyclic voltammetry (Sifuna et al. 2016) on two pharmaceuticals, namely sulfamethoxazole and dichlofenac, and their destruction by electrolysis on platinum electrode and graphite carbon electrode in aqueous medium. Other studies have also posted on the suitability of other electrodes used as anodes in electrochemical degradation of various pollutants (Cañizares et al. 2005). Other compounds such as atrazine that have an active chlorine that can be electrically generated provide an interesting option for organo-chlorine pesticides degradation (Malpass et al. 2010), such as carbaryl (Malpass et al. 2009), and dyes (Malpass et al. 2008), due to their versatile electrocatalytic property of active chlorine electrogeneration, electrochemical stability, and long lifetime.

Use of specialized sorbents

Adsorption is the adhesion of molecules onto the surface of an adsorbent solid. In the case of water treatment, activated carbon has been used as an adsorbent for the adsorption of MPs. Various phyto-sorbents have been applied to successfully remove various MPs from wastewater (Ngeno et al. 2016). Conventional methods that involve physicochemical treatments such as coagulation, flocculation, settling and screening process are generally inefficient in the removal of pharmaceuticals (Santos et al. 2010) and other organic pollutants from water. Adsorption processes do not add undesirable by-products in the environment (Tong et al. 2010), and in addition, have been found to be efficient for MPs (Gupta et al. 2009). Among other materials that have been tested as potential adsorbents for the removal of the emerging contaminants from wastewater, some of them are fly ash, blast furnace slag and sludge, black liquor lignin, red mud, and waste slurry. Different types of adsorbents are classified into natural adsorbents or synthetic adsorbents. Natural adsorbents include charcoal, clays, clay minerals, zeolites, and ores. These natural materials, in many instances, are relatively cheap, abundant in supply and have significant potential for modification and ultimate enhancement of their adsorption capabilities.

Apart from adsorbent potential to remove persistent MPs, they have been used to adsorb trace metals from aquatic ecosystems (Buasri et al. 2012) and do not generate potentially toxic degradation byproducts (Tong et al. 2010).

Ultrafiltration and membrane technology

Filtration can also be used to supplement advanced treatment processes at the tertiary stage. Tertiary filtration treatment traps MPs fixed on suspended solids. Settling and filtration remove MPs from water, mainly by trapping the suspended solids on which they are attached. Ultrafiltration membranes allow small molecules (water and salts) to pass through and stop molecules with a high molar mass, which may be the MPs of concern. Ultrafiltration efficiency works on the principal of reduction of suspended solids, disinfection and removal of the MPs fixed on trapped particle matter. Membrane bioreactors (MBR) can also be applied and it combines advanced clarification through ultrafiltration membranes for biological degradation of pollution. The purification efficiency of a conventional WWTP can drop below 50% while under the same conditions, a WWTP with a MBR has an efficiency of over 80% (Carballa et al. 2006, Clara et al. 2005). Overall, biodegradation is the major removal mechanism for most compounds during the MBR treatment. Ultrafiltration and membrane technology produced effluent is of high quality, compliant with the standards for discharges in sensitive areas or for re-use. Functionalization of Cellulose Nanofiber membranes can be used to purify water by selectively removing unwanted MPs from water media. Luo et al. (2014) observed that for most pharmaceutical MPs removals, efficiency was high using biofilm technologies, such as moving bed biofilm reactors (MBBR) compared to what will be achieved with the conventional WWTPs. Ibuprofen, salicylic acid, Primidone, and Naproxen were efficiently eliminated using this particular process (93.7%, 91.1%, 83.5%, and 81.1% respectively). The high removal efficiency could be ascribed to the presence of strong electron donating (readily biodegradable) functional groups (e.g., eOH) on these compounds. A subsequent study by Luo et al. (2015) showed that the MBBR-membrane coupled system had lower fouling tendency than a conventional membrane, and the compound-specific removal efficiencies varied significantly, ranging from 25.5 to 99.5% with a hydraulic retention time of 24 hours.

Conclusions

The general effect of WWTPs processes is to concentrate the MPs in influent that is received from various sources and later remove them though effluent. The extent of this removal depends on the properties of the MP species. The overall result of this process is to "discharge" the non-degraded MPs, and to act as a "source point" of metabolites and new chemicals generated through biotransformation and reaction processes, into the other environmental media through effluent and sludge. Contamination of natural water by thousands of chemical compounds that are normally detected at very low concentrations (pg^{-1} to $\mu g\ L^{-1}$) raises considerable ecological issues, posing a risk to human health and a major concern for public health almost all around the world (Schwarzenbach et al. 2006). The primary treatment process in a WWTP has a relative removal of MPs in the range of up to 50%. This means that 50% of the MPs in the influent are passed on to the secondary treatment process in a conventional WWTP. Notably 50% MPs that are removed from the WWTP primary process through coagulation and flocculation or sorption on biosolids, are especially those that are hydrophobic. In the second stage, where the process utilizes microorganisms in wastewater treatment, sorption behavior of micro-pollutants influences their availability for biotransformation due to increased exposure to transforming and degrading microorganism. The resultant chemicals in wastewater from the secondary process that are passed to the final treatment stage are non-degradable MPs, metabolites resulting from biodegradation and new chemicals resulting from chemicals biotransformation and reactions. These chemicals contribute to elevated levels of MPs in effluent from WWTPs. However, with the application of required advanced treatment of effluent, the percentage removal of MPs can be maximized. Conventional water treatment is based on the assumption that drinking water is the main exposure route of micro-pollutants to humans and other biota. However, this approach does not consider the critical aspect that leads to the risks posed by transfer of the micro-pollutants to biota, directly from wastewater treatment plants. Therefore, incorporating additional new advanced wastewater treatment technologies such as reverse osmosis, and advanced oxidation, perhaps followed by biological activated carbon, will enhance wastewater reclamation and the elimination of chemical pollutants from wastewater. In addition, these technologies will be a priority in managing micro-pollutants in general. The understanding of physicochemical properties of MPs, such as their hydrophilicity and hydrophobicity, are important considerations for the choice of the advanced wastewater treatment technology that can be applied.

Acknowledgments

The author would like to acknowledge the various funding organizations such as the National Commission for Science, Technology and Innovation of Kenya (NACOSTI), International Foundation for Science (IFS) and the World Academy of Sciences (TWAS). Acknowledgements are also due to the following institutions for collaboration: Lake Victoria North Water Services Board, Lake Victoria South Water Services Board and the Department of Environmental Science and Analytical Chemistry (ACES). Stockholm University staff, especially Zhe Li, Marko Filipovic, Ian Causin and Robin Vestergren. In addition, thanks go to colleagues Natalia Quinete and Prof. Rolf-Dieter Wilken for their assistance.

References

Ahrens, L. 2011. Polyfluoroalkyl compounds in the aquatic environment: A review of their occurrence and fate. J. Environ. Monitor. 13: 20–31.

Benner, J., D.E. Helbling, H.P. Kohler, J. Wittebol, E. Kaiser, C. Prasse et al. 2013. Is biological treatment a viable alternative for micropollutant removal in drinking water treatment processes? Water Res. 15: 47(16): 5955–76.

Bernhard, M., J. Muller and T.P. Knepper. 2006. Biodegradation of persistent polar pollutants in wastewater: Comparison of an optimized lab-scale membrane bioreactor and activated sludge treatment. Water Res. 40: 3419–3428.

Boxall, A.B.A., D.W. Kolpin, B. Halling-Sørensen and J. Tolls. 2003. Are veterinary medicines causing environmental risks? Environ. Sci. Technol. 37(15): 286–294.

Buasri, A., N. Chaiyut, K. Tapang, S. Jaroensin and S. Panphrom. 2012. Biosorption of heavy metals from aqueous solutions using water hyacinth as a low cost biosorbent. Civil and Environmental Research. 2(2): 17–24.

Cañizares, P., J. Lobato, R. Paz, M.A. Rodrigo and C. Sáez. 2005. Electrochemical oxidation of phenolic wastes with boron-doped diamond anodes. Water Res. 39: 2687–2705.

Carballa, M., F. Omil and J.M. Lema. 2004. Removal of cosmetic ingredients and pharmaceuticals in cells. Environ. Sci. Technol. 40(7): 2442–2447.

Carballa, M., F. Omil, A.C. Alder and J.M. Lema. 2006. Comparison between the conventional anaerobic digestion (CAD) of sewage sludge and its combination with a chemical or thermal pre-treatment concerning the removal of Pharmaceuticals and Personal Care Products (PPCPs). Water Sci. Technol. 53(8): 109–117.

Chirikona, F., M. Filipovic, S. Ooko and F. Orata. 2015. Perfluoroalkyl acids in selected wastewater treatment plants and their discharge load within the Lake Victoria basin in Kenyan. Environ. Monit. Assess. 187(5): 4425.

Christen, V., S. Hickmann, B. Rechenberg and K. Fent. 2010. Highly active human pharmaceuticals in aquatic systems: a concept for their identification based on their mode of action. Aquat. Toxicol. 96: 167–81.

Clara, M., B. Strenn, O. Gans, E. Martinez, N. Kreuzinger and H. Kroiss. 2005. Removal of selected pharmaceuticals, fragrances and endocrine disrupting compounds in a membrane bioreactor and conventional wastewater treatment plants. Water Res. 39: 4797–807.

Cloutier, F., L. Clouzot and P.A. Vanrolleghem. 2012. Predicting the fate of emerging contaminants in wastewater treatment plants. pp. 3828–3836. *In*: Proceedings of WEFTEC 2012, 85th Annual Water Environment Federation Technical Exhibition and Conference, New Orleans, Louisiana, USA, 29th September–3rd October 2012.

Comninellis, C., A. Kapalka, S. Malato, S.A. Parson, L. Poulios and D. Mantzavinos. 2008. Perspective advanced oxidation processes for water treatment: Advanced and trends for R&D. J. Chem. Technol. Biotechnol. 83: 769–776.

Conder, J.M., R.A. Hoke, W. Wolf, M.H. Russell and R.C. Buck. 2008. Are PFCAs bioaccumulative? A critical review and comparison with regulatory lipophilic compounds. Environ. Sci. Technol. 42: 995–1003.

Ebert, I., J. Bachmann, U. Kühnen, A. Küster, C. Kussatz, D. Maletzki et al. 2011. Toxicity of the fluoroquinolone antibiotics enrofloxacin and ciprofloxacin to photoautotrophic aquatic organisms. Environ. Toxicol. Chem. 30(12): 2786–2792.

Eggen, R.I.L., J. Hollender, A. Joss, M. Schärer and C. Stamm. 2014. Reducing the discharge of micropollutants in the aquatic environment: The benefits of upgrading wastewater treatment plants. Environ. Sci. Technol. 48(14): 7683–7689.

EUREAU. 2001. Keeping raw drinking water safe from pesticides. EUREAU position paper. http://www.water.org.uk/static/files_archive/Full_report.pdf.

Gillis, P.L., F. Gagné, R. McInnis, T.M. Hooey, E.S. Choy, C. André et al. 2014. The impact of municipal wastewater effluent on field-deployed freshwater mussels in the Grand River (Ontario, Canada). Environ. Toxicol. Chem. 33(1): 134–143.

Gómez, M.J., S. Herrera, D. Solé, E. García-Calvo and A.R. Fernández-Alba. 2012. Spatio-temporal evaluation of organic contaminants and their transformation products along a river basin affected by urban, agricultural and industrial pollution. Sci. Total Environ. 420: 134–45.

Gromaire, M.C., S. Garnaud, M. Saad and G. Chebbo. 2001. Contribution of different sources to the pollution of wet weather flow in combined sewers. Water Res. 35(2): 521–533.

Grung, M., T. Källqvist, S. Sakshaug, S. Skurtveit and K.V. Thomas. 2008. Environmental assessment of Norwegian priority pharmaceuticals based on the EMEA guideline. Ecotoxicol. Environ. Saf. 71(2): 328–340.

Guo, R., W.J. Sim, E.S. Lee, J.H. Lee and J.E. Oh. 2010. Evaluation of the fate of perfluoroalkyl compounds in wastewater treatment plants. Water Res. 44: 3476–3486.

Gupta, V.K., P.J.M. Carrott, M.M.L. Ribeiro Carrott and T.L. Suhas. 2009. Low-cost adsorbents: growing approach to wastewater treatment—a review. Crit. Rev. Env. Sci. Technol. 39: 783–842.

Halden, R. 2005. Secondary Routes of Exposure to Biocides. Presented to the Food and Drug Administration (FDA) Nonprescription Drugs Advisory Committee, Silver Spring, Maryland, on October 20, 2005. https://www.fda.gov/ohrms/dockets/ac/05/slides/2005-4184S1_06_FDA-Halden.ppt.

Hernando, M.D., M. Mezcua, A.R. Fernández Alba and D. Barceló. 2006. Environmental risk assessment of pharmaceutical residues in wastewater effluents, surface waters and sediments. Talanta. 69: 334–342.

Hunga, H., M. MacLeod, R. Guardans, M. Scheringer, R. Barra, T. Harner et al. 2013. Toward the next generation of air quality monitoring: Persistent organic pollutants. Atmospheric Environ. 80: 591–598.

Jarvis, A.L., M.J. Bernot and R.J. Bernot. 2014. The effects of the psychiatric drug carbamazepine on freshwater invertebrate communities and ecosystem dynamics. Sci. Total Environ. 496: 461–470.

Jelic, A., M. Gros, A. Ginebreda, R. Cespedes-Sánchez, F. Ventura, M. Petrovic et al. 2010. Occurrence, partition and removal of pharmaceuticals in sewage water and sludge during wastewater treatment. Water Res. 45(3): 1165–76.

Joss, A., S. Zabczynski, A. Göbel, B. Hoffmann, D. Löffler, C.S. McArdell et al. 2006. Biological degradation of pharmaceuticals in municipal wastewater treatment: proposing a classification scheme. Water Res. 40(8): 1686–1696.

Jurgens, D.M., I.E.K. Holthaus, C.A. Johnson, J.L.J. Smith, M. Hetheridge and J.R. Williams. 2002. The potential for estradiol and ethinylestradiol degradation in English rivers. Environ. Toxicol. Chem. 21(3): 480–488.

Kasprzyk-Hordern, B., R.M. Dinsdale and A.J. Guwy. 2009. The removal of pharmaceuticals, personal care products, endocrine disruptors and illicit drugs during wastewater treatment and its impact on the quality of receiving waters. Water Res. 43(2): 363–380.

Katsoyiannis, A. and C. Samara. 2004. Persistent organic pollutants (POPs) in the sewage treatment plant of Thessaloniki, northern Greece: occurrence and removal. Water Res. 38: 2685.

Khunjar, W.O., S.A. Mackintosh, J. Skotnicka-Pitak, S. Baik, D.S. Aga and N.G. Love. 2011. Elucidating the relative roles of ammonia oxidizing and heterotrophic bacteria during the biotransformation of 17α-ethinylestradiol and trimethoprim. Environ. Sci. Technol. 45(8): 3605–3612.

Kim, Y., K. Choi, J. Jung, S. Park, P. Kim and J. Park. 2007. Aquatic of acetaminophen, carbamazepine, cimetidine, diltiazem and six major sulfonamides, and their potential ecological risks in Korea. Environ. Int. 33: 370–375.

Klenow, S., G. Heinemeyer, G. Brambilla, E. Dellatte, D. Herzke and P. de Voogt. 2013. Dietary exposure to selected perfluoroalkyl acids (PFAAs) in four European regions. Food Addit. Contam. Part A Chem. Anal. Control Expo. Risk Assess. 30(12): 2141–51.

Knepper, T.P., D. Barcelo, K. Lindner, P. Seel, T. Reemtsma, F. Ventura et al. 2004. Removal of persistent polar pollutants through improved treatment of wastewater effluents (P-THREE). Water Sci. Technol. 50(5): 195–202.

Köck-Schulmeyer, M., M. Villagrasa, M. López de Alda, R. Céspedes-Sánchez, F. Ventura and D. Barceló. 2013. Occurrence and behavior of pesticides in wastewater treatment plants and their environmental impact. Sci. Total Environ. 458-460: 466–476.

Kröfges, P., D. Skutlarek, H. Färber, C. Baitinger, I. Gödeke and R. Weber. 2007. PFOS/PFOA contaminated megasites in Germany polluting the drinking-water supply of millions of people. Organohalogen Compd. 69: 877–880.

Kumar, A., B. Chang and I. Xagoraraki. 2010. Human health risk assessment of pharmaceuticals in water: Issues and challenges ahead. Int. J. Environ. Res. Publ. Health. 7: 3929–3953.

Lee, W., S. Park, J. Kim and J. Jung. 2015. Occurrence and removal of hazardous chemicals and toxic metals in 27 industrial wastewater treatment plants in Korea. Desalination Water Treat. 54(4-5): 1141–1149.

Le-Minha, N., S.J. Khana, J.E. Drewesa and R.M. Stuetza. 2010. Fate of antibiotics during municipal water recycling treatment processes. Water Res. 44(15): 4295–4323.

Levine, A.D., M.T. Meyer and G. Kish. 2006. Evaluation of the persistence of micropollutants through pure-oxygen activated sludge nitrification and denitrification. Water Environ. Res. 78(11): 2276–85.

Li, B. and T. Zhang. 2010. Biodegradation and adsorption of antibiotics in the activated sludge process. Environ. Sci. Technol. 44: 3468–3473.

Loonen, H., F. Lindgren, B. Hansen, W. Karcher, J. Niemelä, K. Hiromatsu et al. 1999. Prediction of biodegradability from chemical structure: Modeling of ready biodegradation test data. Environ. Toxicol. Chem. 18: 1763–1768.

Luo, Y., W. Guo, H.H. Ngo, L.D. Nghiem, F.I. Hai, J. Kang et al. 2014. Removal and fate of micropollutants in a sponge-based moving bed bioreactor. Bioresour. Technol. 159: 311–319.

Luo, Y., Q. Jiang, H.H. Ngo, L.D. Nghiem, F.I. Hai, W.E. Price et al. 2015. Evaluation of micropollutant removal and fouling reduction in a hybrid movingbed biofilm reactoremembrane bioreactor system. Bioresour. Technol. 191: 355–359.

Malpass, G.R.P., D.W. Miwa, S.A.S. Machado and A.J. Motheo. 2008. Decolourisation of real textile waste using electrochemical techniques: effect of electrode composition. J. Hazard. Mater. 156: 170.

Malpass, G.R.P., D.W. Miwa, S.A.S. Machado and A.J. Motheo. 2009. Study of photo-assisted electrochemical degradation of carbaryl at dimensionally stable anodes. J. Hazard. Mater. 167: 224.

Malpass, G.R.P., D.W. Miwa, L. Gomes, E.B. Azevedo, W.F.D. Vilela, M.T. Fukunaga et al. 2010. Unexpected toxicity decrease during photoelectrochemical degradation of atrazine with NaCl. Water Sci. Technol. 62: 2729.

Meakins, N.C., J.M. Bubb and J.N. Lester. 1994. The behavior of s-Atrazine herbicides, Atrazine and simazine durng primary and secondary biological wastewater treatment. Chemosphere. 28: 1611.

Melcer, H., G. Klecka, H. Monteith and C. Staples. 2007. Wastewater Treatment of Alkylphenols and their Ethoxylates. Water Environment Federation, Alexandria, VA.

Murray, K.E., S.M. Thomas and A.A. Bodour. 2010. Prioritizing research for trace pollutants and emerging contaminants in the freshwater environment. Environ. Pollut. 158: 3462–3471.

Nakada, N., T. Tanishima, H. Shinohara, K. Kiri and H. Takada. 2006. Pharmaceutical chemicals and endocrine disrupters in municipal wastewater in Tokyo and their removal during activated sludge treatment. Water Res. 40: 3297.

Ngeno, E.C., F. Orata, L.D. Baraza, V.O. Shikuku and S.J. Kimosop. 2012. Adsorption of caffeine and ciprofloxacin onto pyrolitically derived water hyacinth biochar: isothermal, kinetic and thermodynamic studies. J. Chem. Chem. Eng. 10: 185–194.

Onunga, D.O., I.O. Kowino, A.N. Ngigi, A. Osogo, F. Orata, Z.M. Getenga et al. 2015. Biodegradation of carbofuran in soils within Nzoia River Basin, Kenya. J. Environ. Sci. Health, Part B. 50: 387–397.

Orata, F., N. Quinete, A. Maes, F. Werres and R.-D. Wilken. 2008. Perfluorooctanoic acid and perfluorooctane sulfonate in Nile Perch and tilapia from gulf of Lake Victoria (2008). Afr. J. Pure Appl. Chem. 2(8): 075–079.

Orata, F. and F. Birgen. 2016. Fish tissue bio-concentration and interspecies uptake of heavy metals from waste water lagoons journal of pollution effects & control. J. Pollut. Eff. Cont. 4: 2.

Pal, A., K.Y.H. Gin, A.Y.C. Lin and M. Reinhard. 2010. Impacts of emerging organic contaminants on freshwater resources: review of recent occurrences, sources, fate and effects. Sci. Total Environ. 408: 6062–9.

Pasquini, L., C. Merlin, L. Hassenboehler, J.F. Munoz, M.N. Pons and T. Görner. 2013. Impact of certain household micropollutants on bacterial behavior. Toxicity tests/study of extracellular polymeric substances in sludge. Sci. Total Environ. 1; 463-464: 355–65.

Plósz, B.G., H. Leknes, H. Lilved and K.V. Thomas. 2010. Diurnal variations in the occurrence and the fate of hormones and antibiotics in activated sludge wastewater treatment in Oslo, Norway. Sci. The Tot. Environ. 408(8): 1915–1924.

Plósz, B., L. Benedetti, G. Daigger, K.H. Langford, H. Larsen, H. Monteith et al. 2013. Modelling micro-pollutant fate in wastewater collection and treatment systems: Status and challenges. Wat. Sci. Tech. 67(1): 1–15.

Pomati, F., S. Castiglioni, E. Zuccato, R. Fanelli, D. Vigetti, C. Rossetti et al. 2006. Effects of a complex mixture of therapeutic drugs at environmental levels on human embryonic cells. Environ. Sci. Technol. 40(7): 2442–2447.

Powell, M.C., M.P.A. Griffin and S. Tai. 2008. Bottom-up risk regulation? How nanotechnology risk knowledge gap challenge federal and state environmental agencies. Environ. Manage. 42: 426.

Pulgarin, C., M. Invernizzi, S. Parra, V. Sarria, R. Plania and P. Peringer. 1999. Strategy for the coupling of photochemical and biological flows reactors useful in mineralization of biorecalcitrant industrial pollutants. Catalysis Today. 2: 341–352.

Quinete, N., F. Orata, F. Werres, I. Moreira and R.-D. Wilken. 2009. Determination of perfluorooctane sulfonate and perfluooctanoic acid in the rhine river. Germany. 18. F-2009-043.

Rahman, M.F., S. Peldszus and W.B. Anderson. 2014. Behavior and fate of perfluoroalkyl and polyfluoroalkyl substances (PFASs) in drinking water treatment: A review. Water Res. 50: 318–340.

Reemtsma, T., S. Weiss, J. Mueller, M. Petrovic, S. González, D. Barcelo et al. 2006. Polar pollutants entry into the water cycle by municipal wastewater: a European perspective. Environ. Sci. Technol. 40(17): 5451–8.

Ricart, M., H. Guasch, M. Alberch, D. Barceló, C. Bonnineau, A. Geiszinger et al. 2010. Triclosan persistence through wastewater treatment plants and its potential toxic effects on river biofilms. Aquat. Toxicol. 100(4): 346–353.

RIWA. 2012. Evaluatie van de brede screening van stoffen in de Rijn bij Lobith (2010–2011). RIWA, Nieuwegein.

Rogers, H.R. 1996. Sources, behavior and fate of organic contaminants during sewage treatment and in sewage sludges. Sci. Total Environ. 185: 3–26.

Santos, L.H., A.N. Araújo, A. Fachini, A. Pena, C. Delerue-Matos and M.C. Montenegro. 2010. Ecotoxicological aspects related to the presence of pharmaceuticals in the aquatic environment. J. Hazard Mater. 175(1-3): 45–95.

Santos, P.S.M., E.B.H. Santos and A.C. Duarte. 2013. Seasonal and air mass trajectory effects on dissolved organic matter of bulk deposition at a coastal town in South-Western Europe. Environ. Sci. Pollut. Res. Int. 20(1): 227–237.

Schultz, M.M., C.P. Higgins, C.A. Huset, R.G. Luthy, D.F. Barofsky and J.A. Field. 2006. Fluorochemical mass flows in a municipal wastewater treatment facility. Environ. Sci. Technol. 40: 7350–7357.

Schwarzenbach, R.P., B.I. Escher, K. Fenner, T.B. Hofstetter, C.A. Johnson, U. Von Gunten et al. 2006. The challenge of micropollutants in aquatic systems. Science. 313(5790): 1072–1077.

Sepulvado, J.G., A.C. Blaine, L.S. Hundal and C.P. Higgins. 2011. Occurrence and fate of perfluorochemicals in soil following the land application of municipal biosolids. Environ. Sci. Technol. 45: 8106–8112.

Sifuna, F.W., F. Orata, V. Okello and S. Jemutai-Kimosop. 2016. Phosphate and sulfate supporting electrolytes comparative studies in electrochemical degradation of sulfamethoxazole and diclofenac in water using various electrodes. J. Environ. Sci. Health, Part A. 0: 1–8.

Sindiku, O., F. Orata, R. Weber and O. Osibanjo. 2013. Per- and polyfluoroalkyl substances in selected sewage sludge in Nigeria. Chemosphere. 92: 329–335.

Singhal, N. and O. Perez-Garcia. 2016. Degrading organic micropollutants: The next challenge in the evolution of biological wastewater treatment processes. Front. Ecol. Environ. 4. http://dx.doi.org/10.3389/fenvs.2016.00036.

Soares, A., B. Guieysse, B. Jefferson, E. Cartmell and J.N. Lester. 2008. Nonylphenol in the environment: A critical review on occurrence, fate, toxicity and treatment in wastewaters. Environ. Int. 34: 1033–1049.

Song, H., J.W. Addison, J. Hu and T. Karanfil. 2010. Halonitromethanes formation in wastewater treatment plant effluents. Chemosphere. 79(2): 174–9.

Stackelberg, P.E., E.T. Furlong, M.T. Meyer, S.D. Zaugg, A.K. Henderson and D.B. Reissman. 2004. Persistence of pharmaceutical compounds and other organic wastewater contaminants in a conventional drinking-water-treatment plant. Sci. Total Environ. 329: 99–113.

Staples, C.A., P.B. Dorn, G.M. Klecka, S.T. O'Block and L.R. Harris. 1998. A review of the environmental fate, effects, and exposures of bisphenol A. Chemosphere. 36: 2149.

Stasinakis, A.S. 2008. Use of selected Advanced Oxidation Processes (AOPs) for wastewater treatment—A mini review. Global NEST Journal. 10: 376–385.

Stasinakis, A.S., S. Kotsifa, G. Gatidou and D. Mamais. 2009. Diuron biodegradation in activated sludge batch reactors under aerobic and anoxic conditions. Water Res. 43(5): 1471–9.

Stasinakis, A.S., N.S. Thomaidis, O.S. Arvaniti, A.G. Asimakopoulos, V.G. Samaras, A. Ajibola et al. 2013. Contribution of primary and secondary treatment on the removal of benzothiazoles, benzotriazoles, endocrine disruptors, pharmaceuticals and perfluorinated compounds in a sewage treatment plant. Sci. Total Environ. 463-464: 1067–1075.

Stockholm Convention. 2001. UNEP, Stockholm Convention on Persistent Organic Pollutants, Secretariat of the Stockholm Convention Report No., Geneva, Switzerland. p. 43. http://chm.pops.int/Convention/tabid/54/language/en-US/Default.aspx.

Stockholm Convention. 2009. In: Report of the Conference of the Parties of the Stockholm Convention on Persistent Organic Pollutants on the Work of its Fourth Meeting. UNEP/POPS/COP.4/38, 8 May 2009.

Stockholm Convention. 2010. STARTUP GUIDANCE for the 9 New POPs (General Information, Implications of Listing, Information Sources and Alternatives), December 2010.

Suarez, S., J.M. Lema and F. Omil. 2010. Removal of Pharmaceutical and Personal Care Products (PPCPs) under nitrifying and denitrifying conditions. Water Res. 44(10): 3214–3224.

Swartz, C.H., S. Reddy, M.J. Benotti, H.F. Yin, L.B. Barber and B.J. Brownwell. 2006. Steroid oestrogens, nonylphenol ethoxylate metabolites, and other wastewater contaminants in groundwater effected by residential septic system on Cape Cod, MA. Environ. Sci. Technol. 40(16): 4894–4902.

Takatsuki, M., Y. Takayanagi and M. Kitano. 1995. An attempt to SAR of degradation. pp. 67–103. In: Peijnenburg, W.J.M. and W. Karcher (eds.). Proceedings of the Workshop, Quantitative Structure Activity Relationship of Biodegradation. National Institute of Public Health and Environmental Protection (RIVM), Bilthoven, The Netherlands.

Tetreault, G.R., C.J. Bennett, C. Cheng, M.R. Servos and M.E. McMaster. 2012. Reproductive and histopathological effects in wild fish inhabiting an effluent-dominated stream, Wascana Creek, SK, Canada. Aquat. Toxicol. 110-111: 149–161.

Tixier, C., H.P. Singer, S. Oellers and S.R. Müller. 2003. Occurrence and fate of carbamazepine, clofibric acid, diclofenac, ibuprofen, ketoprofen, and naproxen. Environ. Sci. Technol. 37: 1061–1068.

Togola, A. and H. Budzinski. 2008. Multi-residue analysis of pharmaceutical compounds in aqueous samples. J. Chromatogr. A. 1177: 150–158.

Tong, D.S., C.H. Zhou, Y. Lu, H. Yu, G.F. Zhang and W.H. Yu. 2010. Adsorption of acid red G dye on octadecyltrimethylammoniummontmorillonite. Appl. Clay Sci. 50: 427–431.

Treadgold, J. and Q.T. Liu. 2012. Pharmaceuticals and personal-care products. pp. 207–227. In: Plant, J.A., N. Voulvoulis and K.V. Ragnarsdottir (eds.). Pollutants, Human Health and the Environment: A Risk Based Approach, ISBN: 9780470742617.

Tunkel, J., P.H. Howard, R.S. Boethling, W. Stiteler and H. Loonen. 2000. Predicting ready biodegradability in the Japanese ministry of international trade and industry test. Environ. Toxicol. Chem. 19: 2478–2485.

van Beelen, E.S.E. 2007. Municipal waste water treatment plant (WWTP) effluents a concise overview of the occurrence of organic substances. RIWA, Rhine Water Works, the Netherlands, p. 34.

Venkatesan, K.A. and U.R. Halden. 2014. Wastewater treatment plants as chemical observatories to forecast ecological and human health risks of manmade chemicals. Sci. Rep. 4: 3731.

Verlicchi, P., M. Al Aukidy and E. Zambello. 2012. Occurrence of pharmaceutical compounds in Urban wastewater: removal, mass load and environmental risk after a secondary treatment—a review. Sci. Total Environ. 429: 123–155.

Vestergren, R., F. Orata, U. Berger and I.T. Cousins. 2013. Bioaccumulation of perfluoroalkyl acids in dairy cows in a naturally contaminated environment. Environ. Sci. Pollut. Res. 20(11): 7959–7969.

Washington, J.W., H. Yoo, J.J. Ellington, T.M. Jenkins and E.L. Libelo. 2010. Concentrations, distribution, and persistence of perfluoroalkylates in sludge applied soils near Decatur, Alabama, USA. Environ. Sci. Technol. 44: 8390–8396.

Westerhoff, P., Y. Yoon, S. Shane and E. Wert. 2005. Fate of endocrine-disruptor, pharmaceutical, and personal care product chemicals during simulated drinking water treatment processes. Environ. Sci. Technol. 39: 6649–6663.

WHO. 2008. Guideline for drinking water quality. Third edition, incorporating the first and second agenda. Volume 1: Recommendations. World Health Organization. Geneva. pp. 1–668.

Wille, K., F.H. De Brabander, E. De Wulf, P. Van Caeter, R.C. Janssen and L. Vanhaecke. 2012. Coupled chromatographic and mass-spectrometric techniques for the analysis of emerging pollutants in the aquatic environment. Trends Anal. Chem. 35: 87–108.

Wu, C., A.L. Sponberg, J.D. Witter, M. Fang and K.P. Czajkowski. 2010. Uptake of pharmaceuticals and personal care products by soybean plants from soils applied with biosolids and irrigated with contaminated water. Environ. Sci. Technol. 44(16): 6157–6161.

Wu, M., L. Wang, H. Xu and Y. Ding. 2013. Occurrence and removal efficiency of six polycyclic aromatic hydrocarbons in different wastewater treatment plants. Water Sci. Technol. 68(8): 1844 51.

Yamamoto, H., Y. Nakamura, C. Kitani, T. Imari and J. Sekizawa. 2007. Initial ecological risk assessment of eight selected human pharmaceuticals in Japan. Environ. Sci. 14: 177–93.

Yang, L., S. Chen, M. Hu, W. Hao, P. Geng and Y. Zhang. 2011. Biodegradation of carbofuran by Pichia anomala strain HQ-C-01 and its application for bioremediation of contaminated soils. Biol. Fertil. Soils. 47: 917–923.

Yu, J., C. He, X. Liu, J. Wu, Y. Hu and Y. Zhang. 2013. Removal of perfluorinated compounds by membrane bioreactor with powdered activated carbon (PAC): Adsorption onto sludge and PAC. Desalination. 334: 23–28.

12

Monitoring of Two Taste and Odor Causing Compounds in a Drinking Water Reservoir

Hongbo Liu,[1,][*] *Yanhua Li,*[1] *Ding Pan,*[1] *Dong Zhang,*[2] *Yueqing Jin*[3] and *Yonghong Liu*[4]

Introduction

Rapid development has been witnessed in the past decades in China; meanwhile, some environmental problems have also been encountered. One of the main issues is to guarantee the supply of drinking water for increasing urban residents. For example, Shanghai will lack drinking water by about 2.58 billion m^3/d in 2020, if no other water source is developed. Considering this situation, a new drinking water reservoir named Qingcaosha has been constructed in Shanghai, which takes water from the Yangtze River. The size of the reservoir is about 67 km^2, with an operational water depth of 8.6 m. It started to run in 2010 with a daily water supply of more than 7 million m^3 for Shanghai (Ping 2009).

Shanghai is located in the Yangtze River estuary. Due to domestic and industrial pollution of the upper reaches, the average concentrations of total nitrogen (TN)

---

[1] School of Environment and Architecture, University of Shanghai for Science and Technology, 200093 Shanghai China.
[2] National Engineering Research Center of China (South) for Urban Water Development and Utilization 200082 Shanghai China.
[3] China-Singapore Suzhou Industrial Park Environmental technology Co., Ltd., 215000, Suzhou China.
[4] Qingyuan-HongKong & China Water Co. Ltd., 215000, Suzhou China.
[*] Corresponding author: Liuhb@usst.edu.cn

and total phosphorus (TP) are more than 1 mg/L and 0.1 mg/L, respectively. The risk of algae bloom would be stimulated when the water comes into the reservoir and is stored for more than 15 days as in this study (Qin et al. 2014, Tew et al. 2014, Welker et al. 2003, Wood et al. 2010). This increases the worries of algae related water quality problems such as taste and odor (T & O) causing compounds and microcystins (Isaacs et al. 2014, Pawlik-Skowronska et al. 2004, Pestana et al. 2014, Vieira et al. 2005, Wang et al. 2002, Zhang et al. 2010).

Among the T & O causing compounds, 2-methylisoborneol (MIB) and geosmin (GSM) are two model algal-derived odorants that can induce olfactory problems in rivers and lakes, especially when the water is serving as drinking water sources, landscaping, irrigation and other functions (Choi ct al. 2010, Qi et al. 2009, Tung et al. 2008). Reported olfactory threshold is 6–8 ng/L (Salto et al. 2008, Zhang et al. 2010). The quality standard for MIB and GSM specified by the Chinese drinking water standard is less than 10 ng/L.

In this context, the study aims to determine two model odorants, MIB and GSM, in a large and shallow reservoir to improve the safety of drinking water for Shanghai. Spatial and seasonal distribution of the two model compounds were also investigated using the two-year field data; the role of wind in MIB and GSM occurrence was also investigated.

Materials and Methods

Sampling stations

The sampling stations (shown in Fig. 1) are selected as follows: 10 stations inside the reservoir (S1-10) and one outside the reservoir (near the Inlet). Sampling stations inside the reservoir are spatially distributed as reservoir head (S1), island area (S2-4), middle of reservoir (S5-7), rear of reservoir (S8-9) and the pump station area (S10, for raw water). Vertically, 1–3 samples were taken for each station according to water depth. The specific sampling scheme in vertical direction for each station are as follows: the sampling point is chosen as 0.5 meters from the surface when the water depth is not greater than 5 meters (S1-3, S5, S7); the sampling points are chosen as 0.5 meters from the surface and 0.5 meters from the bottom, respectively, when the water depth is greater than 5 meters but not greater than 10 meters (S4, S8, S10); the sampling points are chosen as 0.5 meters from the surface, middle of water depth and 0.5 meters from the bottom, respectively, when the water depth is greater than 10 meters (S6, S9). Water depth of the sampling station outside the reservoir is influenced by tide; contents of the two odorants under both higher and lower tide conditions were sampled and analyzed. Sampling and monitoring frequency in this study was twice a month in summer and once a month in other seasons. The monitoring frequency is going to increase when large scale algae growth occurs.

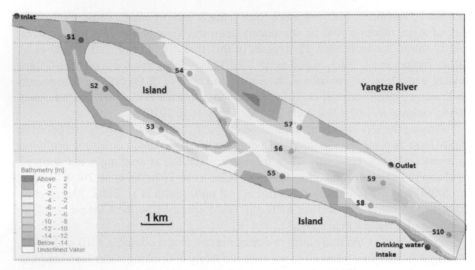

Fig. 1. Profile of the studied reservoir and sampling stations.

Analytical Method

Determination of MIB and GSM

MIB and GSM are determined with HSPME+GC-MS method. The whole analysis was conducted in Agilent 6890/5975 GC/MS system (Agilent, USA). The separation of two odorants was carried out on a HP-5ms (30 m × 0.25 mm × 0.25 μm) column. A SUPELCO HSPME instrument equipped with DVB/Carbone/PDM fiber was used in the study for the HSPME procedure.

Sample preparation: a micro magnetic rotor was put into a 40 ml vial filled with 25 ml water sample, and then 6.25 g of NaCl was dosed and dissolved in the water sample. The vial was sealed immediately with silicone rubber cap coated with PTME. The water sample was then heated to 65°C and maintained. The stainless steel needle was pierced into the silicone rubber pad gently and was moved into the extraction vial before the fiber inside was pushed into the headspace. The magnetic stirring speed was fixed as 200–250 rpm and the speed was maintained for 30 min, during which process the target odorant was extracted into the fiber for analyzing with GC/MS.

The following were GC-MS conditions: the electronic energy was 70 eV, the electron multiplier voltage was 824 V, the head pressure was 50 Kpa, the transmission line temperature was 280°C, and the ion source temperature was 230°C. The temperature program for GC was set as follows: the initial temperature was set as 40°C and holds for 2 min, after which the temperature rises to 240°C with a rate of 10°C/min, and then holds for 3 min. The total temperature program lasts for 25 min. Samples were injected splitless using selected ion mode. Characteristic ions for MIB and GSM are m/z (95, 107, 108) and m/z (112, 111, 125) with m/z 95 and m/z 112 as quantitative ions, respectively.

Determination of general water quality parameters

Total organic carbon (TOC) was determined by a TOC/TN_b analyzer (Multi N/C 3100). Algal density was counted by a Hemocytometer using the microscope technology. The other parameters were determined by standard methods (American Public Health Association (APHA) 1998).

Results and Discussion

Water quality in the reservoir

Water quality, both inside and outside the reservoir after two years of field monitoring, is illustrated in Table 1. The turbidity has been significantly reduced due to precipitation of particulate pollutants inside the reservoir. Although TN and TP were also significantly reduced in the reservoir due to precipitation and other processes such as nutrient uptake by planktons, their concentrations are still much higher than the threshold values triggering eutrophication (Guildford and Hecky 2000, Huang and Zhao 2012). Abundant nutrient, proper temperature and the weak hydraulic conditions inside the reservoir make its algae density almost 10 times higher than outside the reservoir. When the algae density reaches 2 million individual/L (ind./L), the risk of algae derived microcystins as well as occurrence of T & O events is reported to be very high (CAO et al. 2005, Srinivasan and Sorial 2011). Since MIB and GSM are two major algal derived odorants that can induce olfactory problems in water bodies, it is necessary to determine their contents in the studied reservoir.

Table 1. Major water quality parameters both inside and outside the reservoir.

Parameters	Inside the reservoir	Outside the reservoir
TOC (mg/L)	2.38–2.80	3.50–4.19
UV_{254} (cm^{-1})	0.036–0.047	0.044–0.054
Turbidity (NTU)	3.2–14.2	50–100
TN (mg/L)	0.285–0.446	1.71–1.85
NH_3-N (mg/L)	0.077–0.115	0.12–0.25
NO_3-N (mg/L)	0.070–0.167	1.423–1.632
TP	0.03–0.05	0.09–0.11
PO_4^{3-}-P (mg/L)	0.01–0.04	0.02–0.05
Algae density (ind./L)	1–30 million[a]	0.2–2 million[b]

[a] 8–30 million in warmer seasons (June–September); 1–4 million in other seasons
[b] 1–2 million in warmer seasons (June–September); 0.2–1 million in other seasons

Screen of MIB and GSM determination methods

Reported literature mainly used an internal standard method to determine MIB and GSM with response factors to quantify contents of the odorant and standard deviations to determine accuracy of the tests (Fujise et al. 2010, Salto et al. 2008, Zuo et al. 2009). However, the external standard method has the advantages of intuitive quantization and easier data validation. The internal standard method uses Equation 1 for quantization while the external standard method uses standard curve for quantization.

$$C = (A_x)(C_{is})/(RF) \tag{1}$$

Where:

C: Concentration of odorants, ng/L;

A_x: peak area of the target ions;

A_{is}:   peak area of the internal quantitative ion;

C_{is}:   concentration of the internal standard, ng/L;

RF: average responding of the target odorants.

Both quantitative methods were used for comparison in this study by determining MIB and GSM contents of the same serial of standards; concentration of the serial standards were 5, 10, 20, 50, 100 and 200 ng/L, respectively.

(1) The internal standard method

Quantitative parameters of the internal standard method are listed in Table 2. The internal standard is IBMD (2-isopropyl-3-methoxypyrazine). SD (Standard derivation) of responding factors for MIB and GSM are very close (2%), while the RSD (relative standard derivation) of responding factor for MIB is 9.3%, which is much higher than that for GSM, i.e., 5.2%.

Table 2. Quantitative parameters of the internal standard method.

Concentration of standards (ng/L)	Peak area			Responding factor	
	IBMD	MIB	GSM	RF (MIB)	RF (GSM)
5	69342	3845	7892	0.221799198	0.455250786
10	68209	6225	13837	0.182527232	0.405723585
20	67110	13742	27523	0.204768291	0.410117717
50	70899	33643	72325	0.189808037	0.408045247
100	76443	66552	163582	0.174121895	0.427984250
200	74515	15184	336349	0.212284775	0.451384285
		SD (RF)		0.01839423	0.022309703
Statistical parameters		Average (RF)		0.197551571	0.426417645
		RSD (%)		9.3%	5.2%

(2) The external standard method

Quantitative curve for the external standard method is derived from the same standard serial spikes as in the internal standard quantification method. Calibration curve for MIB and GSM were shown in equations 2–3. Square values of the linear regression quotient (R^2) are 0.9936 and 0.9988 for MIB and GSM, respectively.

MIB	$Y = 0.0013X + 3.5767$	$R^2 = 0.9936$	(2)
GSM	$Y = 0.0006 X + 2.4898$	$R^2 = 0.9988$	(3)

Where

    X: peak area of the internal quantitative ion;

    Y: concentration of MIB and GSM, ng/L.

The recovery rates of spike tests for both internal and external standard methods are listed in Table 3. Table 3 shows that the recovery rate of the internal standard method is higher than the external standard method. Thus the internal standard method is employed in this work.

Leaving the shortcomings on the parameters mentioned aside, however, the external method was also proved to be a viable quantification method as a monitoring case in July 2010. The MIB and GSM contents both inside and outside the reservoir were determined using the established external standard method in July 2010; the results are shown in Table 4. The results are proved to be consistent with actual T & O reports by the drinking water plants during the same period. The major odorant was MIB both inside and outside the reservoir. MIB contents in S2, S10 (bottom) and Inlet (lower tide) in July 2010 were higher than 8 ng/L, which was higher than

Table 3. The recovery rates of spike adding tests for both internal and external standard method.

Item		Concentration in the reservoir water (ng/L)	Concentration of spikes (ng/L)	Concentration after spikes (ng/L)	Recovery rate (%)
Internal standard method	MIB	5.6	5.0	10.6	100.1
		5.6	10.0	17.1	109.7
		5.6	15.0	24.5	118.9
	GSM	2.1	5.0	6.9	98.0
		2.1	10.0	13.2	109.2
		2.1	15.0	19.6	114.9
External standard method	MIB	5.7	5.0	10.7	99.9
		5.7	10.0	12.9	81.9
		5.7	15.0	15.9	76.7
	GSM	2.6	5.0	7.1	94.2
		2.6	10.0	9.9	78.6
		2.6	15.0	12.5	71.5

Table 4. MIB and GSM contents of the reservoir water in July 2010.

Samples	MIB (ng/L)	GSM (ng/L)
S1-surface	ND[a]	0.34
S2-surface	9	0.74
S3-surface	6.92	0.35
S4-surface	6.65	0.2
S4-bottom	7.91	0.25
S5-surface	4.65	0.65
S6-surface	0	0.69
S6-middle	6.2	0.23
S6-bottom	7.79	2.15
S8-surface	11.35	1.63
S8-bottom	5.25	2.02
S10-surface	5.72	0.92
S10-bottom	8.1	1.16
Inlet (Lower tide)	9.72	2.42
Inlet (Higher tide)	7.60	2.40

ND[a] = not detected

the risk threshold concentration specified by reports (Lin et al. 2009, Matsui et al. 2010), while MIB contents in S8 was even higher than that specified by the Chinese drinking water standard (10 ng/L).

Spatial distribution of MIB and GSM in the reservoir

MIB and GSM were continuously detected during the whole monitoring period. Generally, GSM concentrations were lower than 10 ng/L from July 2010 to July 2012 (Fig. 4), while MIB concentrations varied dramatically, especially during warm months. For example, MIB concentration reached more than 30 ng/L in summer and autumn in 2011 (Fig. 3), while in majority of the monitoring period, MIB concentrations were lower than 30 ng/L from July 2010 to July 2012. Spatial distribution of MIB and GSM along the reservoir from July 2010 to February 2011 are illustrated in Fig. 2, where the reservoir head is represented by S1, island area by S3, middle of reservoir by S5, rear of reservoir by S8, the pump station area (for raw water) by S10 and outside the reservoir by the Inlet. Figure 2A illustrates that MIB and GSM outside the reservoir was 0.2 times higher than specified by the Chinese drinking water standard in July 2010; and the level of MIB and GSM follows the order, the rear of the reservoir > island area > the pump station area. MIB contents in December 2010 decreased to below the standard level (Fig. 2B); the algae density kept dropping because of the low temperature during the time. Figure 2C

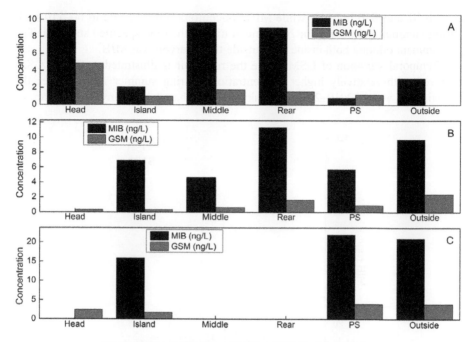

Fig. 2. Spatial distributions of MIB and GSM in the reservoir.

indicated that MIB was much higher than specified by the Chinese standard outside the reservoir in February 2011, which increased MIB levels inside the reservoir, especially in the area near the island and the pump station and brought about risk of T & O events for drinking water plants. It can be extrapolated form the Fig. 2 that the reasons for the spatial distributions of MIB and GSM were far more complicated. First, algal derived compounds are the main cause of odorants. Water temperature varied during months, and the light intensity changed in different months; these are the two essentially important factors of algal growth, which directly influence the distributions of MIB and GSM. Besides, hydrodynamic environment around the algal community also impacts a lot. More details about the variations of MIB and GSM in this newly constructed reservoir, such as algal density and nutrients, are shown in the reported article of Liu (Liu et al. 2015).

Table 4 also indicates that MIB and GSM contents at the bottom of water column were higher than at the surface with S8 as an exception, which could be explained by algae decay and fungus activities from the sediment that induced odor releasing (Chen et al. 2010, Eaton and Sandusky 2009, Fujise et al. 2010, Srinivasan and Sorial 2011, Zuo et al. 2010).

Seasonal variation of MIB and GSM

Figure 3 showed seasonal variation of MIB concentrations at the head and the rear positions of the reservoir (S1 and S10) in 2011. The MIB concentration was less than 10 ng/L specified by the Chinese drinking water standard during spring and winter at both S1 and S10 in 2011, while MIB concentration reached up to 60–110 ng/L during summer and autumn in 2011, much higher than the specified standard. The predominant odorant both inside and outside the reservoir was MIB.

Temporal variation of GSM inside the reservoir is illustrated in Fig. 4. GSM occurred with relatively higher concentrations during summer months over the investigated years (2010–2012), a risky period shared by many other lakes or

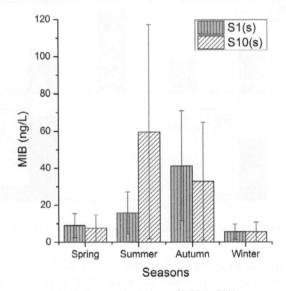

Fig. 3. Seasonal variations of MIB in 2011.

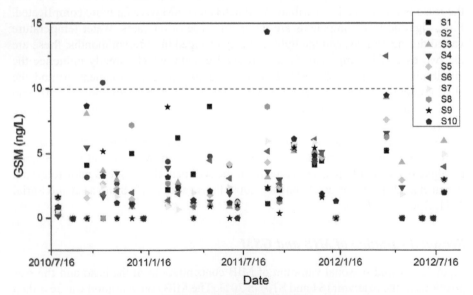

Fig. 4. Seasonal variation of GSM.

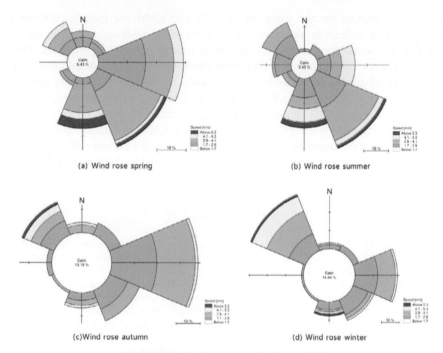

(a) Wind rose spring (b) Wind rose summer

(c)Wind rose autumn (d) Wind rose winter

Fig. 5. Seasonal wind rose profiles in year 2011.

reservoirs (Anderson and Quartermaine 1998). Spatial distribution of GSM varied with temporal changes. During the warmer months, GSM concentrations in S10 (the rear part of the reservoir) and S2 (shallow area near the island) were much higher than at other locations, which could be explained by weak hydrodynamic conditions that tended to enhance phytoplankton growth in warm months and thus increase secondary algal metabolites such as MIB and GSM (Barr et al. 2008).

Seasonal variations of GSM were apparently associated with the water temperature and light intensity. In spring and winter, algal growth was maintained at a low level due to the restrictions of soft light and low temperature, which led to a low MIB level. In summer and autumn, due to the strong light and high temperature, MIB concentration increased intensely. Wind also played an important role in influencing MIB and GSM occurrence. Figure 5 indicates that the prevailing wind directions are SE (southeast) and S (south) near the reservoir, while in the autumn, the prevailing wind directions are NW (northwest) and E (east), which explained the different MIB and GSM levels between S1 and S10, both in the summer and in the autumn of 2011. In spring and winter, influence of wind was insignificant as the original MIB concentration was also low.

Conclusions

Compared to external method, MIB and GSM are more scientific to be quantified by the internal standard method. As these two odors mainly results from algal derived compounds, reasons for the variation of MIB and GSM are mainly ascribed to the factors that influences algal growth. In the studied reservoir, wind as well as hydrodynamic conditions played an important role in influencing MIB and GSM occurrence, while temperature and light were two essential factors. Algal growth rate was maintained at a low level due to the restrictions of soft light and low temperature during spring and winter when MIB and GSM was kept at lower level, while in summer and autumn, MIB concentration increased intensely up to 60 ng/L, mainly due to the strong light and high temperature. Besides,MIB and GSM in influent of the reservoir was 0.2 times higher than that specified by the Chinese drinking water standard; therefore, there was a probability of risk caused by MIB and GSM inside the reservoir.

References

American Public Health Association (APHA), American Water Works Association (AWWA), Water Environment Federation (WEFW) 1998. Standard Methods for the Examination of Water and Wastewater. Washington, DC.

Anderson, B.C. and L.K. Quartermaine. 1998. Tastes and odors in kingston's municipal drinking water: A case study of the problem and appropriate solutions. Journal of Great Lakes Research. 24: 859–867.

Barr, N., A. Kloe, T. Rees, C. Scherer, R. Taylor and A. Wenzel. 2008. Wave surge increases rates of growth and nutrient uptake in the green seaweed Ulva pertusa maintained at low bulk flow velocities. Aquatic Biology. 3: 179–186.

Cao, X.H., G.Y. Liu, D.M. Wang and Y. An. 2005. Monitoring and control of algae toxins in surface water. Energy Research and Information. 21: 192–196.

Chen, Y.M., P. Hobson, M.D. Bruch and T.F. Lin. 2010. *In situ* measurement of odor compound production by benthic cyanobacteria. Journal of Environmental Monitoring. 12: 769–775.

Choi, Y., H. Oh, S. Lee, Y. Choi, T. Hwang, J. Jeon et al. 2010. Removal of taste and odor model compounds (2-MIB and geosmin) with the NF membrane. Desalination and Water Treatment. 15: 141–148.

Eaton, R.W. and P. Sandusky. 2009. Biotransformations of 2-methylisoborneol by camphor-degrading bacteria. Applied and Environmental Microbiology. 75: 583–588.

Fujise, D., K. Tsuji, N. Fukushima, K. Kawai and K. Harada. 2010. Analytical aspects of cyanobacterial volatile organic compounds for investigation of their production behavior. Journal of Chromatography A. 1217: 6122–6125.

Guildford, S.J. and R.E. Hecky. 2000. Total nitrogen, total phosphorus, and nutrient limitation in lakes and oceans: Is there a common relationship? Limnology and Oceanography. 45: 1213–1223.

Huang, W. and L.J. Zhao. 2012. Identification model of significant impact factors for cyanobacterial bloom. Journal of University of Shanghai for Science and Technology. 34: 435–440.

Isaacs, D.J., W.K. Strangman, A.E. Barbera, M.A. Mallin, M.R. McIver and J.L.C. Wright. 2014. Microcystins and two new micropeptin cyanopeptides produced by unprecedented *Microcystis aeruginosa* blooms in North Carolina's Cape Fear River. Harmful Algae. 31: 82–86.

Lin, T.F., D.W. Chang, L. Shaokai, T. Yunshen, C. Yiting and Y.S. Wang. 2009. Effect of chlorination on the cell integrity of two noxious cyanobacteria and their releases of odorants. Journal of Water Supply Research and Technology-Aqua. 58: 539–551.

Liu, H., D. Pan, M. Zhu and D. Zhang. 2015. Occurrence and emergency response of 2-methylisoborneol and geosmin in a large shallow drinking water reservoir. CLEAN—Soil, Air, Water. n/a–n/a.

Matsui, Y., Y. Nakano, H. Hiroshi, N. Ando and T. Matsushita. 2010. Geosmin and 2-methylisoborneol adsorption on super-powdered activated carbon in the presence of natural organic matter. Water Science and Technology. 62: 2664–2668.

Pawlik-Skowronska, B., T. Skowronski, J. Pirszel and A. Adamczyk. 2004. Relationship between cyanobacterial bloom composition and anatoxin-A and microcystin occurrence in the eutrophic dam reservoir (SE Poland). Polish Journal of Ecology. 52: 479–490.

Pestana C.J, P.K.J. Robertson, C. Edwards, W. Wilhelm, C. McKenzie and L.A. Lawton. 2014. A continuous flow packed bed photocatalytic reactor for the destruction of 2-methylisoborneol and geosmin utilising pelletised TiO$_2$. Chemical Engineering Journal. 235: 293–298.

Ping, L.-S., UNEP Environmental Assessment, EXPO 2010, Shanghai, China. Produced by the UNEP Division of Communications and Public Information, China, 2009.

Qi, F., B.B. Xu, Z.L. Chen, J. Ma, D.Z. Sun and L.Q. Zhang. 2009. Efficiency and products investigations on the ozonation of 2-methylisoborneol in drinking water. Water Environment Research. 81: 2411–2419.

Qin, H.P., S.T. Khu and C. Li. 2014. Water exchange effect on eutrophication in landscape water body supplemented by treated wastewater. Urban Water Journal. 11: 108–115.

Saito, K., K. Okamura and H. Kataoka. 2008. Determination of musty odorants, 2-methylisoborneol and geosmin, in environmental water by headspace solid-phase microextraction and gas chromatography-mass spectrometry. Journal of Chromatography A. 1186: 434–437.

Srinivasan, R. and G.A. Sorial. 2011. Treatment of taste and odor causing compounds 2-methyl isoborneol and geosmin in drinking water: A critical review. Journal of Environmental Sciences. 23: 1–13.

Tew, K.S., P.J. Meng, D.C. Glover, J.T. Wang, M.Y. Leu and C.C. Chen. 2014. Characterising and predicting algal blooms in a subtropical coastal lagoon. Marine and Freshwater Research. 65: 191–197.

Tung, S.C., T.F. Lin, F.C. Yang and C.L. Liu. 2008. Seasonal change and correlation with environmental parameters for 2-MIB in Feng-Shen Reservoir, Taiwan. Environmental Monitoring and Assessment. 145: 407–416.

Vieira, J.M.D.S., M.T.D.P. Azevedo, R.Y. Honda and B. Correa. 2005. Toxic cyanobacteria and microcystin concentrations in a public water supply reservoir in the Brazilian Amazonia region. Toxicon. 45: 901–909.

Wang, X.F., Preeda Parkpian, Naoshi Fujimoto, K. Mathurosruchirawat, R.D. Delaune and A. Jugsujinda. 2002. Environmental conditions associating microcystins production to Microcystis aeruginosa in a reservoir of Thailand. Journal of Environmental Science and Health Part a-Toxic/Hazardous Substances & Environmental Engineering. 37: 1181–1207.

Welker, M., H. Tauscher, S. Cew and M. Erhard. 2003. Toxic microcystis in shallow lake Muggelsee (Germany)—dynamics, distribution, diversity. Archiv. Fur Hydrobiologie. 157: 227–248.

Wood, S.A., M.J. Prentice, K. Smith and D.P. Hamilton. 2010. Low dissolved inorganic nitrogen and increased heterocyte frequency: precursors to Anabaena planktonica blooms in a temperate, eutrophic reservoir. Journal of Plankton Research. 32: 1315–1325.

Zhang, T., L. Li, Y.X. Zuo, Q. Zhou and L.R. Song. 2010. Biological origins and annual variations of earthy-musty off-flavours in the Xionghe Reservoir in China. Journal of Water Supply Research and Technology-Aqua. 59: 243–254.

Zuo, Y.X., L. Li, Z.X. Wu, L.R. Song and M. Suffet. 2009. Isolation, identification and odour-producing abilities of geosmin/2-MIB in actinomycetes from sediments in Lake Lotus, China. Journal of Water Supply Research and Technology-Aqua. 58: 552–561.

Zuo, Y., L. Li, T. Zhang, L. Zheng, G. Dai, L.M. Song et al. 2010. Contribution of Streptomyces in sediment to earthy odor in the overlying water in Xionghe Reservoir, China. Water Research. 44: 6085–6094.

13

Biomarkers of Susceptibility for Human Exposure to Environmental Contaminants

Thaís de A. Pedrete* and *Josino C. Moreira*

Introduction

Life is a complex and risky process. It is necessary to understand and consider its complexity and risks in order to improve human well-being.

Risk can be defined as a threat from either an identified hazard to which a significant exposure may occur or from an unexpected new hazard or increased significant exposure and/or susceptibility to a known hazard. A process called risk assessment (RA) was developed with the aim of decreasing and/or eliminating risks, and is defined as an estimate of the probability of risk to individuals or populations associated with that hazard (Park and Choi 2009).

Thus, risk can be expressed by the following equation:

$$Risk = Hazard \times Exposure \times Susceptibility \qquad (1)$$

Hazard identification is one of the first steps of this methodology, and is usually readily available. Specifically in the case of hazardous chemicals, knowledge regarding the exposure assessment and toxicological properties of a certain substance are essential for a RA process. Exposure assessment requires the understanding of hazard routes (such as air, water, food, soil, and workstations), frequency and

Escola Nacional de Saúde Pública, Fundação Oswaldo Cruz, Rua Leopoldo Bulhões, 1480, Manguinhos, CEP: 21041-210, Rio de Janeiro, RJ, Brazil.
 E-mail: josinocm@fiocruz.br
* Corresponding author: tha.pedrete@gmail.com

duration of exposure and the evaluation of the probability of any adverse effect. Although RA is most often based on cause-effect and dose-response data (Park and Choi 2009), workers and the general population are frequently exposed not only to an isolated substance but to complex mixtures. The possible interactions of components of these mixtures (e.g., addictive, synergistic or antagonistic actions) increases the complexity of a risk assessment determination even more (DeBord et al. 2015, Park and Choi 2009).

In addition to risk assessments, it is also very important to develop risk management and risk communication procedures, thereby providing a scientific basis to support decision-making in risk management. This aids in determining the means of eliminating or controlling exposure in any unsafe situation (DeBord et al. 2015). However, even under risk management policies, unexpected toxicity and adverse events can be observed generally in hypersensitive individuals or in a relatively small, undetected, susceptible population group (Lin and Chen 2012). These susceptible groups must be considered in risk assessments in order to improve the effectiveness of any risk management policy. However, the most difficult component of the risk equation to evaluate is indeed, susceptibility, which is generally set aside.

Once the basis of our understanding of effective risk assessment is ascertained, an important question that should be answered is, how do we identify these susceptible groups? The answer to this question is not easy because, usually, several of these health effects are complex and may have multifactorial causes. New strategies for risk assessment have been described to enable more accurate assessments and to prevent or avoid any adverse effect, evaluating individual responses through the increased use of more elaborated biomonitoring procedures (DeBord et al. 2015). Thus, RA can now improve dose-response estimations and measure the severity of human exposure to chemicals, their potential biochemical effects, and individual susceptibility. Identification of specific biomarkers, however, is necessary for improving diagnostics and risk prediction assessments. Biomonitoring approaches and, especially, the use of "omics" technologies are, increasingly, being used to achieve more precise exposure assessments, allowing simultaneous measurement of macromolecules such as DNA, RNA, and proteins biomarkers. The set of data obtained from "omics" approaches are providing new insights on modes of action and dose-response relationships (DeBord et al. 2015).

Monitoring Tools, Susceptibility and Biomarkers

Humans are continuously exposed to a diversity of chemical threats, some of them with carcinogenic and/or mutagenic properties, which may significantly contribute to the causation of some human cancers or other chronic diseases. The full understanding of the potential implications of various levels of exposure in both occupation and environmental settings, and the identification of population subgroups with increased susceptibility to such exposure are of great importance to public health.

Measurements of the concentrations of chemical substances in human body fluids and tissues, known as biomonitoring, have been frequently applied in various health inquiries, leading to a rise in knowledge on the effects and mechanisms of human exposure to chemical substances, improving human health risk assessments through investigation of relations among low-level exposures, adverse health effects and potentially vulnerable population groups. On the other hand, the use of such data creates a number of challenges, since it often deals with non-homogeneous results. Therefore, increased attention has been given to personalized exposure information, in which specific adverse health effects are attributed to environmental exposure to chemicals at individual level (Boogaard and Money 2008). However, further studies are necessary to define how biomarkers of effect and susceptibility could be reliably inserted in individual risk assessments.

The need to include complex interactions between environmental exposures and genetic factors in these studies has been increasingly acknowledged, since environmental elements not only interact with genes and damaged DNA but may also modulate genetic effects and influence phenotypes and alter gene expression through epigenetic mechanisms that could be reversible (Spitz and Bondy 2009).

Although experimental studies are ideal for evaluating biological processes, these usually do not take into account the etiology of health problems. Intrinsic factors like diet, aging, exposure history, genetic susceptibility and health status can influence the toxicity of chemicals and individual responses to these compounds (Boogaard and Money 2008). In addition, other factors can significantly affect the use of experimental data for health risk assessments, such as target organ responses, extrapolation from experimental dose to human exposure conditions, interactions with other toxic chemicals and, differences in exposure conditions (e.g., chronic and acute exposures, inhalation and ingestion, among others). Taken together, this will be useful to identify information gaps and prioritize topics for investigation, improving the knowledge in the environmental health and toxicology fields (Au et al. 2002).

Fields of knowledge that generate information about the genome (such as toxicogenomics) are being increasingly used to investigate changes in gene expression and proteins following exposure to chemicals, increasing our knowledge in toxicological mechanisms and modes of action. Also, these fields would enhance the identification and characterization of sensitive life stages, subpopulations and individuals. One possibility involves molecular fingerprinting, a way of encoding the structure of a molecule that allows the determination of the degree of similarity between two molecules, which can be used to categorize chemicals and mixtures into different modes of action groups, contributing to the understanding of effects regarding different levels of dose exposure (Oberemm et al. 2005).

Recently, several authors have also discussed the application of systems biology to address risk assessment issues. Sauer et al. (2015) established that there is a need for more predictive and accurate approaches to risk assessment requiring a mechanistic understanding of the process by which a xenobiotic perturbs biological systems. Sauer et al. (2016) recommend that the use of systems toxicology with advanced analytical and computational tools should be integrated with classical toxicology. They also suggest that quantitative analysis of large networks of molecular and functional changes occurring across multiple levels of biological organization should be carried out. In this context, Wetmore and Merrick (2004) defended the toxicoproteomic approach, which is positioned towards an expanded understanding of protein expression during toxicity and environmentally-induced disease, for the advancement of public health. Titz et al. (2014) point out the fact that protein alterations could be a close reflection of biological effects and Sturla et al. (2014) discuss the identification of how biological networks are perturbed by exposure to xenobiotic and enable the development of predictive mathematical models of toxicological processes.

Clearly, the use of systems biology/toxicology will produce a great amount of data facilitating a more complete understanding of the overall biological processes. However, in order for this data to be used for risk assessment in a significant number of persons, the cost will be very high. Hence, the identification of susceptibility biomarkers could provide the development of cheap and useful tools that can be applied worldwide (Pedrete et al. 2016).

In this regard, studies of individual susceptibility to toxicants, gene gene and gene-environment interactions have emerged as important components of molecular epidemiology, which has established molecular markers for most chronic diseases of public health importance (Dougherty et al. 2008, Thier et al. 2003). In human health risk assessment, the phenotypes/genotypes should be evaluated in a characterized population in relation to environmental exposures and it might be considered how these phenotypes/genotypes affect the xenobiotic biotransformation or the disease processes (Thier et al. 2003). Regarding these facts, the combination of classical toxicology and epidemiology provides information for scientific risk assessments and will improve the understanding of more complex gene-environment interactions and their role in human health (Fig. 1).

Research employing molecular biomarkers suggest that individuals may differ in their susceptibility to xenobiotic induced diseases, and genetic polymorphisms may contribute to this variability (Orphanides and Kimber 2003). Thus, a better understanding of genomic expression will enable a greater insight into variability in susceptibility to chemical exposure (Oberemm et al. 2005, Wogan et al. 2004). In addition, the use of increasingly accurate biological-based markers of exposure,

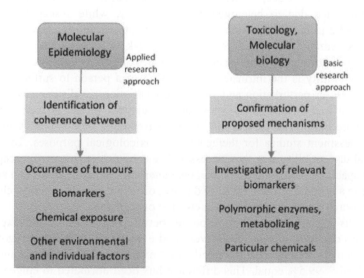

Fig. 1. Different approaches for risk assessments to human exposure.

intermediate effect, outcome, and susceptibility and their correlations will facilitate the process of identification of variants that act as effect modifiers. For this, new paradigms for interdisciplinary research that involve large-scale studies and the development of an integrated database that links new findings on exposures, etiologic pathways, relevant genes, proteins and their polymorphisms and functions will be required. This integrated database would guide the design of new studies as well as data analysis and interpretation of results (Boffetta and Islami 2013).

In this regard, environmental toxicology has been revealed to be an important tool to link polymorphisms to susceptibility to cancer and other adverse health outcomes related to occupational or environmental exposure (Ginsberg et al. 2010). Polymorphisms are a potential source of interindividual variability in internal dose of a parent compound or its active metabolites and, thus, may affect the distribution of risk across the population. Nevertheless, there is a lack of genotype-phenotype information of these polymorphisms for risk assessment that can be incorporated into pharmacokinetic/dynamic predictive models. In fact, genes involved in response of an individual to chemical agent can also be polymorphic (Ginsberg et al. 2010), altering the pharmacodynamics of a chemical substance, indicating that genes are responsible for xenobiotic metabolism and cellular defense, which can be polymorphic in the same individual, leading to a cumulative impact on biological response.

To address susceptibility to environmental stressors, it is important to take into account individual variability. With emerging molecular techniques, it is possible to acquire new understanding of inherent differences among people, which can then be used to predict how they differ in susceptibility to environmental stressors improving the accuracy of risk assessments in a public health context.

But, what is this susceptibility after all?

It is easy to mix up susceptibility with variability and/or vulnerability. Variability is the difference due to heterogeneity or diversity, while susceptibility is the capacity to be affected. Variation in risk reflects susceptibility. According to the National Research Council (2009), individual risk will depend on the person's characteristics prior to exposure, such as age, genetic attributes and sex. On the other hand, vulnerability is the intrinsic predisposition of a person to suffer harm from external stress or perturbation and is based on variations in disease susceptibility, psychological and social factors, exposures, and adaptive measures to anticipate and reduce future harm. The recognition of such susceptible groups is very important in risk assessment studies for therapeutic or toxicological purposes. To evaluate individual susceptibility, it is, thus, necessary to establish biomarkers of susceptibility that are capable of indicating the natural characteristics of an organism that are more sensitive to a specific adverse effect or disease, or responsive to a specific chemical/drug exposure (e.g., polymorphisms in enzyme or carriers).

There is a great variability in responses between individuals when exposed to a hazardous chemical at same dose levels, and even twins (mono or dizygotic) and isogenic animals may respond differently after exposure to a xenobiotic, since their DNA is "only" 99.5% equal. This difference has been attributed to epigenetic and environmental factors (Bell and Spector 2011). It is apparently clear that chromosomal DNA alone cannot completely determine the susceptibility of an individual. DNA interacts with the environment and this interaction can predispose or protect the organism from a disease or other health hazards (Turner 2009, Wong et al. 2005). Furthermore, individual responses can also differ in chronic diseases such as cancer and neurodegenerative and cardiovascular disorders, which have been investigated and also related to genetic variability.

In fact, susceptibility results from complex interactions, among several factors. In addition to genetic factors, experiments in animals reveal that 20–30% of observed individual differences are due to environmental influences, while the remaining 70–80% are attributed to a third component, creating biological random variability. This is the most important component of the phenotypic random variability, fixing its range and dominating the genetic and the environmental component (Gärtner 2012, Wong et al. 2005).

It is important to state that a particular cellular environment is determined by the physiology and metabolism of the entire organism and of the cells in their immediate neighborhood (Turner 2009). Signals from this local environment lead to gene expression appropriate for replication, differentiation, quiescence, or apoptotic death, depending on the cell type and developmental context (Turner 2009). In humans, cells are genetically homogeneous but can be structurally and functionally diverse, owing to different gene expression. Therefore, identification of the proteins produced by these different tissues or group of cells may be an important tool to understand the complex cellular processes or even the impact of a toxicant on an exposed organism (Jaenisch and Bird 2003).

Biomarkers

Biomonitoring is a tool to evaluate chemical exposure and/or its subsequent impacts on toxicity pathways that lead to adverse health outcomes through biomarker determinations. As established by WHO, biomarker is any substance, structure, or process that can be measured in the body or its products and influence or predict the incidence of outcome or disease (WHO 2001). To evaluate any alteration in the structure or function of an organism, biomarkers have been used to obtain information about exposure, internal dose, early biological effects, and susceptibility, as displayed in Fig. 2. Determination of biomarkers can aid in outlining the continuity of events, occurring from exposure to the response time. Certain biomarkers can provide qualitative and quantitative indices of the status of individuals at different stages of the toxicological process, from exposure to disease, especially in diseases with a long latency period (Chen et al. 2015, Park and Choi 2009). A new era for biomarker discovery may result from the application of "omics" technologies (e.g., genomics, proteomics, metabolomics), which are completely modifying our understanding of medicine and biology.

Biomarkers can elucidate the cause-effect and dose-response relationships in health risk assessments, in both clinical diagnostic and biological monitoring studies. Biomarkers are classified mostly into three types: (i) biomarkers of exposure (a substance or its metabolites in biological fluids, protein and DNA adducts);

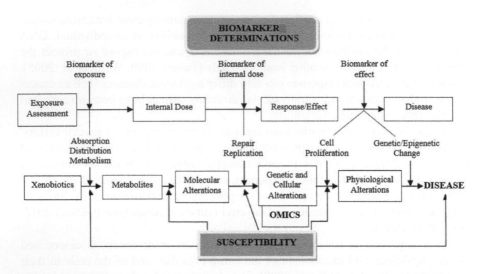

Fig. 2. Important factors in the relationship between exposure and disease and susceptibility affecting from exposure to response time, along a xenobiotic disposition (Pedrete et al. 2016).

(ii) biomarkers of effect (chromosome aberrations, sister chromatid exchanges, micronuclei and comet assay), which are evaluated according to different genotypes/phenotypes of activating/detoxifying metabolic activities; and (iii) biomarkers of susceptibility, which can identify a toxic substance or an adverse condition before any damage to health is evidenced (Boogaard and Money 2008, DeBord et al. 2015, Pavanello and Clonfero 2000). In particular, genetic markers play an important role in understanding disease risk, since it is known that chronic diseases arise not only from single gene-variants or single exposures, but rather from multiple genetic and environmental factors (e.g., susceptibility, personal exposure history) (Kelly and Vineis 2014).

A biomarker of susceptibility is an indicator of an inherent (genetic) or acquired factor that may increase or decrease an individual risk and ability to respond to the effect of exposure to a specific xenobiotic or to the effects of a group of such compounds. These markers indicate individual or population differences that affect their response to that chemical substance. Such markers may include inborn differences in metabolism, variations in immunoglobulin levels, low organ-reserve capacity, or other identifiable genetically determined or environmentally induced variations in absorption, metabolism, and response to environmental agents (Hocquette 2005). Other factors that may affect individual susceptibilities include the nutritional status of the organism, the role of the target site in overall body function, condition of the target tissue (present or prior to disease) and compensation by homeostatic mechanisms during and after exposure (Pielaat et al. 2013). This means that variations in xenobiotic responses by individuals are closely related to specific genotypes and phenotypes, which is the basis of individual clinical toxicology (Cimino et al. 2013).

According to Zanger and Schwab (2013), the polymorphism of activating and detoxicating systems are the most significant biomarkers of susceptibility.

In this regard, the measurements of the activity of certain polymorphs of detoxicating enzymes such as CYP, glutathione-S-transferases, acetyltransferases, sulfotransferases, glucuronyltransferases and paraoxonase, among others, have been used as biomarkers of susceptibility. For example, predisposition to certain types of cancer (e.g., bladder) has been correlated with genetic polymorphisms of N-acetyltransferases, enzymes involved in the deactivation of aromatic amines (Zanger and Schwab 2013). Moreover, organophosphates can be inactivated (hydrolyzed) by paraoxonase (PON1), which exhibits an important polymorphism (Agúndez 2008).

The use of such susceptibility biomarkers enables the identification of the severity of individual responses to a chemical exposure. In fact, two kinds of susceptibility biomarkers are possible: those used for prognosis and those used for prediction purposes. Prognostic biomarkers are biological measurements capable of indicating an individual's susceptibility to develop an adverse effect in a clinical treatment; in other words, they may predict the progress of the disease. Predictive biomarkers are used to indicate the possibility of an adverse effect on health when a xenobiotic is administered to an individual in a particular condition, evaluating the response to treatment (Chen et al. 2015). In both cases, susceptibility biomarkers are indicators of individual differences in the development of an adverse effect in response to a specific chemical exposure and are used to differentiate patients according to the degree of susceptibility (Chen et al. 2014).

Biotransformation

The biological action of a xenobiotic in any organism, requires the substance to reach its target. Hence, after absorption, the xenobiotic and its metabolites will be distributed within the organism and will cross biological membranes to reach their site of action.

To prevent any deleterious effect, after absorption of an exogenous and toxic substance, the organism should eliminate it. The compound can be excreted either in its original form or as a biotransformed metabolite form, resulting from enzymatic action on the xenobiotic molecule by a wide array of enzymes that are present within the organism. In general, the metabolism produces less toxic and more soluble products than the parent compound, facilitating excretion. Additionally, these metabolites may serve as substrates for other enzymes. Occasionally, the produced metabolites (reactive metabolites) may react with cellular macromolecules, such as DNA and proteins. The overall balance between activation and detoxification differs among individuals and determines the dose of a biological active toxicant, thereby influencing the risk of health effects (Thier et al. 2003, Zanger and Schwab 2013).

Xenobiotic detoxification is usually conducted by certain enzyme families, such as CYP450, aldehyde dehydrogenase (ALDH), myeloperoxidase (MPO), epoxide hydrolase (EPH) N-acetyltransferase (NAT), sulfotransferase (SULT), glucuronosyltransferase (GLUT), and glutathione-S-transferase (GST). One of the families very frequently involved in the toxicity of several xenobiotics is the Cytochrome P450 enzyme family. These enzymes differ substantially in their amino acid sequences and are encoded by distinct genes. Although the great majority of xenobiotics can be metabolized by CYP enzymes, producing inactive metabolites, some environmental and industrial chemicals undergo an oxidative metabolism by these enzymes, forming chemically reactive electrophiles (phase I) that are able to react with DNA, which may, eventually, lead to a carcinogenic response. Other enzyme families also metabolize chemicals by inactivation pathways (phase II), conjugating the metabolites with glutathione (GSTs), for example, to produce readily excretable hydrophilic products.

The connection between chemical exposure, individual disposition and biological/clinical effect, taking cancer as an example, is displayed in Fig. 3. If a carcinogen does not undergo a metabolic detoxification and is not excreted by the organism, either in its parent form or activated metabolite, the cells will be subject to various events (adduct formation, DNA modification, DNA repair, cell death, cell proliferation, among others), leading to cancer.

A diversity of genes encoding enzymes involved in biotransformation of toxicants and in cellular defense has been identified, leading to increased knowledge of allelic variants of genes and genetic defects that may result in a differential susceptibility regarding environmental toxicants (Thier et al. 2003). Furthermore, some enzymes influence important diseases indirectly, by metabolizing a number of endogenous compounds such as sex hormones, corticosteroids and bile acids. Mutations in the corresponding genes may promote carcinogenesis and progression of tumors (Bozina et al. 2009, Zhou et al. 2008).

According to Gresner et al. (2007), the enzyme-coding genes remain in gene–gene and gene–environment interactions characterized by different degree of complexity. Therefore, polymorphism in only one enzyme-coding gene to evaluate a disease risk is not sufficient to explain inter-individual differences in susceptibility caused by exposure to xenobiotics (Gresner et al. 2007). The ideal approach should be based on simultaneous study of several enzyme-coding genes and their combined

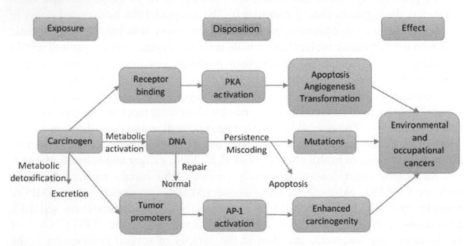

Fig. 3. Biological actions of a carcinogenic xenobiotic in humans from exposure to effect. Modified from Wogan et al. (2004).

effect to generate a more comprehensive relation cause-effect-susceptibility (Gresner et al. 2007, Pedrete et al. 2016).

In parallel, the distribution mechanism of the xenobiotic and/or its metabolites within the organism is regulated by a series of endocrine substances such as carriers (transporters) and receptors. It has been widely shown that transporters have great significance in the disposition of a xenobiotic to its active sites where it ultimately displays its effect (Kusuhara and Sugiyama 2002).

Generally, simple diffusion is the most common pathway by which chemicals cross the cellular membranes. Physicochemical properties such as hydrophobicity, size, and charge are very important factors that govern the crossing of chemicals by both active and passive mechanisms (Klaassen and Aleksunes 2010). In addition, to crossing the biological membranes, exogenous substances can use a set of specialized proteins called transporters. These proteins are involved in both absorption and excretion of substrates by the cells. Certain genetic differences, such as polymorphisms in these transporters, which result in altered transport rates, can cause individual differences in response to xenobiotic exposure, exhibiting variations in toxicity or effect. For example, differences in genes encoding potential Hg-transporters may affect uptake and elimination of Hg in persons working or living in mining areas producing high urinary Hg concentrations (U-Hg) (Engström et al. 2013). Another polymorphism, DMT1 IVS4.44C/A, is associated with inter-individual variations in blood iron, lead and cadmium levels (Kayaaltı et al. 2015). Individuals with the DMT1 IVS4.44 CC genotype thus seem to be more susceptible to metal toxicity when compared to those with AC and AA genotypes, suggesting that individuals with the DMT1 IVS4.44 CC genotype should be more careful in protecting their health against the toxic effects of the heavy metals (Kayaaltı et al. 2015).

Currently, more than 400 membrane transporters have been identified and are classified into two super families: ABC (ATP-binding cassette) and SLC (solute carrier) (Consortium TIT 2010). The SLC group of transporters is composed of proteins comprising 300–800 amino acids with molecular masses ranging from 40 to 90 kDa, while ABC transporters are proteins comprising 1,200 to 1,500 amino acids and molecular mass from 140 to 200 kDa (Sai et al. 2010, 2008). The ABC superfamily, for example, has been associated with drug pharmacokinetics and individual susceptibility to side effects, interactions, and treatment efficacy of several drugs, according to clinical evidence (Consortium 2010, Klaassen and Aleksunes 2010, Sai et al. 2010).

The expression levels of xenobiotic metabolizing enzymes are regulated by a specific receptor/transcription factor that may be polymorphic, resulting in variability of expression levels and binding affinities (Fig. 4). The most studied receptors in the xenobiotic metabolism are the aryl hydrocarbon receptor (AhR), the pregnane X receptor (PXR) and the peroxisome proliferator activating receptor (PPAR). A complex receptor-gene interaction may be located in the promotor region of genes, where polymorphisms can occur. Thus, allelic variants of a receptor may have an impact on their expression and, consequently, in xenobiotic effects (Bozina et al. 2009, Thier et al. 2003).

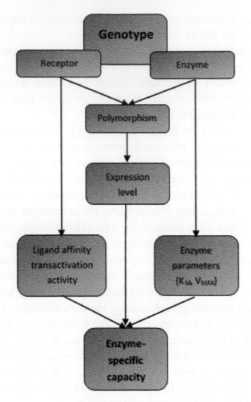

Fig. 4. Molecular background between metabolic enzymes and polymorphisms in enzyme and receptor-coding genes, showing variability in expression levels, transactivation activity and binding affinities. Adapted from Thier et al. (2003).

Enzyme Polymorphisms: Characteristics, Abundance and Mode of Action

Sequence variations in the genes encoding enzymes and proteins result from genetic processes and may accumulate in the population. If the frequency of a specific sequence variant reaches 1% or more in a given population, it is referred to as a polymorphism, and a frequency of 10% or more is typically thought of as common, and less likely to exhibit a greater polymorphism magnitude of effect (Kelada et al. 2003).

A polymorphism may either have no effect, in other words, be "silent", or may be considered functional. Functional polymorphisms include: (i) point mutations in coding regions of genes, resulting in amino acid substitutions, which may alter catalytic activity, enzyme stability, and/or substrate specificity; (ii) duplicated or expanded genes, resulting in higher enzyme levels; (iii) completely or partially deleted genes, resulting in no gene product; and (iv) splice site variants that result in truncated or alternatively spliced protein products. Furthermore, polymorphisms in the regulatory regions of genes may also affect the amount of protein expression and mRNA stability or mRNA splicing (Kelada et al. 2003, Li and Bluth 2011).

Polymorphisms in enzymes can affect the balance of metabolic intermediates but the overall metabolism suffers the influence of genetic and environmental factors as diet, smoking, alcohol ingestion, drug administration, age, sex, hormones, exposure to environmental pollutants and disease states. Therefore, assessment of an individual's ability to metabolically activate and detoxify environmental xenobiotics requires both phenotyping and genotyping methods, since individuals may display different responses even when under identical exposure conditions, such as, for example, in the degree of severity of an effect or even with regard to which individuals become ill or not, which may be explained by genetic polymorphisms. For example, if CYP2D6 has two null alleles, it will be unable to metabolize chemicals. It can be caused by the production of an inactive or unstable protein resulting from gene deletion, gene conversion, or single-base-pair mutations (Orphanides and Kimber 2003). Consequently, the time of permanence of the toxicant into the organism will be higher, facilitating the appearance of undesirable health effects. In case of gene amplification, increased levels of CYP2D6 can occur, resulting in a rapid metabolization of chemicals.

Some polymorphic phase I and phase II metabolic enzyme genes, their characteristics and their related biological activities are displayed in Table 1.

Polymorphisms play an important role in enzymatic efficiency, since the extent of a metabolic reaction and the kinetics of the reaction are regulated by the chemical structure/spatial configuration of the involved enzyme (Bozina et al. 2009). For example, 57 human genes encoding for the previously cited CYP superfamily have been reported with regard to drug metabolism, where enzymes are grouped in 17 families. Among these, the CYP2B6 (48 alleles), 2C9 (32 alleles), 2D6 (92 alleles), and 3A4 (34 alleles) are the most polymorphic (Rodriguez-Antona and Ingelman-Sundberg 2006). In general, the majority of these polymorphs present enzymatic activity lower than their wild type (Thier et al. 2003). Single nucleotide polymorphisms (SNPs) predominantly occur in three polymorphic CYPs (Preissner et al. 2013): CYP2D6 (114 SNPs), CYP2A6 (68 SNPs), and CYP2B6 (57 SNPs), and CYP2D6 has been reported as one of the most drug-metabolizing CYPs (Table 2).

Genotyping for CYP polymorphisms provides important genetic information that helps to understand the effects of xenobiotics in the human body. For drug metabolism, the most important polymorphisms are those of the genes coding for CYP2C9, CYP2C19, CYP2D6, and CYP3A4/5, which can result in therapeutic failure or severe adverse reactions. Genes coding for CYP1A1, CYP1A2, CYP1B1, and CYP2E1 are the most responsible for the metabolic activation of carcinogens (Bozina et al. 2009, Kohlrausch et al. 2014). Moreover, most CYP enzymes can metabolize multiple substrates and catalyze multiple reactions. Therefore, CYP2C19 is suspected to play an important role in either detoxication or inactivation of potential carcinogens, or the bioactivation of some environmental carcinogens to toxic DNA-binding metabolites. Consequently, CYP2C19 polymorphism associated with metabolic activity could cause a susceptibility to several forms of cancer, but the mechanism and the target carcinogen have not been elucidated (Isomura et al. 2010).

Many polymorphic genes show also considerable ethnic differences in allelic distribution (e.g., rare alleles, gene amplifications, pseudogenes), i.e., the expression

Table 1. Polymorphic enzymes for assessment of susceptibility in biomonitoring studies.

Function	Polymorphic enzymes	Allele[a]	Enzymatic activity[a]	Endpoint	References
	ADH1	*1	Null	Telomere	
		*2 *3	Increased	Mean corpuscular volume of erythrocytes	Pavanello et al. (2011)
	ALDH2	*1	Normal	Sister chromatid exchanges	Wong et al. (2003)
		*2	Decreased	DNA adducts	Yukawa et al. (2012)
	CYP1A1	*1	Normal	1-hydroxypyrene	Ada et al. (2007)
		*2	Increased		
		*3	Increased	DNA adducts	Rojas et al. (2000)
		*4	Increased		
Phase I reactions	CYP1A2	*1	Normal	Urinary metabolites	Gross-Steinmeyer and Eaton (2012)
		*2	Inducible	Amino-dimethylimidazol	Stillwell et al. (1997)
	CYP2A6	*1 *8	Normal	3-hydroxycotinine	Nagano et al. (2010)
		*7 *9	Decreased		
	CYP2D6	*1	Normal	S-phenyl mercapturic acid	Rossi et al. (1999)
		*3 o A	Null		
		*4 o B	Null	Comet assay	Singh et al. (2011)
		*5 o D	Null	Acetyl cholinesterase	
		*6 o E	Null		
	CYP2E1	*1	Normal	Sister chromatid exchanges	Wong et al. (2003)
		*3	Increased	Micronuclei	Jiy et al. (2010)
				Trans, trans-muconic acid	Chanvaivit et al. (2007)
	EPHX	R o 1*	Normal	Steroidogenesis	Knag et al. (2013)
		H	Decreased		
		Y	Increased	DNA adducts	Sram et al. (2004)
	NAT2	*4	Rapid	N-acetylbenzidine-hemoglobin adduct	Beyerbach et al. (2006)
		*5A	Slow		
		*5B	Slow		
		*5C	Slow		
		*6A	Slow	Comet assay	Cebulska-Wasilewska et al. (2007)
		*7B	Slow		
Phase II reactions	NQO1	*1	Normal	Plasma prolactin	Vinayagamoorthy et al. (2010)
		*2	Null		
	PON1	A	Low	Enzyme activity levels	Sözmen et al. (2002)
		B	High		
	GSTM1	*1	Normal	DNA adducts	Pavanello et al. (2008)
				Albumin adduct	Wu et al. (2009)
		*0	Null	Micronuclei	Angelini et al. (2008)
	GSTT1	*1	Normal	Hydroxyethyl-valine	Yong et al. (2001)
					Fennell et al. (2000)
		*0	Null	Micronuclei	Angelini et al. (2008)
	GSTP1	A	Normal	Amino-methylimidazol	Koutros et al. (2009)
		B	Low	Amino-dimethylimidazol	
		C	Low	Amino-trimethylimidazol	

ADH1–alcohol dehydrogenase 1 (class I); *ALDH2*–aldehyde dehydrogenase 2 family; *CYP1A1*–cytochrome P450, family 1, subfamily A, polypeptide 1; *CYP1A2*–cytochrome P450, family 1, subfamily A, polypeptide 2; *CYP2A6*–cytochrome P450, family 2, subfamily A, polypeptide 6; *CYP2D6*–cytochrome P450, family 2, subfamily D, polypeptide 6; *CYP2E1*–cytochrome P450, family 2, subfamily E, polypeptide 1; *EPHX*–epoxide hydrolase; *NAT2*–arylamine N-acetyltransferase 2; *NQO1*–NAD(P) H: quinone oxidoreductase; *PON1*–paraoxonase; *GSTM1*–glutathione S-transferase mu 1; *GSTT1*–glutathione S-transferase theta 1; *GSTP1*–glutathione S-transferase pi 1. [a]Pavanello and Clonfero (2000).

Table 2. Number of SNPs and drugs metabolized per CYP, according to Preissner et al. (2013).

Enzyme CYP	Number of single nucleotide polymorphisms	Number of drugs metabolized
2D6	114	223
2A6	68	51
2B6	57	74
3A4	46	434
1A2	41	165
2C9	39	163
2C19	29	140
1B1	28	17
3A5	26	128

of these genetic polymorphisms may modulate the susceptibility of an ethnic group. Therefore, variations in phenotypes and genotypes among different ethnic and/or geographic groups is a growing field of research (Thier et al. 2003). Indeed, the prevalence of certain polymorphs varies according to ethnicity and even within the same ethnic group. For example, reported frequencies of CYP2A6*2 (*2 polymorphism of CYP2A6) differ significantly between ethnicities, with values at 28%, 62%, and 8%, respectively in Asian, African, and Caucasian populations. In another example, one study demonstrated that approximately half of the Japanese population lacks aldehyde dehydrogenase 2 (ALDH2) activity, causing the accumulation of acetaldehyde in their body (Pavanello and Clonfero 2000), while 34 polymorphic alleles in four major CYPs (1A2, 2D6, 2C9, and 2C19) with significant impact on drug metabolism were identified in Caucasians, with CYP2D6 being the greatest contributor of polymorphic alleles in this ethnic group (Preissner et al. 2013).

In a study on 15 polymorphisms in the CYP superfamily in the South of Brazil involving African and European Brazilian descendants (Kohlrausch et al. 2014), the most influential polymorphic variants in this population and their frequencies were in agreement with most descriptions of CYP allele frequencies in other populations of European and African origins. The most frequent alleles found were CYP3A5*3, CYP1A2*1F, CYP3A4*1B, and CYP2C19*2. Significant differences in allelic distribution between African and European descendants were observed for CYP3A4 and CYP3A5 genes. CYP3A4*1B presented higher frequency in African descendants while CYP3A5*3 was seen in European descendants (Kohlrausch et al. 2014).

It has been recognized that gender may also have an influence on polymorphic genes of the metabolism, affecting susceptibility to carcinogens, suggesting that women may be more susceptible to effects than men. Indeed, gender differences have been observed in the expression of phase I and II metabolizing enzymes. For example, for non-Hodgkin lymphoma, the H139R polymorphism within the gene EPHX1 confers a protective effect only in females, while the protective effect associated with the Y113H polymorphism was apparent only in males (Kelly and Vineis 2014).

Genotyping is also important regarding drug pharmacokinetics, since polymorphism in genes coding for drug metabolism can interfere in the treatment efficacy of several drugs (Pedrete et al. 2016). An interesting example of such a relationship is the codeine-morphine effect. Codeine is metabolized by CYP2D6 to morphine in the human body. CYP2D6 is a highly polymorphic enzyme with 5–10% of the Caucasian population carrying a poor metabolizer allelic variant (Samer et al. 2013). The activity of this enzyme is important since, in the case of poor metabolizers, reduced, or absence of morphine after administration of codeine results in low or no analgesic effect. In contrast, the presence of ultra-rapid metabolizing variants results in a quicker analgesic effect and some undesirable effects, including deaths. Morphine and codeine may permeate cell membranes by passive diffusion of their non-charged forms. But only morphine can be a OCT1-dependent transport (Tzvetkov et al. 2013). As OCT1 is highly polymorphic, the pharmacokinetics of morphine are greatly dependent on the activity of OCT1 variants. In humans possessing low or absent OCT1 activity, the administration of codeine will result in high morphine plasma concentrations and in case of ultra-rapid CYP2D6 metabolism, may result in severe morphine toxicity (Tzvetkov et al. 2013).

GSTs are responsible for the detoxification of various reactive toxic and mutagenic compounds; thus, it is likely that null genotypes are associated with health consequences (Angelini et al. 2008). The GST family also appears to form part of a protective mechanism against the development of cancer after carcinogen exposure. In addition, molecular epidemiology studies indicate that the lung cancer risk for an individual is high when interactions with GST polymorphisms and other risk factors (e.g., cigarette smoking) occur. The most studied polymorphic GSTs are deletion in the GSTM1 and GSTT1 genes, resulting in a reduced or total lack of the enzymes' activities in individuals with one or both alleles deleted, respectively.

Examples of Effects of Selected Polymorphisms

Benzene is an example of a ubiquitous toxic environmental pollutant of concern, and population may potentially suffer ill health effects after exposure. Even at relatively low levels of benzene exposure, workers may have an increased risk for genotoxicity that is due to a decrease in repair capacity (Chanvaivit et al. 2007). Moreover, an association with cancer induction may depend on genetic susceptibility and exposure levels. Polymorphisms in genes involved in benzene metabolism influence individual susceptibility to various levels of exposure (Dougherty et al. 2008, McHale et al. 2012). These genetic markers should be considered for studying the biological effects in susceptible populations, monitoring levels of benzene to identify workers who are at risk.

Detoxification can protect cells against oxidative stress and toxic quinones by converting benzene to less toxic compounds. Benzene is metabolized by phase I enzymes, mainly CYP2E1, into intermediate metabolites including phenol, hydroquinone, catechol and 1,2,4-benzenetriol (Au et al. 2002). The toxicity of benzene is mediated by its toxic metabolites, but there is a great concern in elucidating the genetic susceptibility to benzene toxicity, especially regarding the inheritance of polymorphic genes related to metabolism. CYP2E1 polymorphisms have been found to have a significant effect in benzene toxicity, gene expression and disease risk (Buthbumrung et al. 2008, Ginsberg et al. 2010). Polymorphisms have been reported in the DraI, RsaI and PstI restriction sites in the promoter region of the gene and may be associated with both increased and decreased enzymatic activity of CYP2E1 (Dougherty et al. 2008).

Genetic polymorphisms in genes encoding CYP2E1, NQO1, and GSTs might be responsible for human susceptibility to benzene toxicity. It has been found that susceptible genotypes for CYP1A1 and GSTT1 are significantly associated with shortened gestation among women exposed to low benzene levels (Wang et al. 2000). The association between variant metabolizing genes CYP2E1 (activating) and NQO1 (detoxifying) has been investigated (Au et al. 2002). NQO1 is responsible for the reduction of benzoquinones to less toxic dihydroquinones, thus preventing oxidative damage, while conjugation with GSTs is responsible for the production of less toxic compounds (Ginsberg et al. 2010). The NQO1 C609T polymorphism is associated with loss of enzyme activity in the TT homozygous variant, while heterozygotes exhibit an intermediate activity (Dougherty et al. 2008). The NQO1 C465T polymorphism can also cause a reduction of enzyme activity. Both glutathione S-transferase T1 (GSTT1) and glutathione S-transferase M1 (GSTM1) are involved in the detoxification of benzene oxide to S-phenylmercapturic acid, but only the polymorphic chemical metabolizing gene GSTT1 was reported to influence the benzene-induced sister chromatid exchanges (Dougherty et al. 2008, Maestri et al. 2005, Pavanello and Clonfero 2000). Moreover, the variation consisting in the complete deletion of GST genes has been associated with different types of leukemia, including acute myeloid leukemia (Dougherty et al. 2008). It has been reported that GSTM1*2/*2 and GSTT1*2/*2 genotypes in workers increase susceptibility to benzene, causing DNA damage and myelodysplastic syndrome (Buthbumrung et al. 2008).

Reduced susceptibility to certain diseases has also been ascribed to polymorphisms. For example, myeloperoxidase (MPO) converts intermediate metabolites into toxic quinones, which promote the formation of protein and DNA adducts and produces reactive oxygen species (ROS). The G > A polymorphism at the 463 position of the myeloperoxidase molecule decreases enzyme activity through loss of a transcription-binding site (Zhang et al. 2007). Thus, the MPO G463A variant genotype has been associated with a reduced risk of acute leukemia due to the diminished activation of carcinogens by this variant (Zhang et al. 2007).

The opposite is also true, that polymorphisms have been linked to increased susceptibility to certain conditions. For instance, epidemiological studies have reported that single-nucleotide polymorphisms in genes associated with the base excision repair (BER) pathway, such as XRCC1, AP endonuclease 1 (APE1) and 8-oxoguanine DNA glycosylase 1 (OGG1), are associated to increased risk of malignancy, including breast cancer (Kelada et al. 2003, Sigounas et al. 2010). Aberrations in breast cancer susceptibility genes, such as TP53, BRCA1, BRCA2, and ATM, which are also implicated in DNA repair, occur early in sporadic breast tumors and potentially play a role in the immortalization of breast epithelial cells (Sigounas et al. 2010).

Another type of disease that can be influenced by susceptibility and affected by polymorphisms is occupational contact dermatitis (OCD), caused mainly by contact allergic dermatitis. It is one of the most common work-related diseases and tends to become chronic, causing impaired quality of life and loss of work ability.

Workers with higher incidence of OCD usually work in health care, hairdressing, food sectors and the metal industry. Genes involved in the skin barrier, inflammatory response and biotransformation of xenobiotics provide more insight in the individual susceptibility for OCD. Information about the factors which predispose to OCD is useful in occupational health for the application of preventive measures and for career guidance for workers (Kezic et al. 2009).

Increased susceptibility to sensitization may be acquired, and susceptibility to elicitation may be increased by allergen or by co-factors such as irritation of the skin. Moreover, body homeostasis may be influenced by endocrinological or pharmacological factors causing increased or decreased susceptibility to contact allergy. An approach to evaluate the genetics of contact allergy is the study of candidate genes. Polymorphisms and mutations affecting the proteins like N-acetyltransferase (NAT) 1 and 2, glutathione-S-transferase (GST) M and T, angiotensin-converting enzyme (ACE), tumor necrosis factor (TNF) and interleukin-16 (IL-16), have been related to an increased risk of contact allergy (Schnuch et al. 2011).

Adduct formation is the result of the covalent bonding between reactive electrophilic substances and nucleophilic DNA and protein sites. Preferred sites for adduct formation are guanine with nucleophilic sites in the DNA and the sulfhydryl groups of cysteine, the histidine nitrogen, and valine N-terminal in proteins (Törnqvist et al. 2002). Metabolic activation may result in the formation of DNA adducts, when the carcinogen bounds covalently to DNA, the main role of a carcinogenic process. If their formation is inhibited or blocked, it is a way to carcinogenesis (Wogan et al. 2004), which is a complex multistage process that includes initiation, promotion, and progression. Each step depends on a number of factors that can promote or prevent carcinogenesis (Belitsky and Yakubovskaya 2008). If DNA adducts skip cellular repair mechanisms and persist, they may lead to miscoding, resulting in permanent mutations, as seen in Fig. 3. Cells with damaged DNA may be removed by apoptosis, or programmed cell death. If a permanent mutation occurs in a critical region of an oncogene or tumor suppressor gene, it can lead to activation of the oncogene or deactivation of the tumor suppressor gene (Belitsky and Yakubovskaya 2008, Wogan et al. 2004).

A current interest is to elucidate the genetic susceptibility to toxicity of chemicals, especially on the inheritance of polymorphic genes and formation of adducts. Potential genetically based susceptibility factors capable of modulating individual response to low genotoxic exposure and the consequent risk of cancer have been studied through analysis of adducts in lymphocytes of workers with different exposures, using 32P-postlabelling and immunoassay methods (Gyorffy et al. 2008, Koivisto and Peltonen 2010, Pavanello et al. 2008). In addition, differences in susceptibility to cigarette smoke exposure in the formation of DNA adducts can be observed between exposed and controls (Chuang et al. 2013).

Non-specific adducts of hemoglobin and serum albumin, like 8-hydroxyguanine, have been measured after exposure to a variety of electrophilic carcinogens (e.g., PAHs, polychlorinated biphenyls, dibenzodioxins, benzene), and their measurement has advantages that include the amount of protein present in blood which is larger than that of nuclear DNA, and the stability of protein adducts. Moreover, in the case of hemoglobin adducts, they represent a measure of short-term cumulative exposure, given the lifespan of about 120 days of red blood cells (Gyorffy et al. 2008, Törnqvist et al. 2002). Nevertheless, it should be made clear that these proteins do not represent the target of carcinogenic substances.

Other studies have adopted mass spectrometry detection to analyze DNA adducts, such as N7-alkylguanine, O-6-methylguanine and N7-(2-hydroxyethyl)guanine (Zarth et al. 2014). Examples of chemical-specific DNA adducts in lymphocyte and urine that have been measured by mass spectrometry are: anti-BPDE-DNA, BP-6-N7Gua, BP-6-N7Ade e AFB-N7-Gua (Gyorffy et al. 2008, Koivisto and Peltonen 2010, Wang et al. 2007). The major advantage of measuring chemical-specific DNA adducts is to offer an assessment of the dose of carcinogens close to the molecular target.

Mutation x Cancer x Susceptibility

Several possible factors, including gene flow due to population migration, homologous recombination or crossing over during meiosis, polyploidy (presence of more than two homologous chromosomes), and mutations, might contribute to the genetic variability in the population. Of these possibilities, mutations are the primary source for genetic variation. The genotype is the total sum of all the genetic information of an individual. It is often applied more narrowly to the set of alleles present at one or more specific loci. In a population, individuals differ from each other due to their genotypes and their interactions with environment. These differences in the genetic traits are referred to as genetic variability, which in response to the genetic and environmental influences determines the susceptibility of the individual to toxicant injury or disease (Thier et al. 2003). Genetic susceptibility represents an increased likelihood of developing a disease, otherwise known as genetic predisposition (Hong and Oh 2010).

Mutations consist in a change in the nucleotide sequence as a result of DNA damage which may be caused by exogenous agents such as chemicals, viruses and irradiation, or caused by reactive molecules generated by normal cellular processes, which can damage DNA by the generation of reactive oxygen and nitrogen species, alkylation, depurination, and cytidine deamination (Wogan et al. 2004).

Mutagenesis by reactive oxygen species (ROS) can also contribute to the initiation of cancer, in the promotion and progression phases, causing structural alterations in DNA. ROS can produce chromosomal alterations, and thus could be involved in the inactivation or loss of the second wild-type allele of a mutated proto-oncogene or tumor-suppressor gene that can occur during tumor promotion and progression, allowing expression of the mutated phenotype. Moreover, ROS can affect cytoplasmic and nuclear signal transduction pathways, and modulate the activity of the proteins and genes related to cell proliferation, differentiation and apoptosis (Belitsky and Yakubovskaya 2008, Sigounas et al. 2010, Wang et al. 2012).

Many cancers and other chronic diseases may develop in consequence of more complex gene-gene and gene-environment interactions. Thus, it is important to identify relevant environmental factors and respective genetic modulators.

Many genes have been identified that are likely to be important factors in genetic susceptibility and these genes are involved in important functions in organisms, including cell cycle control, DNA repair, regulation of cell division, cell signaling, apoptosis and metabolism (Waters et al. 2003).

Cancers must exhibit a mutator phenotype, which refers to the increase in mutation rate of cancer cells. This term is used to account for the disparity between the rarity of spontaneous mutations in normal cells and the large numbers of mutations observed in human tumors (Wogan et al. 2004). The main consequences of these mutations are chromosomal alterations that involve translocations, deletions, amplifications and aneuploidy, and point mutations that involve only a few nucleotide substitutions. Multiple mutations in human tumors have important implications, since they provide a monitor for the malignant state of a tumor and may be used to measure the susceptibility of an individual to different carcinogens after chronic exposure (Wogan et al. 2004).

The study of cancer risk should consider genetic predisposition and environmental and occupational exposure to carcinogens owing to individual susceptibility to carcinogens. Genetic predisposition originates the differences in metabolism of xenobiotics and mechanisms in DNA repair, possibly due to polymorphisms. Indeed, genetic differences in expression and activity of the xenobiotic metabolizing enzymes are due to the existence of polymorphic alleles encoding these enzymes (Bozina et al. 2009, Gresner et al. 2007).

A number of studies have investigated associations between polymorphisms of metabolizing enzymes and cancer risk (Seide et al. 2011, Song et al. 2009, Thier et al. 2003). Several CYP2E1 genotypes seem to be associated with different levels of expression of enzyme activity. Genetic polymorphisms of GSTM1 may be linked to the occurrence of human bladder cancer, for example, supporting the hypothesis that exposure to PAH might be involved in urothelial cancers (Thier et al. 2003). Conjugator and non-conjugator phenotypes are coincident with the presence and absence of the GSTT1 gene, a catalyzing polymorphic variant (Seide et al. 2011, Song et al. 2009).

Allelic variants of genes and genetic defects may result in a differential susceptibility toward environmental toxicants. Low penetrating genes are those that occur in only a portion of the genotype carriers that presents the corresponding phenotype and they tend to be much more common in the population than allelic variants of high penetrating cancer genes. For example, an association between breast cancer and the high penetrating BRCA1 or BRCA2 tumor suppressor genes has been demonstrated (Sigounas et al. 2010). Moreover, positive associations between cancer in the aerodigestive tract and CYP1A1 alleles were found and the effect of the variant CYP1A1 allele becomes apparent in connection with the GSTM1 null allele (Thier et al. 2003). The CYP1B1 codon 432 polymorphism (CYP1B1*3) has also been identified as a susceptibility factor in cancer risk and has been associated with the frequency of somatic mutations of the p53 gene (Bozina et al. 2009, Thier et al. 2003). Combined genotype analysis of CYP1B1 and GSTM1 or GSTT1 has also pointed to interactive effects (Thier et al. 2003).

"Omics" Technologies

To improve the necessary understanding of disease mechanisms and identification of molecular targets and specific biomarkers, a new wide range of analytical tools have been developed, named "omics" technologies. Their application has become feasible in recent years due to lower costs, and increase in the sensitivity, resolution and throughput of -omics based assays, for example, examining impacted gene functions and pathways. The development of these -omics technologies has contributed greatly to our understanding of the living organisms at a molecular level. These technologies are able to generate a great set of data (genes, transcripts, proteins and metabolites) simultaneously in a short period of time, improving our understanding of cellular responses, tissue damage, and of functional perturbations caused by exposure to a xenobiotic, thus making it possible to study not only genotypic but also, and especially, the phenotypic behavior (Aardema and MacGregor 2002, Pesce et al. 2013, Sung et al. 2012). Therefore, the development of "omics" technologies for measuring global molecular expression changes is providing insights for establishing the molecular basis of pharmacological and toxicological responses.

The fields and tools of toxicogenomics, for instance, are particularly useful in this regard. Toxicogenomics comprehends the application of genomic technologies (for example, genetics, genome sequence analysis, gene expression profiling, proteomics, metabolomics, and related approaches) to study the adverse effects of environmental and pharmaceutical chemicals on human health and the environment. This branch of science combines toxicology with information obtained by genomic technologies to integrate toxicant-specific alterations in gene, protein, and metabolite expression patterns with phenotypic responses of cells, tissues, and organisms leading to more predictive, and sensitive information to evaluate toxic exposure or predict effects on human health (NRC 2007).

In genomics/transcriptomics, DNA array technologies allow thousands of genes to be surveyed in parallel, both for expression monitoring under various physiological conditions and in polymorphism analyses (McHale et al. 2012, Oberemm et al. 2005). A key element related to all tools of toxicogenomics is bioinformatics. All "omics" data are being used for constitution of databases containing a great variety of genetic sequences, epigenomics, proteomics, and metabolomics data, as well as clinical and toxicological information. Altogether, "omics" data will allow the study of interrelations among these data and retrieval of significant biological information for predictive toxicology, demonstrating a huge potential to predict toxic responses (Waters et al. 2003). Transcriptomics, proteomics, and epigenomics, in particular, can each provide a "molecular signature" or "fingerprint" of exposure or early effect, which can be compared with the profiles associated with carcinogens to inform hazard identification (McHale et al. 2012, Sung et al. 2012).

A molecular signature is a set of biomolecular features, such as a DNA sequence, mRNA and protein expression. In conjunction with computational procedures, they can aid in predicting a phenotype of clinical interest (Sung et al. 2012), based on single or multiple data types, for example, the prediction of any health risk or organic response to toxic xenobiotic exposure and its physiological actions.

The identification of molecular signatures from "omics" data for diverse clinical applications consists of four stages: (i) definition of the scientific and clinical context for the molecular signature; (ii) data acquisition; (iii) feature selection and modeling; and (iv) evaluation of the molecular signature from independent datasets (Ginsburg and Willard 2009, Sung et al. 2012).

The -omic signatures and the risk induced by exposure can also characterize the exposome (encompass all environmental exposures from conception), responsome (early effect) and outcome of individual susceptibility, facilitating the examination of gene-environment interactions. Thus, these technologies facilitate in depth approaches in understanding the relationship between chemical structure-activity-effects and molecular mechanisms of action. They also aid in the understanding of the adverse effects of xenobiotic on exposed organisms (Aardema and MacGregor 2002, Waters et al. 2003).

The proteome is closer to the phenotype than the genome or the transcriptome, and, as such, may be more directly responsive to natural selection, and, thus, is strictly linked to adaptation (Diz et al. 2012). As displayed in Fig. 5, proteomics is the most appropriate technique of choice in order to identify susceptible groups prior to effects due to an exposure. The "omic", from the potentiality of 'what can happen' (genome) through 'what appears to happen' (transcriptome) and 'what makes it happen' (proteome) to 'what has happened' (metabolome), embodies the paradigm of what needs to be modelled (Pesce et al. 2013).

Proteomics is devoted to the study of the dynamics of protein expression, regulation and interactions. According to Wetmore and Merrick (2004), "proteomics

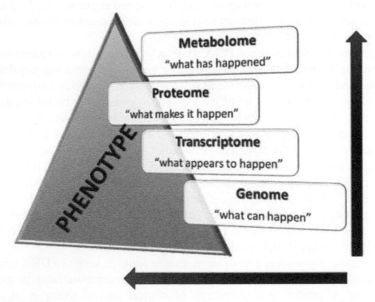

Fig. 5. Relationship between some "omics" technologies and the kind of questions answered related to effects resulting from exposure to a xenobiotic that aids in decoding the phenotype. Modified from Pesce et al. (2013).

is in a unique position to contribute to new protein discovery for the betterment of public health and in linking toxicology and pathology to a systems biology view of protein dysfunction in toxicity and environmental disease".

The investigation of proteomic patterns could, thus, be a powerful tool for the identification of intermediate changes that link environmental exposures to disease (Vineis and Perera 2007).

Mechanisms such as alternative splicing of mRNA precursors, cleavage and processing of polypeptide chains and post-translational modifications may generate multiple protein isoforms (Fig. 6). In addition to these mechanisms, developmental processes and environmental factors may cause proteomic differentiation across tissues and organs, resulting in a distinct phenotype for each level. Hence, it is not possible to have information regarding protein properties from a static DNA alone (Ahmad and Lamond 2014, Diz et al. 2012).

In metabolomics, endogenous metabolites in tissues and body fluids are measured to continuously analyze treatment-induced changes and to demonstrate toxicity-related affection of metabolic pathways. Therefore, the differences between unperturbed and perturbed pathways could provide an insight into the underlying disease pathology and disease prognosis and diagnosis. In fact, this tool provides clinical biomarkers useful for identification of early stage diseases (Wheelock et al. 2013, Zhang et al. 2015).

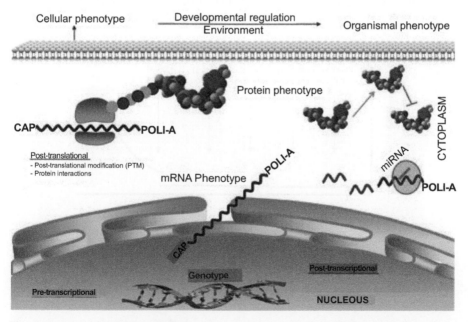

Fig. 6. Phenotype formation according to the expression of mRNA and its corresponding protein, regulated by diverse mechanisms. Adapted from Diz et al. (2012).

Personalized Clinical Toxicology

Technological development has led us to an era of individualized therapy (Silberring and Ciborowski 2010). According to Hocquette (2005), we will be able to predict the probability for developing specific diseases through scientific results and applied biotechnologies that arise from proteomics, metabolomics, transcriptomics, epigenomics, and genomics, through the association of gene expression patterns with diagnoses, treatment, and clinical data. This is especially clear when observing that, during the progression from a healthy to a disease state (Fig. 7), there are important time points at which several molecular and clinical tools are essential to assess disease risk, screening, diagnosis, prognosis, and therapeutic strategy (Ginsburg and Willard 2009, Hong and Oh 2010).

Thus, the use of "omics" and medicine together will certainly produce new diagnostic tools to determine individual risk factors and personalized medical treatments. It is clear that "omics" are the pillars of personalized clinical toxicology, which is based on knowledge of individual characteristics, and requires an understanding of the factors that influence organic variability, as well as the specific factors that cause predisposition to diseases (Tremblay and Hamet 2013). Thus, prevention and treatment strategies will take into account individual variability, with great potential for improving health (Khoury et al. 2016, Rubin 2015).

In order to increase the effectiveness of omics-based risk assessments, these techniques must be standardized and integrated into health systems (Hayes et al. 2014, Hong and Oh 2010). For example, the identification of patients who would have no

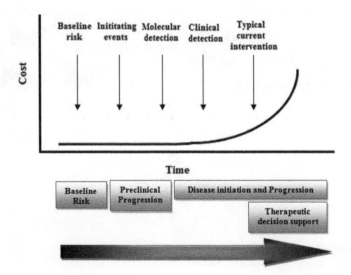

Fig. 7. Progression of a chronic disease and time points at which -omics can be applied to personalize health care. Adapted from Ginsburg and Willard (2009).

beneficial effect or have the risk of developing adverse effects from an unnecessary treatment could save great cost in the healthcare system and clinical trials (Chen et al. 2015, Lin and Chen 2012). It is very challenging to conduct large scale, prospective studies to establish causal associations between genetic variations and drug response or to evaluate the utility and cost-effectiveness of genomic medicine. Overcoming these challenges is, thus, ideal for achieving the goal of effective, safe and adequate medication to targeted patients with appropriate genotypes (Seide et al. 2011).

Genomics, for example, has rapidly advanced, serving as the basis for many medical decisions and public health initiatives. The identification of genetic variants associated with individual response may help to predict the occurrence of health events in susceptible individuals. Individual attributes, such as resistance, regimens, and dosing, interfere in the results of toxicological trials. Genetic, phenotypic and environmental factors should be taken into account in order to provide biomarkers with analytical validity and clinical utility to optimize the effectiveness of a specific treatment (Cimino et al. 2013, Hayes et al. 2014).

Conclusions

The biological diversity among humans can regulate (improve or decrease) the effect of xenobiotics. In fact, no two humans are equal and DNA alone cannot be responsible for susceptibility. The previous generation of biomarkers has contributed greatly to our understanding of risk and susceptibility related largely to genotoxic chemicals. More recently, developed biomarkers have considerable potential in molecular epidemiology because they reflect another important mechanism of certain diseases, such as cancer, namely, epigenetic alterations that affect the expression of genes and proteins.

It might be expected that the continuous development of high-throughput genotyping techniques capable of analyzing multiple polymorphisms within a gene as well as several genes along the same metabolic pathway, appropriate data stratification and evaluation of the multiple levels of gene-gene and gene-environment interactions will contribute towards the assessment of an individual's susceptibility and risk. Current and future efforts to identify new polymorphisms in genes involved in environmental response will broaden the scope of potential genetic effect.

The expectancy brought by the "omics" technologies in relation to personalized toxicology and individual health conditions are still far away from its myriad possibilities. Indubitably, the development of genomics and the new "omics" technologies derived from it, represented a very big step to a better understanding of human organisms and their similarities and individual differences, making it possible to study individual susceptibilities. In addition, as proteomics is the "omics" technology closer to phenotype, proteomic biomarkers will be of great value for risk assessment studies, since this field allows for the evaluation of susceptible individuals or population groups. Furthermore, the application of newly analytical tools in identifying biomarkers of susceptibility, or individual susceptibility will help in generating data that can be used in any risk assessment procedure. Such a scenario will certainly contribute in improving public health.

Acknowledgments

The authors thank the National Research Council (CNPq), the Rio de Janeiro Agency for Research Support (FAPERJ) and Coordination for the Improvement of Higher Education Personnel (CAPES) for financial support.

References

Aardema, M.J. and J.T. MacGregor. 2002. Toxicology and genetic toxicology in the new era of "toxicogenomics": Impact of "-omics" technologies. Mutat. Res. 499: 13–25.

Ada, A.O., M. Yilmazer, S. Suzen, C. Demiroglu, A.E. Demirbag, S. Efe et al. 2007. Cytochrome P450 (CYP) and glutathione S-transferases (GST) urinary levels of 1-hydroxypyrene in Turkish coke oven workers. Evaluation. 519: 511–519.

Agúndez, J.A.G. 2008. Polymorphisms of human N-acetyltransferases and cancer risk. Curr. Drug Metab. 9: 520–31.

Ahmad, Y. and A.I. Lamond. 2014. A perspective on proteomics in cell biology. Trends Cell Biol. 24: 257–264.

Angelini, S., R. Kumar, F. Carbone, J.L. Bermejo, F. Maffei, G. Cantelli-Forti et al. 2008. Inherited susceptibility to bleomycin-induced micronuclei: Correlating polymorphisms in GSTT1, GSTM1 and DNA repair genes with mutagen sensitivity. Mutat. Res. 638: 90–97.

Au, W.W., B. Oberheitmann and C. Harms. 2002. Assessing DNA damage and health risk using biomarkers. Mutat. Res. 509: 153–163.

Belitsky, G.a. and M.G. Yakubovskaya. 2008. Genetic polymorphism and variability of chemical carcinogenesis. Biochem. Biokhimii a. 73: 543–54.

Bell, J.T. and T.D. Spector. 2011. A twin approach to unraveling epigenetics. Trends Genet. 27: 116–125.

Beyerbach, A., N. Rothman, V.K. Bhatnagar, R. Kashyap and G. Sabbioni. 2006. Hemoglobin adducts in workers exposed to benzidine and azo dyes. Carcinogenesis. 27: 1600–1606.

Boffetta, P. and F. Islami. 2013. The contribution of molecular epidemiology to the identification of human carcinogens: current status and future perspectives. Ann. Oncol. 24: 901–908.

Boogaard, P. and C. Money. 2008. A proposed framework for the interpretation of biomonitoring data. Environ. Heal. 7: S12.

Bozina, N., V. Bradamante and M. Lovrić. 2009. Genetic polymorphism of metabolic enzymes P450 (CYP) as a susceptibility factor for drug response, toxicity, and cancer risk. Arh. Hig. Rada Toksikol. 60: 217–242.

Buthbumrung, N., C. Mahidol, P. Navasumrit, J. Promvijit, P. Hunsonti, H. Autrup et al. 2008. Oxidative DNA damage and influence of genetic polymorphisms among urban and rural schoolchildren exposed to benzene. Chem. Biol. Interact. 172: 185–194.

Cebulska-Wasilewska, A., B. Binkova, R.J. Sram, I. Kalina, T. Popov and P.B. Farmer. 2007. Repair competence assay in studies of the influence of environmental exposure to c-PAHs on individual susceptibility to induction of DNA damage. Mutat. Res. 620: 155–164.

Chanvaivit, S., P. Navasumrit, P. Hunsonti, H. Autrup and M. Ruchirawat. 2007. Exposure assessment of benzene in Thai workers, DNA-repair capacity and influence of genetic polymorphisms. Mutat. Res. Genet. Toxicol. Environ. Mutagen. 626: 79–87.

Chen, J.J., W.-J. Lin and T.-P. Lu. 2014. Biomarkers of susceptibility: Pharmacogenomics and toxicogenomics. pp. 975–982. In: Gupta, R.C. (ed.). Biomarkers in Toxicology. Academic Press, Boston.

Chen, J.J., T. Lu and Y. Chen. 2015. Predictive biomarkers for treatment selection: statistical considerations. Biomark. Med. 9: 1121–1135.

Chuan, C.-Y., J.-N. Tung, M.-C. Su, B.-C. Wu, C.-H. Hsin and Y.-J. Chen. 2013. BPDE-like DNA adduct level in oral tissue may act as a risk biomarker of oral cancer. Arch. Oral Biol. 58: 102–109.

Cimino, G., C. Pan and P. Henderson. 2013. Personalized medicine for targeted and platinum-based chemotherapy of lung and bladder cancer. Bioanalysis. 5: 369–391.

Consortium, T.I.T. 2010. Membrane transporters in drug development. Nat. Rev. Drug Discov. 9: 215–236.

Dancey, J. 2012. Genomics, personalized medicine and cancer practice. Clin. Biochem. 45: 379–381.

DeBord, D.G., L. Burgoon, S.W. Edwards, L.T. Haber, M.H. Kanitz, E. Kuempel et al. 2015. Systems biology and biomarkers of early effects for occupational exposure limit setting. J. Occup. Environ. Hyg. 12: S41–S54.

Di Palma, S., M.L. Hennrich, A.J.R. Heck and S. Mohammed. 2012. Recent advances in peptide separation by multidimensional liquid chromatography for proteome analysis. J. Proteomics. 75: 3791–3813.

Diz, A.P., M. Martínez-Fernández and E. Rolán-Alvarez. 2012. Proteomics in evolutionary ecology: Linking the genotype with the phenotype. Mol. Ecol. 21: 1060–1080.

Dougherty, D., S. Garte, A. Barchowsky, J. Zmuda and E. Taioli. 2008. NQO1, MPO, CYP2E1, GSTT1 and GSTM1 polymorphisms and biological effects of benzene exposure—a literature review. Toxicol. Lett. 182: 7–17.

Fennell, T.R., J.P. MacNeela, R.W. Morris, M. Watson, C.L. Thompson and D.A. Bell. 2000. Hemoglobin adducts from acrylonitrile and ethylene oxide in cigarette smokers: Effects of glutathione s-transferase T1-null and M1-null genotypes. Cancer Epidemiol. Biomarkers Prev. 9: 705–712.

Gärtner, K. 2012. A third component causing random variability beside environment and genotype. A reason for the limited success of a 30 year long effort to standardize laboratory animals? Int. J. Epidemiol. 41: 335–341.

Ginsberg, G., K. Guyton, D. Johns, J. Schimek, K. Angle and B. Sonawane. 2010. Genetic polymorphism in metabolism and host defense enzymes: Implications for human health risk assessment. Crit. Rev. Toxicol. 40: 575–619.

Ginsburg, G.S. and H.F. Willard. 2009. Genomic and personalized medicine: foundations and applications. Transl. Res. 154: 277–287.

Gresner, P., J. Gromadzinska and W. Wasowicz. 2007. Polymorphism of selected enzymes involved in detoxification and biotransformation in relation to lung cancer. Lung Cancer. 57: 1–25.

Gross-Steinmeyer, K. and D.L. Eaton. 2012. Dietary modulation of the biotransformation and genotoxicity of aflatoxin B1. Toxicology. 299: 69–79.

Gyorffy, E., L. Anna, K. Kovács, P. Rudnai and B. Schoket. 2008. Correlation between biomarkers of human exposure to genotoxins with focus on carcinogen-DNA adducts. Mutagenesis. 23: 1–18.

Hayes, D.F., H.S. Markus, R.D. Leslie and E.J. Topol. 2014. Personalized medicine: risk prediction, targeted therapies and mobile health technology. BMC Med. 12: 37.

Hocquette, J.F. 2005. Where are we in genomics? J. Physiol. Pharmacol. 56 Suppl. 3: 37–70.

Hong, K.-W. and B.-S. Oh. 2010. Overview of personalized medicine in the disease genomic era. BMB Rep. 43: 643–648.

Isomura, Y., Y. Yamaji, M. Ohta, M. Seto, Y. Asaoka, Y. Tanaka et al. 2010. A genetic polymorphism of CYP2C19 is associated with susceptibility to biliary tract cancer. J. Gastroenterol. 45: 1045–1052.

Jaenisch, R. and A. Bird. 2003. Epigenetic regulation of gene expression: how the genome integrates intrinsic and environmental signals. Nat. Genet. 33 Suppl.: 245–254.

Jiy, F., W. Wangy, Z.L. Xia, Y.J. Zheng, Y.L. Qiu, F. Wu et al. 2010. Prevalence and persistence of chromosomal damage and susceptible genotypes of metabolic and DNA repair genes in Chinese vinyl chloride-exposed workers. Carcinogenesis. 31: 648–653.

Kelada, S.N., D.L. Eaton, S.S. Wang, N.R. Rothman and M.J. Khoury. 2003. The role of genetic polymorphisms in environmental health. Environ. Health Perspect. 111: 1055–1064.

Kelly, R.S. and P. Vineis. 2014. Biomarkers of susceptibility to chemical carcinogens: the example of non-Hodgkin lymphomas. Br. Med. Bull. 111: 89–100.

Kezic, S., M.J. Visser and M.M. Verberk. 2009. Individual susceptibility to occupational contact dermatitis. Ind. Health. 47: 469–478.

Khoury, M.J., M.F. Iademarco and W.T. Riley. 2016. Precision public health for the era of precision medicine. Am. J. Prev. Med. 50: 398–401.

Klaassen, C.D. and L.M. Aleksunes. 2010. Xenobiotic, bile acid, and cholesterol transporters: function and regulation. Pharmacol. Rev. 62: 1–96.

Knag, A.C., S. Verhaegen, E. Ropstad, I. Mayer and S. Meier. 2013. Effects of polar oil related hydrocarbons on steroidogenesis *in vitro* in H295R cells. Chemosphere. 92: 106–115.

Kohlrausch, F.B., Á. Carracedo and M.H. Hutz. 2014. Characterization of CYP1A2, CYP2C19, CYP3A4 and CYP3A5 polymorphisms in South Brazilians. Mol. Biol. Rep. 41: 1453–1460.

Koivisto, P. and K. Peltonen. 2010. Analytical methods in DNA and protein adduct analysis. Anal. Bioanal. Chem. 398: 2563–2572.

Koutros, S., S.I. Berndt, R. Sinha, X. Ma, N. Chatterjee, M.C.R. Alavanja et al. 2009. Xenobiotic metabolizing gene variants, dietary heterocyclic amine intake, and risk of prostate cancer. Cancer Res. 69: 1877–1884.

Kusuhara, H. and Y. Sugiyama. 2002. Role of transporters in the tissue-selective distribution and elimination of drugs: transporters in the liver, small intestine, brain and kidney. J. Control. Release. 78: 43–54.

Li, J. and M.H. Bluth. 2011. Pharmacogenomics of drug metabolizing enzymes and transporters: implications for cancer therapy. Pharmgenomics. Pers. Med. 4: 11–33.

Lin, W.J. and J.J. Chen. 2012. Biomarker classifiers for identifying susceptible subpopulations for treatment decisions. Pharmacogenomics. 13: 147–157.

Maestri, L., S. Negri, M. Ferrari, S. Ghittori and M. Imbriani. 2005. Determination of urinary S-phenylmercapturic acid, a specific metabolite of benzene, by liquid chromatography/single quadrupole mass spectrometry. Rapid Commun. Mass Spectrom. 19: 1139–44.

McHale, C.M., L. Zhang and M.T. Smith. 2012. Current understanding of the mechanism of benzene-induced leukemia in humans: implications for risk assessment. Carcinogenesis. 33: 240–52.

Nagano, T., H. Yamazaki, M. Shimizu, K. Kiyotani, T. Kamataki, R. Takano et al. 2010. Biomonitoring of urinary cotinine concentrations associated with plasma levels of nicotine metabolites after daily cigarette smoking in a male Japanese population. Int. J. Environ. Res. Public Health. 7: 2953–2964.

National Research Council. 2007. Applications of Toxicogenomic Technologies to Predictive Toxicology and Risk Assessment. The National Academies Press, Washington, DC, USA.

National Research Council (US) Committee on Improving Risk Analysis Approaches Used by the U.S. EPA. 2009. Uncertainty and variability: The recurring and recalcitrant elements of risk assessment. pp. 93–126. *In*: NRC (ed.). Science and Decisions: Advancing Risk Assessment. The National Academies Press, Washington, DC, USA.

Neverova, I. and J.E. Van Eyk. 2005. Role of chromatographic techniques in proteomic analysis. J. Chromatogr. B Anal. Technol. Biomed. Life Sci. 815: 51–63.

Oberemm, A., L. Onyon and U. Gundert-Remy. 2005. How can toxicogenomics inform risk assessment? Toxicol. Appl. Pharmacol. 207: 592–598.

Orphanides, G. and I. Kimber. 2003. Toxicogenetics: applications and opportunities. Toxicol. Sci. 75: 1–6.

Park, S.K. and J.-Y. Choi. 2009. Risk assessment and pharmacogenetics in molecular and genomic epidemiology. J. Prev. Med. Public Health. 42: 371–6.

Pavanello, S. and E. Clonfero. 2000. Biological indicators of genotoxic risk and metabolic polymorphisms. Mutat. Res. 463: 285–308.

Pavanello, S., A. Pulliero and E. Clonfero. 2008. Influence of GSTM1 null and low repair XPC PAT+ on anti-B[a]PDE-DNA adduct in mononuclear white blood cells of subjects low exposed to PAHs through smoking and diet. Mutat. Res. 638: 195–204.

Pavanello, S., M. Hoxha, L. Dioni, P.A. Bertazzi, R. Snenghi, A. Nalesso et al. 2011. Shortened telomeres in individuals with abuse of alcohol consumption. Int. J. Cancer. 129: 983–992.

Pedrete, T. de A., C. de L. Mota, E.S. Gonçalves and J.C. Moreira. 2016. Towards a personalized risk assessment for exposure of humans to toxic substances. Cad. Saúde Coletiva. 24: 262–273.

Pesce, F., S. Pathan and F.P. Schena. 2013. From -omics to personalized medicine in nephrology: integration is the key. Nephrol. Dial. Transplant. 28: 24–8.

Pielaat, A., G.C. Barker, P. Hendriksen, P. Hollman, A. Peijnenburg and B.H. Ter Kuile. 2013. A foresight study on emerging technologies: State of the art of omics technologies and potential applications in food and feed safety. REPORT 1: Review on the state of art of omics technologies in risk assessment related to food and feed safety. EFSA Support. Inf. EN-495: 1–126.

Preissner, S.C., M.F. Hoffmann, R. Preissner, M. Dunkel, A. Gewiess and S. Preissner. 2013. Polymorphic cytochrome P450 enzymes (CYPs) and their role in personalized therapy. PLoS One. 8: 1–12.

Rodriguez-Antona, C. and M. Ingelman-Sundberg. 2006. Cytochrome P450 pharmacogenetics and cancer. Oncogene. 25: 1679–1691.

Rojas, M., I. Cascorbi, K. Alexandrov, E. Kriek, G. Auburtin, L. Mayer et al. 2000. Modulation of benzo[a]pyrene diolepoxide–DNA adduct levels in human white blood cells by CYP1A1, GSTM1 and GSTT1 polymorphism. Carcinog. 21: 35–41.

Rossi, A.M., C. Guarnieri, C. Rovesti, F. Gobba, S. Ghittori, G. Vivoli et al. 1999. Genetic polymorphisms influence variability in benzene metabolism in humans. Pharmacogenet. Genomics. 9.

Rubin, R. 2015. Precision medicine: The future or simply politics? JAMA J. Am. Med. Assoc. 313: 1089–1091.

Sai, K., Y. Saito, M. Itoda, H. Fukushima-Uesaka, T. Nishimaki-Mogami, S. Ozawa et al. 2008. Genetic variations and haplotypes of ABCC2 encoding MRP2 in a Japanese population. October. 23: 139–147.

Sai, K., Y. Saito, K. Maekawa, S.R. Kim, N. Kaniwa, T. Nishimaki-Mogami et al. 2010. Additive effects of drug transporter genetic polymorphisms on irinotecan pharmacokinetics/pharmacodynamics in Japanese cancer patients. Cancer Chemother. Pharmacol. 66: 95–105.

Samer, C.F., K.I. Lorenzini, V. Rollason, Y. Daali and J.A. Desmeules. 2013. Applications of CYP450 testing in the clinical setting. Mol. Diagnosis Ther. 17: 165–184.

Sauer, J.M., T. Hartung, M. Leist, T.B. Knudsen, J. Hoeng and A.W. Hayes. 2015. Systems toxicology: The future of risk assessment. Int. J. Toxicol. 34: 346–348.

Sauer, J.M., A. Kleensang, M.C. Peitsch and A.W. Hayes. 2016. Advancing Risk Assessment through the Application of Systems Toxicology. 32: 5–8.

Schnuch, A., G. Westphal, R. Mössner, W. Uter and K. Reich. 2011. Genetic factors in contact allergy-review and future goals. Contact Dermatitis. 64: 2–23.

Seide, F., G. Li and D. Yu. 2011. Conversational speech transcription using context-dependent deep neural networks. Proc. Annu. Conf. Int. Speech Commun. Assoc. INTERSPEECH. 63: 437–440.

Sigounas, G., J.W. Hairr, C.D. Cooke, J.R. Owen, A.S. Asch, D.A. Weidner et al. 2010. Role of benzo[alpha]pyrene in generation of clustered DNA damage in human breast tissue. Free Radic. Biol. Med. 49: 77–87.

Silberring, J. and P. Ciborowski. 2010. Biomarker discovery and clinical proteomics. TrAC—Trends Anal. Chem. 29: 128–140.

Singh, S., V. Kumar, K. Vashisht, P. Singh, B.D. Banerjee, R.S. Rautela et al. 2011. Role of genetic polymorphisms of CYP1A1, CYP3A5, CYP2C9, CYP2D6, and PON1 in the modulation of DNA damage in workers occupationally exposed to organophosphate pesticides. Toxicol. Appl. Pharmacol. 257: 84–92.

Song, D.K., D.L. Xing, L.R. Zhang, Z.X. Li, J. Liu and B.P. Qiao. 2009. Association of NAT2, GSTM1, GSTT1, CYP2A6, and CYP2A13 gene polymorphisms with susceptibility and clinicopathologic characteristics of bladder cancer in Central China. Cancer Epidemiol. 32: 416–423.

Sözmen, E.Y., B. Mackness, B. Sözmen, P. Durrington, F.K. Girgin, L. Aslan et al. 2002. Effect of organophosphate intoxication on human serum paraoxonase. Hum. Exp. Toxicol. 21: 247–252.

Spitz, M.R. and M.L. Bondy. 2009. The evolving discipline of molecular epidemiology of cancer. Carcinogenesis. 31: 127–134.

Sram, R.J., O. Beskid, B. Binkova, P. Rossner and Z. Smerhovsky. 2004. Cytogenetic analysis using fluorescence *in situ* hybridization (FISH) to evaluate the impact of environmental exposure to PAHs. Cancer Res. 64: 455–456.

Stillwell, W.G., L.C. Kidd, J.S. Wishnok, S.R. Tannenbaum and R. Sinha. 1997. Urinary excretion of unmetabolized and phase II conjugates of 2-amino-1-methyl-6-phenylimidazo[4,5-b]pyridine and 2-amino-3,8-dimethylimidazo[4,5-f]quinoxaline in humans: relationship to cytochrome P4501A2 and N-acetyltransferase activity. Cancer Res. 57: 3457–3464.

Sturla, S.J., A.R. Boobis, R.E. Fitzgerald, J. Hoeng, R.J. Kavlock, K. Schirmer et al. 2014. Systems toxicology: From basic research to risk assessment. Chem. Res. Toxicol. 27: 314–329.

Sung, J., Y. Wang, S. Chandrasekaran, D.M. Witten and N.D. Price. 2012. Molecular signatures from omics data: From chaos to consensus. Biotechnol. J. 7: 946–957.

Thier, R., T. Brüning, P.H. Roos, H.-P. Rihs, K. Golka, Y. Ko et al. 2003. Markers of genetic susceptibility in human environmental hygiene and toxicology: the role of selected CYP, NAT and GST genes. Int. J. Hyg. Environ. Health. 206: 149–171.

Titz, B., A. Elamin, F. Martin, T. Schneider, S. Dijon, N.V. Ivanov et al. 2014. Proteomics for systems toxicology. Comput. Struct. Biotechnol. J. 11: 73–90.

Törnqvist, M., C. Fred, J. Haglund, H. Helleberg, B. Paulsson and P. Rydberg. 2002. Protein adducts: Quantitative and qualitative aspects of their formation, analysis and applications. J. Chromatogr. B Anal. Technol. Biomed. Life Sci. 778: 279–308.

Tremblay, J. and P. Hamet. 2013. Role of genomics on the path to personalized medicine. Metabolism. 62 Suppl. 1: S2–5.

Turner, B.M. 2009. Epigenetic responses to environmental change and their evolutionary implications. Philos. Trans. R. Soc. B Biol. Sci. 364: 3403–3418.

Tzvetkov, M.V., J.N. Dos Santos Pereira, I. Meineke, A.R. Saadatmand, J.C. Stingl and J. Brockmöller. 2013. Morphine is a substrate of the organic cation transporter OCT1 and polymorphisms in OCT1 gene affect morphine pharmacokinetics after codeine administration. Biochem. Pharmacol. 86: 666–678.

Vinayagamoorthy, N., K. Krishnamurthi, S.S. Devi, P.K. Naoghare, R. Biswas, A.R. Biswas et al. 2010. Genetic polymorphism of CYP2D6*2 C → T 2850, GSTM1, NQO1 genes and their correlation with biomarkers in manganese miners of Central India. Chemosphere. 81: 1286–1291.

Vineis, P. and F. Perera. 2007. Molecular epidemiology and biomarkers in etiologic cancer research: The new in light of the old. Cancer Epidemiol. Biomarkers Prev. 16: 1954–1965.

Wang, H., W. Chen, H. Zheng, L. Guo, H. Liang, X. Yang et al. 2007. Association between plasma BPDE-Alb adduct concentrations and DNA damage of peripheral blood lymphocytes among coke oven workers. Occup. Environ. Med. 64: 753–758.

Wang, L., X. He, Y. Bi and Q. Ma. 2012. Stem cell and benzene-induced malignancy and hematotoxicity. Chem. Res. Toxicol. 25: 1303–15.

Waters, M.D., K. Olden and R.W. Tennant. 2003. Toxicogenomic approach for assessing toxicant-related disease. Mutat. Res. 544: 415–424.

Wetmore, B. and B. Merrick. 2004. Toxicoproteomics: Proteomics applied to toxicology and pathology. Toxicol. Pathol. 32: 619–642.

Wheelock, C.E., V.M. Goss, D. Balgoma, B. Nicholas, J. Brandsma, P.J. Skipp et al. 2013. Application of omics technologies to biomarker discovery in inflammatory lung diseases. Eur. Respir. J. 42: 802–25.

Wogan, G.N., S.S. Hecht, J.S. Felton, A.H. Conney and L.A. Loeb. 2004. Environmental and chemical carcinogenesis. Semin. Cancer Biol. 14: 473–486.

Wong, A.H.C., I.I. Gottesman and A. Petronis. 2005. Phenotypic differences in genetically identical organisms: The epigenetic perspective. Hum. Mol. Genet. 14: 11–18.

Wong, R.-H., J.-D. Wang, L.-L. Hsieh and T.-J. Cheng. 2003. XRCC1, CYP2E1 and ALDH2 genetic polymorphisms and sister chromatid exchange frequency alterations amongst vinyl chloride monomer-exposed polyvinyl chloride workers. Arch. Toxicol. 77: 433–440.

Wu, H.-C., Q. Wang, H.-I. Yang, H. Ahsan, W.-Y. Tsai, L.-Y. Wang et al. 2009. Aflatoxin B(1) exposure, hepatitis B virus infection and hepatocellular carcinoma in taiwan. Cancer Epidemiol. Biomarkers Prev. 18: 846–853.

Yekta, R.F., M. Koushki and N.A. Dashatan. 2015. Advances in proteomics analytical techniques. J. Paramed. Sci. 6: 135–144.

Yong, L.C., P.A. Schulte, J.K. Wiencke, M.F. Boeniger, L.B. Connally, J.T. Walker et al. 2001. Hemoglobin adducts and sister chromatid exchanges in hospital workers exposed to ethylene oxide: Effects of glutathione S-transferase T1 and M1 genotypes. Cancer Epidemiol. Biomarkers Prev. 10: 539–550.

Yukawa, Y., M. Muto, K. Hori, H. Nagayoshi, A. Yokoyama, T. Chiba et al. 2012. Combination of ADH1B*2/ALDH2*2 polymorphisms alters acetaldehyde-derived DNA damage in the blood of Japanese alcoholics. Cancer Sci. 103: 1651–1655.

Zanger, U.M. and M. Schwab. 2013. Cytochrome P450 enzymes in drug metabolism: Regulation of gene expression, enzyme activities, and impact of genetic variation. Pharmacol. Ther. 138: 103–141.

Zarth, A.T., G. Cheng, Z. Zhang, M. Wang, P.W. Villalta, S. Balbo et al. 2014. Analysis of the benzene oxide-DNA adduct 7-phenylguanine by liquid chromatography-nanoelectrospray ionization-high resolution tandem mass spectrometry-parallel reaction monitoring: application to DNA from exposed mice and humans. Chem. Biol. Interact. 215: 40–5.

Zhang, A., H. Sun, G. Yan, P. Wang and X. Wang. 2015. Metabolomics for biomarker discovery: Moving to the clinic. Biomed. Res. Int. 2015: 1–6.

Zhou, S.-F., Y.M. Di, E. Chan, Y.-M. Du, V.D.-W. Chow, C.C. Xue et al. 2008. Clinical pharmacogenetics and potential application in personalized medicine. Curr. Drug Metab. 9: 738–84.

Index

‖‖

Printed and bound by CPI Group (UK) Ltd, Croydon, CR0 4YY

01/11/2024

01782623-0005